Causes of Diabetes

Causes of Diabetes

Genetic and Environmental Factors

Edited by R. D. G. Leslie
St Bartholomew's Hospital, London, UK

JOHN WILEY & SONS
Chichester · New York · Brisbane · Toronto · Singapore

Other Wiley Editorial Offices

John Wiley & Sons, Inc., 605 Third Avenue,
New York, NY 10158-0012, USA

Jacaranda Wiley Ltd, G.P.O. Box 859, Brisbane,
Queensland 4001, Australia

John Wiley & Sons (Canada) Ltd, 22 Worcester Road,
Rexdale, Ontario M9W 1L1, Canada

John Wiley & Sons (SEA) Pte Ltd, 37 Jalan Pemimpin #05-04,
Block B, Union Industrial Building, Singapore 2057

Library of Congress Cataloging-in-Publication Data

Causes of diabetes : genetic and environmental factors / edited by
R.D.G. Leslie
p. cm.
Includes bibliographical references and index.
ISBN 0 471 94040 2
1. Diabetes—Etiology. 2. Diabetes—Genetic aspects. 3. Non-insulin-dependent diabetes—Etiology. 4. Non-insulin-dependent
diabetes—Genetic aspects. I. Leslie, R.D.G.
[DNLM: 1. Diabetes Mellitus, Insulin-Dependent—etiology.
2. Diabetes Mellitus, Non-Insulin-Dependent—etiology. WK 810 C374
1993]
RC660.C36 1993
616.4′62071—dc20
DNLM/DLC
for Library of Congress   93-11222
                                                            CIP

British Library Cataloguing in Publication Data

A catalogue record for this book is available from the British Library

ISBN 0 471 94040 2

Typeset in 10/12pt Times by Acorn Bookwork, Salisbury, Wiltshire
Printed and bound in Great Britain by Biddles Ltd, Guildford, Surrey

Contents

List of Contributors

K. G. M. M. ALBERTI *The Medical School, University of Newcastle upon Tyne, UK*

R. ASSAN *Diabetes Department, Bichat Hospital, Paris, France*

D. J. P. BARKER *MRC Environmental Epidemiology Unit, Southampton General Hospital, UK*

A. H. BARNETT *Department of Medicine, University of Birmingham, Birmingham B15 2TH, UK*

P. J. BINGLEY *Department of Diabetes and Metabolism, St Bartholomew's Hospital, London EC1, UK*

D. A. CAVAN *Department of Medicine, University of Birmingham, Birmingham B15 2TH, UK*

E. L. CONNOR *Department of Pathology and Laboratory Medicine, University of Florida College of Medicine, Gainesville, Florida, USA*

J. COOK *John Radcliffe Hospital, Headington, Oxford, UK*

G. DAHLQUIST *Department of Paediatrics, University of Umeå, Sweden*

R. B. ELLIOTT *Department of Paediatrics, University of Auckland, New Zealand*

E. A. M. GALE *Department of Diabetes and Metabolism, St Bartholomew's Hospital, London EC1, UK*

G. A. HITMAN *Medical Unit, The Royal London Hospital, London E1 1BB, UK*

W. C. KNOWLER *Diabetes and Arthritis Epidemiology Section, National Institute of Diabetes and Digestive and Kidney Diseases, Phoenix, Arizona, USA*

R. E. LAPORTE *Department of Epidemiology, Graduate School of Public Health, Pittsburgh, Pennsylvania, USA*

E. LARGER *Diabetes Department, Bichat Hospital, Paris, France*

R. D. G. LESLIE *Department of Diabetes and Metabolism, St Bartholomew's Hospital, London EC1, UK*

D. R. MCCANCE *Diabetes and Arthritis Epidemiology Section, National Institute of Diabetes and Digestive and Kidney Disease, Phoenix, Arizona, USA*

M. MCCARTHY *Medical Unit, The Royal London Hospital, London E1 1BB, UK*

N. K. MACLAREN *Department of Pathology and Laboratory Medicine, University of Florida College of Medicine, Gainesville, Florida, USA*

J. E. MANSON *Department of Medicine, Harvard Medical School and Brigham and Women's Hospital, Boston, Massachusetts, USA*

M. MATSUSHIMA *Department of Epidemiology, Graduate School of Public Health, Pittsburgh, Pennsylvania, USA*

E. J. MAYER *Kaiser-Permanente Division of Research, Oakland, California, USA*

D. K. NAGI *Diabetes and Arthritis Epidemiology Section, National Institute of Diabetes and Digestive and Kidney Diseases, Phoenix, Arizona, USA*

B. NEWMAN *The University of North Carolina at Chapel Hill, North Carolina, USA*

K. O'DEA *Deakin University, Geelong, Victoria, Australia*

Y. H. PARK *Faculty of Medicine, The University of Calgary, Alberta T2N 4N1, Canada*

D. J. PETTITT *Diabetes and Arthritis Epidemiology Section, National Institute of Diabetes and Digestive and Kidney Diseases, Phoenix, Arizona, USA*

D. I. W. PHILLIPS *MRC Environmental Epidemiology Unit, Southampton General Hospital, UK*

D. A. PYKE *Royal College of Physicians, London NW1 4LE, UK*

J. V. SELBY *Kaiser-Permanente Division of Research, Oakland, California, USA*

A. SPELSBERG *Department of Medicine, Harvard Medical School and Brigham and Women's Hospital, Boston, Massachusetts, USA*

N. TAJIMA *Third Department of Internal Medicine, Jikei University School of Medicine, Tokyo, Japan*

R. TURNER *John Radcliffe Hospital, Headington, Oxford, UK*

M. WALKER *The Medical School, University of Newcastle upon Tyne, UK*

J. W. YOON *Faculty of Medicine, The University of Calgary, Alberta T2N 4N1, Canada*

P. ZIMMET *International Diabetes Institute, Alfred Group of Hospitals, Melbourne, Victoria, Australia*

Foreword

To someone who has studied diabetes for 40 years this is an extraordinary book—extraordinary because of the enormous range of research it reflects. Less than 20 years ago diabetes was thought of as a single disease more or less severe. The insulin-dependent type 1 (IDDM), the more 'severe', was thought (by some at least) to result from a double genetic dose: the non-insulin requiring type 2 (NIDDM) was due to a single genetic factor. The *clinical* distinction between the two types had been recognized for many years but the fundamental difference in their causes was appreciated only when IDDM was found to be closely associated with certain HLA types and NIDDM was not. Since then the nature of the genetic predisposition to IDDM has been refined with the detailed clarification of the loci involved, a process which continues at an increasing pace and is reviewed by Cavan and Barnett in Chapter 1.

But genetics is not all. Studies of identical twins have shown that no more than one third of pairs are concordant for IDDM. Concordance does not prove a genetic cause—identical twins share environments as well as genes. A concordance rate therefore sets an upper limit on genetic causes no more. These results from twin studies have shown that non-genetic factors are likely to be highly important, initiating the destruction of β cells in those who are genetically susceptible.

Although the importance of environmental factors in causing IDDM has been known for about 20 years we still have little idea what the actual trigger factors may be. An early suspicion that viruses, especially the Coxsackie virus, might be involved—a brilliant and unorthodox idea at the time—now seems less likely. If viruses cause this type of diabetes it seems that they do so only occasionally and in unusual circumstances; or perhaps we simply do not know what viruses to look for or how to look for them. The search is on for other possible causes.

An encouraging finding is that the immune changes of early diabetes may remit spontaneously. The fact that islet cell antibodies may disappear without apparently doing, or reflecting, lasting islet cell damage makes it more difficult to predict the appearance of IDDM diabetes, but it raises the hope that if we could discover what causes this benign course of events we could learn how to imitate it, that is to abort diabetes in its earliest stage.

All these lines of research are included here and at much greater length and depth than those into genetic causes. That is deliberate. The emphasis is on *non*-genetic factors. There have to be such factors. If they can be identified we might approach the Holy Grail of all diabetic researchers: the *prevention* of diabetes.

We seem to be a long way from that, but the scene is set at last for real progress towards that goal. It is a goal worth achieving: for all the improvements in the treatment of IDDM, diabetes can still be a devastating disorder, crippling and killing people in the prime of life.

But not all diabetes is insulin-requiring. The commoner NIDDM is produced by a different mechanism from IDDM. We do not know what that mechanism is, but we do know that there is no autoimmune destruction of the pancreatic β cells in this disorder, only a gradual insufficiency of insulin secretion and partial resistance to its action.

The genetic predisposition here is quite different. The degree of concordance in identical twins with this type of diabetes is nearly complete. Presumably this means that genetic causes are very powerful, but again concordance does not prove genetic aetiology. These twins too share environments, so factors such as diet, inactivity and obesity could account for the findings. These possibilities are considered in a review by Newman, Mayer and Selby in Chapter 13. They point out that for all the suggestive evidence we still have not demonstrated complete concordance between twins and that concordance rates vary in different studies. So that even here, in this seemingly genetic disorder, there is room for a major role to be played by environmental causes—causes which we might be able to influence, even eliminate. NIDDM can be just as destructive as IDDM, so prevention is just as alluring a goal. Perhaps dietary change can cause diabetes. For example, it could explain the apparent increase in the incidence of NIDDM in the Australian Aborigines who have adopted a Western lifestyle as suggested by Zimmet and O'Dea in Chapter 14, and what a pleasant surprise that the condition in them seems to be rapidly reversible; there was a striking metabolic improvement on reverting to a traditional hunter/gatherer diet after only 7 weeks. It hardly seems likely that a similar treatment would have such an effect on 'ordinary' NIDDM of Caucasians, but as Spelsberg and Manson point out in Chapter 17 there are considerable possibilities, largely untested, of preventing NIDDM by modifying diet, alcohol intake and exercise.

There has been a recent revival of interest in the concept of the 'thrifty genotype' put forward by James Neel more than 30 years ago. At that time the two types of diabetes were not clearly separated, and ideas of their causation were by today's standards primitive. It was difficult to understand the biological advantage of the commoner NIDDM, whose incidence is predominantly after the end of reproductive life. But Zimmet and O'Dea (Chapter 14) point out that the advantage might appear earlier in life. The metabolic changes of NIDDM are gradual and may be detected many years before the clinical picture emerges, so those who will later become diabetic could have survival advantage. The more understandable mechanism of survival of this type of diabetes might be that proposed by Phillips and Barker (Chapter 15) of a thrifty phenotype, based on the remarkable finding that low birth weight babies have a greater chance of developing impaired glucose tolerance about 60 years later.

There can be no doubt about the genetic cause of one type of diabetes—non-insulin diabetes appearing in early life and seemingly inherited in a simple Mendelian dominant manner (MODY). Here brilliant work in England, France and the USA has shown single gene defects, but there are different defects in different families; in most cases we still have not demonstrated any gene abnormality. It is tempting to think that single defects affecting the glucokinase gene or others will be found to explain these cases. But if so, where does that get us with regard to NIDDM generally? Is that disease completely separate from MODY? Is it one disease or many?

The encouraging feature of this book is that it can be written at all, and to realize that there is such a momentum behind present-day research into the causes of diabetes. It is the rate of progress that is exhilarating. At last we can hope that we may learn how to control, reduce or prevent diabetes—a distant goal perhaps but one end worth striving for.

David Pyke

_____Part I

Insulin-dependent Diabetes Mellitus

Chapter One

Genetic Causes of Insulin-dependent Diabetes Mellitus

David A. Cavan and Anthony H. Barnett

Department of Medicine, University of Birmingham, Birmingham, UK

INTRODUCTION

Insulin-dependent diabetes mellitus (IDDM) is a T cell-dependent autoimmune disease characterized by infiltration and destruction of the pancreatic islets, leading to absolute dependence on exogenous insulin[1]. It is predominantly a Caucasoid disease, affecting about 2 per 1000 population in the UK. The highest prevalence rates occur in northern European countries[2], with a north–south gradient of prevalence rates, which range from 2.2 per 1000 population in Finland[3] to 0.24 per 1000 in France[4]. Although only scanty data are available in some cases, evidence suggests that the prevalence is low in most other races, including Asian Indians[5], Chinese[6], Japanese and black Africans[2]. The prevalence of the disease in black Americans and Afro-Caribbeans is, however, intermediate between that seen in white Caucasians and black Africans[7]. This may result from admixture of Caucasian genes in the Negroid genome (estimated to be around 21% in black Americans). Both genetic and environmental factors have been implicated to explain the differences in prevalence between different races and within the same race.

Causes of Diabetes. Edited by R. D. G. Leslie

Pancreatic β cell destruction depends on activation of $CD4^+$ T cells following presentation of antigen bound to class II human leucocyte antigen (HLA) molecules. The latter occur on the surface of antigen-presenting cells such as macrophages, B lymphocytes and activated T lymphocytes. An early clue to the nature of the genetic susceptibility was the demonstration that IDDM is associated with certain HLA types. Antigen presentation, and hence disease susceptibility, may be influenced by the nature of the HLA molecules. The genes encoding these molecules are thus good candidate susceptibility genes and have been extensively studied. Although strong disease associations have been demonstrated with HLA genes, these alone cannot account for the genetic susceptibility to the disease. Non-HLA genes which may be implicated include the T cell receptor genes, insulin gene and immunoglobulin genes.

Despite the strong evidence for inherited susceptibility, studies of identical twins suggest that this accounts for only 30–40% of disease susceptibility[8]. Environmental factors must, therefore, also play an important role. Seasonal variation in the onset of disease has been reported in many different populations, indicating a possible viral aetiology[9]. Migrants from low to high-risk areas assume the higher risk of their host country, e.g. Japanese migrants to Hawaii and French migrants to Canada, suggesting that disease susceptibility may be influenced by the host environment[10]. Temporal changes in disease incidence have also occurred, with a reported doubling in incidence in 3 years in an area of western Poland[11]. One possible explanation is that disease is initiated in genetically susceptible individuals following exposure to an unidentified environmental agent such as a virus which triggers autoimmune β cell destruction.

METHODS OF ESTABLISHING DISEASE ASSOCIATIONS WITH SUSCEPTIBILITY GENES

POPULATION ASSOCIATIONS

These involve identification of polymorphic genes and comparison of their frequency in patients versus controls (association analysis). A significant association with disease suggests a causative role for the gene polymorphism or linkage between the marker allele and the disease susceptibility allele. Unless the marker is very close to a susceptibility locus, recombination events are likely to have occurred in many members of the population and a significant association between two loci will not be detected. It is important that patients and controls are precisely matched for ethnic background. This may be difficult since unrecognized population stratification may exist.

Varying disease frequencies within these strata may result in spurious associations.

LINKAGE DISEQUILIBRIUM AND TRANS-RACIAL STUDIES

Linkage disequilibrium defines the co-occurrence of two or more alleles on the same chromosome more frequently than expected by chance and is partly dependent on their close proximity to each other. Thus a disease association with a particular allele may either reflect a true association with that allele or may be secondary to linkage disequilibrium with the true susceptibility allele. Rare recombination events during evolution have resulted in inter-racial differences in linkage disequilibrium. Assuming genetic susceptibility to the disease to be identical in all races, any allele consistently associated with disease in all races studied, despite differences in linkage disequilibrium, is likely to be a primary disease determinant. Trans-racial analysis, therefore, helps to distinguish primary disease associations from associations secondary to linkage disequilibrium.

FAMILY STUDIES

Linkage analysis estimates genetic distance between a susceptibility locus and a marker locus from the study of the inheritance of both the disease and marker in family pedigrees. Recombination is less likely than in a population enabling detection of linkage between much more widely separated loci.

ANIMAL MODELS

The short time between birth and fecundity and the potential for inbreeding experiments have allowed close study of linkage and segregation of marker genes with various diseases. Animal models may identify candidate genes or candidate areas of particular chromosomes which can then be targeted in the human genome.

THE GENES OF THE HLA REGION

The genes encoding HLA molecules are located within the major histocompatibility complex (MHC) (Figure 1) located on the short arm of chromosome 6. The class I genes include those encoding the respective α chains which combine with β_2-microglobulin to form the HLA-A, B and C molecules. These occur on all cell types and present antigen to cytotoxic T cells. Class II genes include DR, DQ and DP, each subdivided into A and B loci. They express class II molecules, which consist of an α and β chain, encoded by

6

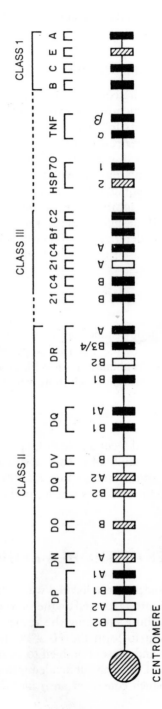

Figure 1 Diagrammatic representation of the major histocompatibility complex on chromosome 6. Expressed genes are shown as filled bars, pseudogenes (not expressed) as open bars and genes of undetermined status as hatched bars

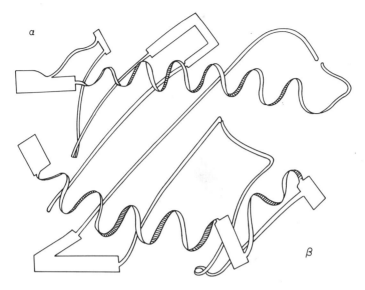

Figure 2 Structural model of a class II molecule. The α and β chains enclose an antigen-binding cleft. Antigen bound intracellularly is presented in this cleft on the cell surface, where it interacts with the T cell receptor

the respective A and B genes. A model of HLA molecular structure suggests that the α and β chains enclose an antigen-binding cleft formed by their tertiary structure[12] (Figure 2).

These molecules are expressed by antigen-presenting cells. The first domains of the extracellular portion of class II molecules bind foreign antigen and present it to CD4$^+$ T cells[13]. Many of the class II genes are highly polymorphic, resulting in great variation in the class II molecules possessed by different individuals. There is strong linkage disequilibrium within the HLA region, both between class I and class II genes and between genes within each class; this has hindered accurate mapping of susceptibility determinants of IDDM.

The class III region includes the genes which encode complement molecules. Genes encoding tumour necrosis factor and heat shock protein lie between the class I and class III genes.

HLA ASSOCIATIONS WITH IDDM

Early serological typing showed positive associations between the class I antigens B8 and B15 and IDDM[14,15]. Stronger disease associations were later shown with the DRB1 alleles encoding the class II antigens DR3 and DR4[16], which are in linkage disequilibrium with those encoding B8 and B15 respectively. This suggests that class II genes, or closely linked genes, may be primary susceptibility determinants and that the class I associations are secondary to linkage disequilibrium. Ninety-five per cent of Caucasian insulin-dependent diabetic subjects possess one or both of DR3 and DR4, which are positively associated with disease in all races in which they are common (Table 1). DR3/4 heterozygosity confers even greater disease susceptibility, and the genes encoding these types, or closely associated genes, may act synergistically in predisposing to disease. DR3 or DR4 also occur in up to 60% of non-diabetic Caucasians and cannot therefore be regarded as primary susceptibility determinants, regardless of the penetrance of the disease susceptibility alleles[17]. Attention has therefore focused on other class II genes, particularly the DQ loci, in the search for susceptibility genes. The DR, DQA1 and DQB1 associations with disease in different races are shown in Table 1.

The first evidence that DR-associated susceptibility might be DQ-encoded was the finding that 90% of a Caucasian DR4-positive diabetic population possessed the DQB1*0302 allele and only 10% the DQB1*0301 allele, whereas both alleles were equally represented in a DR4-positive control population[18]. Although a similar finding was observed in DR4-positive north

Table 1 HLA class II associations with type I diabetes in five races

	Caucasian	Negroid	N I Asian	S Chinese	Japanese
DR2	−	−	−	N	N
DR3	+	+	+	+	R
DR4	+	+	+	N+	+
DR6	−	N−	N−	N	N−
DR7	N−	+	N	N	N
DR9	N	+	N	N	+
DQA1:					
*0102	−	−	N−	N−	N−
*0103	−	R	−	R	N−
*0201	−	N−	−	R	R
*0301	+	+	+.	N	+
DQB1:					
*0201	+	+	+	N	N
*0302	+	+	+	N+	N
*0602	−	−	−	R	N−
*0603	−	−	−	R	R

+ denotes positive association, − negative association and N neutral association. N+/N− denotes inconsistent or non-significant positive or negative associations respectively. R = race in which marker is rare.

Indian Asians[19], this association was not confirmed in southern Chinese[20] or Japanese[21] populations, and DQB1*0302 is therefore unlikely to be a primary disease susceptibility determinant.

The Caucasian DR3 haplotype is associated with DQB1*0201, which also occurs on disease-predisposing haplotypes in other races. This allele was not, however, significantly associated with disease in a southern Chinese population and may therefore not be a primary susceptibility allele[20]. It also occurs on about 30% of Caucasian DR7 haplotypes which are not associated with disease[22].

The DR7-DQB1*0201 haplotype is, however, positively associated with disease in Negroids. This illustrates how the same DQB1 allele may have differing disease associations in different races and suggests that loci other than DRB1 and DQB1 must be involved in determining disease susceptibility. The contribution of DQA1 was demonstrated by comparison of Caucasian and Negroid DR7-DQB1*0201 haplotypes by sequencing the first domain-coding portions of their DRB1, DQA1 and DQB1 genes. While the DRB1 and DQB1 alleles were identical, the DQA1 alleles were different. The Caucasian haplotype possessed the DQA1*0201 allele whereas the Negroid haplotype possessed the DQA1*0301 allele, which also occurs on DR4 haplotypes[23].

The frequency of DQA1*0301 has now been studied in several races. It was found to be positively associated with IDDM in Caucasian[22,24], north Indian Asian[25], Japanese[21] and Negroid populations[26]. It was also present in 66% of a southern Chinese insulin-dependent diabetic population but this was not significantly different from the control population (56%)[20]. Furthermore, DQA1*0301 occurs on all DR4 haplotypes whether or not they are diabetogenic. These data suggest, therefore, that disease associations with this allele may be secondary to linkage disequilibrium with an as yet undetermined susceptibility allele. An alternative explanation is that DQA1*0301 is a susceptibility allele whose effects are modified by other factors. One such factor might be levels of gene expression, determined by the gene promoter region, which contains sequences which interact with transcription factors to initiate gene transcription. Polymorphism within the promoter region might be associated with different levels of gene expression and hence disease susceptibility. The sequence of the DQA1 promoter region has recently been determined in Caucasian diabetic and control subjects homozygous for the DQA1*0301 allele. The promoter sequence was identical in both diabetic and control subjects which suggests that differential expression of DQA1*0301 is unlikely to be important in determining susceptibility to Type 1 diabetes[27].

Evidence from other workers suggests, however, that levels of expression of DQ molecules may be important in determining susceptibility to insulin-dependent diabetes. The promoter regions of DQB1*0301 (neutral/protective) and DQB1*0302 (predisposing) have been shown to have different promoter strengths[28] and it is possible that overall DQ molecular density, rather than specific DQ type alone, is important in determining disease susceptibility.

DR3 is in strong linkage disequilibrium with DQA1*0501 on both diabetic and non-diabetic haplotypes[22]. Restriction fragment length polymorphism (RFLP) analysis using the restriction enzyme BglII and a DQA probe has been shown to distinguish disease-associated DR3 haplotypes in a small Caucasian population[29]. As the first-domain coding region of DQA1*0501 is not known to be polymorphic, confirmation of this finding in a larger population may indicate that DR3-associated disease susceptibility is determined by polymorphism in non-coding or regulatory regions.

OTHER HLA GENES

The DP loci lie centromeric to the DQ loci (Figure 1). The DPB1 gene is highly polymorphic and, although certain disease associations have been reported[30], there is little evidence for susceptibility alleles occurring at this locus. The genes which encode tumour necrosis factor (TNF) lie telomeric to the DR genes. Heterozygosity for a TNF-β gene RFLP is associated with disease in Caucasians but not in north Indian Asians, and this association is probably secondary to linkage disequilibrium with class II genes which directly confer susceptibility.[31]

PATTERNS OF INHERITANCE

The synergistic effect of DR3 and DR4 suggests that more than one gene is involved in susceptibility. The use of computer models of disease inheritance has suggested that DR3 is linked with a gene which acts recessively in the absence of DR4, and DR4 is linked with a gene which acts dominantly in the absence of DR3[32]. IDDM does not, therefore, follow a simple Mendelian pattern of inheritance. Analysis of inheritance in multiplex families (families with at least two diabetic siblings) has shown furthermore that the parental origin of DR3 and DR4 is important in determining disease susceptibility[33]. There is preferential transmission of maternal DR3 and paternal DR4 to affected offspring. Furthermore the offspring of diabetic fathers are at increased risk of disease than those of diabetic mothers[34]. This, together with the increased transmission of DR4 from diabetic parents to diabetic offspring, suggests dominant transmission of the DR4-associated gene.

PROTECTIVE HLA GENES

DR15 (a split of DR2) protects from IDDM in a number of races[24-26]. Analysis of our large Caucasian population showed that DR13 (a split of DR6) was also strongly protective; DR7 was observed to have a weaker protective effect[22]. The strength of the association with DR13 had not been reported previously and reflected the negative association of both DR13 (Dw18) and DR13 (Dw19) subtypes in this study. In another large population study, DR13 was positively associated with disease[35]; others have yielded conflicting results[16,36]. There is evidence that DR13 types are more frequent in British subjects than in some other European populations, but this alone would not explain the marked difference in frequency between diabetic and control subjects[37]. Confusion between DR3 and DR13 using older serological typing reagents may account for some of the discrepancies between these studies.

Both DR13 (Dw19) and DR15 carry DQA1*0102, which occurs on over 40% of non-diabetic haplotypes and is the single most frequent DQ allele in the non-diabetic population[22]. This indicates that the DQA1 locus may have a role in conferring protection from disease. The only haplotype carrying DQA1*0102 which has been shown to predispose to disease is DR16-DQA1*0102-DQB1*0502, which is very rare[15]. It is possible that the protective effect of DQA1*0102 is modified by a strong predisposing effect of the DQB1 allele on this haplotype. DQA1*0102 is reduced in diabetic compared with control subjects in Afro-Caribbeans[26], north Indian Asians[25] and southern Chinese[20], as well as in Caucasians. DQA1*0103 is associated with protection from disease in Caucasians[22], Japanese[38] and north Indian Asians[19]. The α chains encoded by DQA1*0102 and DQA1*0103 are very similar, differing at only two amino acid residues[39].

No single DQB1 allele occurs on both DR13 and DR15 haplotypes: DR13 is associated with DQB1*0603 and DQB1*0604, and DR15 with DQB1*0602. All have been shown to be significantly protective in Caucasians[22], although others have shown only weak protective or neutral effects of DQB1*0604[24,35]. DQB1*0602 and DQB1*0603 are very similar alleles and are protective in Negroids and north Indian Asians. One study showed both alleles to be absent in a southern Chinese diabetic population[20], and DQB1*0602 is reduced in Japanese diabetic subjects[21].

Further evidence for the role of the DQA1 locus comes from the protective association of Caucasian DR7 haplotypes[22]. This is despite the occurrence on 70% of these haplotypes of DQB1*0201, which is positively associated with disease. Almost all DR7 haplotypes carry DQA1*0201, which is significantly protective and which may counter the predisposing effect of DQB1*0201 on DR7 haplotypes. This is in contrast to the Negroid DR7 haplotype, which carries DQA1*0301 and DQB1*0201 and is positively associated with disease[23]. The protective effect of DQA1*0201 is also seen in north Indian Asians but this allele is rare in other races[25].

It is noteworthy that the protective DR and DQ types are very rare, or absent, in diabetic populations. This contrasts with the high frequency of predisposing types in non-diabetic populations and suggests that HLA status may be more important in conferring protection from disease rather than susceptibility to it. This is supported by the demonstration that the effect of a protective HLA type is dominant in subjects heterozygous for a protective and predisposing allele at either the DRB1, DQA1 or DQB1 locus[22].

STRUCTURAL CONSIDERATIONS OF DQ MOLECULES

Sequence studies of the DQB1 alleles led to the observation that those alleles negatively associated with disease in Caucasians encode aspartate at position 57, whereas those positively associated with disease do not. This position is at one end of the antigen-binding cleft and it was suggested that the amino acid at this position was directly involved in determining disease susceptibility[12].

While there is a significant association between Asp57-negative DQB1 alleles and IDDM in Caucasians, the occurrence of an Asp57 allele on a haplotype does not always protect from disease. Conversely, DQB1*0604 is protective despite encoding valine at position 57[22]. In the Japanese, Asp57 alleles predispose to disease[40], and further evidence against the Asp57 hypothesis has come from an animal model, the non-obese diabetic (NOD) mouse. Expression of a protective MHC gene in these mice prevented insulitis, regardless of its Asp57 status[41].

More recently it has been reported that the DQA1 alleles associated with disease in Caucasians encode arginine at position 52. It has been postulated that disease susceptibility correlates with expression of a DQ molecule bearing Arg52 on the α chain and lacking Asp57 on the β chain[24]. The only common Arg52-positive DQA1 alleles in Caucasians are those associated with DR3 and DR4, and it is possible that the disease correlation with Arg52 merely reflects the known predisposing effects of these haplotypes. Furthermore, the Arg52-negative allele DQA1*0102, although strongly associated with protection in most cases, is positively associated with disease when it occurs with DQB1*0502.

DQ molecules may be encoded by DQA1 and DQB1 alleles on the same haplotype (in *cis* position) or on different haplotypes (in *trans* position). It has been demonstrated that cells which express a particular DQ heterodimer encoded in *cis* stimulate T cell clones identical to those activated by cells encoding the same heterodimer in *trans*[42]. DQ molecules encoded in both *cis* and *trans* may therefore be important in determining susceptibility to IDDM. Indeed it has been suggested that the synergistic effect of DR3 and DR4 on disease susceptibility may be due to a heterodimer encoded in *trans* by DQA1*0301 (on the DR4 haplotype) and DQB1*0201 (on the DR3 haplotype).

Attempts have been made to quantify disease susceptibility by calculating the number of possible 'diabetogenic' DQ heterodimers (i.e. DQA Arg52-positive and DQB Asp57-negative) that could be expressed in either *cis* or *trans* in individual subjects[43]. Although the maximum possible, four heterodimers, is associated with a high relative risk for disease, subjects with two possible heterodimers are equally represented in diabetic and non-diabetic populations, and the relative risks associated with zero or one diabetogenic heterodimer are very similar[44]. This argues against a simple correlation between possible 'diabetogenic' heterodimers and disease susceptibility. This is not unexpected as genotyping data alone cannot take into account any differences in the level of expression between DQ molecules encoded in *cis* and *trans* or between different DQ molecules. Furthermore the relative risk of disease associated with DR3/4 heterozygosity is greater than with DR3 or DR4 homozygosity even though four 'diabetogenic' heterodimers are possible with each of these genotypes[45]. This is further evidence that while individual amino acid residues on the DQ molecule may be associated with disease susceptibility, it is likely that it is the overall structure of the molecule which is important in determining susceptibility. Further studies are required to demonstrate the existence of molecules expressed in *trans* before conclusions can be drawn about their putative protective effect in IDDM.

FUNCTIONAL CONSIDERATIONS OF DQ MOLECULES

There are a number of mechanisms by which DQ molecules may influence susceptibility to IDDM and thus explain the observed HLA associations. Class II molecules are critical to antigen presentation to CD4$^+$ T cells, which then proliferate and initiate an immune response. Both predisposing and protective disease associations have been demonstrated, which suggests that particular DQ molecules may be more effective either in binding a diabetogenic antigen, or in interacting with the T cell receptor, thereby increasing disease susceptibility. Alternatively, protective DQ molecules may bind antigen and present it to suppressor T cells, thus inhibiting the immune response which leads to β cell destruction. A further possibility is that the structure of protective molecules inhibits binding of diabetogenic antigen which is thus not presented to CD4$^+$ cells.

Our understanding of the link between DQ associations and disease pathogenesis is limited. Further studies into the structural configuration of different DQ molecules and whether this correlates either with disease or with subsequent T cell response (or both) are required. Such studies may also provide a likely structural model of a diabetogenic antigen. The nature of such antigen is not known although a viral antigen is a possible candidate.

VIRAL INFECTION AND IDDM

The strong evidence for environmental effects on disease susceptibility points to involvement of viral infection. Such a trigger may lead to disease in genetically susceptible individuals if presentation of viral antigen with homology with a β cell antigen results in proliferation of T cell clones directed against β cells. There is animal evidence for virally induced diabetes[46], and mumps and rubella infection in man may be associated with the development of islet cell antibodies[47]. Damage to islet cells has been demonstrated following fatal viral infections with Coxsackie B, cytomegalovirus and rubella[48], although in few cases has such infection been associated with the development of diabetes[49]. Aberrant expression of class II molecules on β cells is a feature of diabetic islet cells and may be virally induced[50]. There is no evidence, however, that such aberrant expression leads to autoimmune islet cell destruction.

Toxins may also predispose to disease although it is unlikely that genetic factors predispose to toxin-induced damage. Animal evidence suggests, however, that toxins can potentiate the diabetogenic effect of viruses[51].

DQ MOLECULES AS PROTECTIVE DETERMINANTS

The similarity of the amino acid sequence of the protective DQ molecules DQ6 and DQ1.18 (encoded by DQA1*0102/DQB1*0602 and DQA1*0103/DQB1*0603 respectively) provides an opportunity to investigate the potential contribution of these molecules to protection from disease. An identical T cell response to interaction with these two molecules would suggest that the small differences in their structure are functionally insignificant, and that they may be considered as having the same protective effect. This, together with the consistent protective association of one or both of these molecules in all racial groups studied, might be evidence of a primary protective effect conferred by the respective DQ alleles.

Class II-associated protection from disease may result from their effect on T cell repertoire. This function is unrelated to antigen presentation and occurs via the clonal deletion of T cell populations in the developing thymus. Failure to remove β cell-specific T cells from the circulation may predispose to disease. Autoimmune insulitis is prevented in the NOD mouse by expression of the I-E MHC molecule[52]. One effect of this molecule is to facilitate the clonal deletion of autoreactive T cells[53]. A similar mechanism in man may explain the consistent protective effect of certain HLA genes.

NON-HLA GENETIC ASSOCIATIONS WITH IDDM

A significant component of inherited susceptibility to IDDM is encoded by genes outside the MHC. Until recently the search for non-HLA susceptibility genes was unrewarding, with few consistent disease associations with candidate genes. The use of animal models has recently identified regions associated with disease susceptibility, and the availability of large groups of multiplex families[54] allows targeting of syntenous regions within the human genome. Apart from the insulin gene, the non-HLA genes which have been studied are involved with the immune response.

5' INSULIN REGION

The failure of insulin secretion in IDDM makes the insulin gene a candidate susceptibility determinant. It lies on the short arm of chromosome 11. The major polymorphism is located upstream (5') to the transcription region. There are two alleles in Caucasians which differ in the size of variable-number tandem repeats (VNTR). The class I alleles are of approximately 40 repeats and the larger class 3 alleles of 170 repeats. Most population studies have shown an increase in the frequency of the class I allele in patients compared with controls but this was not confirmed in early linkage studies.[55] A recent study of multiplex families has confirmed linkage between the insulin gene and disease and suggested that this was dependent both on HLA type (DR4) and parental origin of the insulin gene[56]; a further study, however, showed that the association between 5' insulin (INS) and IDDM was independent of parental transmission and HLA type[57].

T CELL RECEPTOR GENES

The HLA complex interacts with a T cell receptor (TCR). This heterodimer comprises an α and β chain and occurs on the surface of CD4$^+$ T cells. It is possible that variation within the TCR might affect antigen presentation and hence disease susceptibility. The genes encoding the α and β chains (TCRA and TCRB) are located on chromosomes 14 and 7 respectively. Despite early reports of a disease association with TCRB heterozygosity[58], there is no convincing evidence that TCR genes influence susceptibility to IDDM, either directly or through interaction with HLA genes[59].

IMMUNOGLOBULIN HEAVY CHAIN REGIONS

Antibody production against islet cells, insulin and glutamic acid decarboxylase is a feature of IDDM. Available data suggest that these antibodies are a secondary phenomenon and not primarily involved in disease susceptibility. Certain immunoglobulin heavy chain (Gm) allotypes are, however, associated with susceptibility to a number of autoimmune diseases[60]. The genes encoding immunoglobulin heavy chains, located on the long arm of chromosome 14, have been studied for evidence of association with IDDM. Several studies have failed to demonstrate a direct disease association, and linkage studies have yielded negative results[60]. There is evidence that genes encoding Gm allotypes may contribute to disease susceptibility through interaction with HLA, TCRB and INS[59]. Many of the reported associations are only weakly statistically significant and require verification from larger studies. Confirmation of these interactions would, however, demonstrate the complex nature of inherited susceptibility to the disease.

THE NOD MOUSE

The NOD mouse spontaneously develops diabetes similar to human IDDM. Like the human disease, there is autoimmune β cell destruction, autoantibody formation and associations with MHC genes.

These animals have been used to search for co-segregation between polymorphic markers and disease. Using this strategy, three regions in the NOD genome have been located which are associated with disease susceptibility: IDD3, IDD4 and IDD5[61]. Two syntenous regions of the human genome are of particular interest. IDD4 lies on mouse chromosome 11, which is homologous with human chromosome 17. Analysis of multiplex families has demonstrated weak evidence of linkage with areas of chromosome 17 (unpublished data). IDD5 on mouse chromosome 1 is homologous with human chromosome 2, which carries two genes involved in immune response and which are thus potential candidate susceptibility genes: the interleukin 1 receptor gene and Lsh/Ity/Bcg, which influences macrophage activation[62].

Candidate genes identified in this way can be tested in association and linkage studies in man. Despite similarity with human MHC susceptibility loci, however, not all susceptibility genes may be shared in both species; furthermore, susceptibility genes identified in the NOD mouse may lie outside the syntenous region and may therefore be located on other chromosomes in man.

SUMMARY AND CONCLUSIONS

Rapid progress has been made in the last decade in furthering understanding of the genetic susceptibility to IDDM. The disease is T cell-dependent and strongly associated with HLA–DQ genes. These encode cell surface DQ molecules which present antigen to T cells. The occurrence of both positive and protective DQ associations suggests that different DQ molecular structures may influence disease susceptibility by effects on antigen binding or presentation. These effects may either promote or inhibit the process which leads to disease. The consistent protective effects of particular DQ molecules in different races suggest they may be more important in conferring protection than predisposition; such protection may ensue from effects on T cell repertoire as well as antigen presentation. Further studies are required to determine whether levels of expression of DQ molecules are important in disease susceptibility. The functional significance of DQ molecular structure also requires further definition.

T cell receptor and immunoglobulin genes are unlikely to have an important effect on disease susceptibility. There is evidence, however, that the recently identified susceptibility genes in the NOD mouse are also immune response genes, and further studies of these candidate genes in human populations are required to determine their role in disease susceptibility. The evidence that the insulin gene is associated with disease, however, emphasizes the complex interactive nature of inherited susceptibility to the disease.

It is likely that an environmental agent triggers the immune response which leads to disease in genetically susceptible individuals. Despite the occurrence of certain features of the disease in association with some viral infections, no virus has been proven to cause disease in man, and the nature of the environmental agent remains a mystery.

Elucidation of further susceptibility genes and thus identification of a high-risk genotype will make genetic screening feasible, at least in high-risk subjects such as siblings of patients. This may be of predictive value in association with surveillance to detect the appearance of immune markers such as islet cell antibodies. If the critical gene product(s) are known, agents could be designed to block or counteract their effect. These possibilities are becoming increasingly likely, with the long-term goal of disease prevention in genetically susceptible individuals.

ACKNOWLEDGEMENTS

D.A.C. is an MRC Training Fellow. We thank Karen Jacobs for preparing figures. We gratefully acknowledge financial support from the British Diabetic Association, the Wellcome Trust, the West Midlands Regional Health Authority and Eli Lilly (UK).

REFERENCES

1 Todd JA. Genetic control of autoimmunity in type I diabetes. *Immunol Today* 1990; **11**: 122–9.
2 Odugbesan O, Barnett AH. Racial differences. In: *Immunogenetics of Insulin Dependent Diabetes* (ed AH Barnett) MTP Press Lancaster, 1987, pp 91–101.

3 Koivisto VA, Åkerblom HK, Wasz-Höckert O. The epidemiology of juvenile diabetes mellitus in Northern Finland. *Nord Council Arct Med Res* 1976; **15**: 58–65.
4 Lestradet H, Besse J. Prevalence and incidence of juvenile insulin-dependent diabetes in France. *Diabete Metab* 1977; **3**: 229–34.
5 Vaishnava H, Bashin RC, Galati PO. Diabetes mellitus with onset under 40 years in North India. *J Assoc Physicians India* 1974; **22**: 879–88.
6 Shanghai Diabetes Research Cooperative Group. Diabetes mellitus survey in Shanghai. *Chin Med J* 1980; **93**: 663–7.
7 Lorenzi M, Cagliero E, Schmidt JJ. Racial differences in incidence of juvenile onset type I diabetes: epidemiologic studies in southern California. *Diabetologia* 1980; **28**: 734–8.
8 Barnett AH, Eff C, Leslie RDG, Pyke DA. Diabetes in identical twins: a study of 200 pairs. *Diabetologia* 1981; **20**: 87–93.
9 Gamble DR, Taylor KW. Seasonal incidence of diabetes mellitus. *Br Med J* 1969; **iii**: 631–3.
10 Diabetes Epidemiology Research International. Preventing insulin-dependent diabetes mellitus: the environmental challenge. *Br Med J* 1987; **295**: 479–81.
11 Rewers M, LaPorte RE, Walczak M, Dmochowski K, Bogaczynska E. An apparent 'epidemic' of youth onset insulin-dependent diabetes mellitus in Western Poland. *Diabetes* 1987; **36**: 106–13.
12 Todd JA, Bell JI, McDevitt HO. HLA-DQβ gene contributes to susceptibility and resistance to insulin-dependent diabetes mellitus. *Nature* 1987; **329**: 599–604.
13 Schwartz RH. T-lymphocyte recognition of antigen in association with gene products of the major histocompatibility complex. *Annu Rev Immunol* 1985; **3**: 237–61.
14 Singal DP, Blajchman MA. Histocompatibility (HL-A) antigens, lymphocytotoxic antibodies and tissue-specific antibodies in patients with diabetes mellitus. *Diabetes* 1973; **22**: 429–32.
15 Nerup J, Platz P, Andersen OO, et al. HL-A antigens in diabetes mellitus. *Lancet* 1974; **ii**: 864–6.
16 Wolf E, Spencer KM, Cudworth AG. The genetic susceptibility to type I (insulin-dependent) diabetes: analysis of the HLA-DR association. *Diabetologia* 1983; **24**: 224–30.
17 Jenkins D, Mijovic C, Fletcher J, et al. Indentification of susceptibility loci for type I (insulin-dependent) diabetes by trans-racial gene mapping. *Diabetologia* 1990; **33**: 387–95.
18 Nepom BS, Palmer J, Kim SJ, et al. Specific genomic markers for the HLA-DQ subregion discriminate between DR4 + insulin-dependent diabetes mellitus and DR4 + seropositive juvenile rheumatoid arthritis. *J Exp Med* 1986; **164**: 345–50.
19 Fletcher J, Odugbesan O, Mijovic C, et al. Class II HLA DNA polymorphisms in type I (insulin-dependent) diabetic patients of North Indian origin. *Diabetologia* 1988; **31**: 343–50.
20 Penny MA, Jenkins D, Mijovic CH, et al. Susceptibility to insulin-dependent diabetes mellitus in a Chinese population: role of HLA class II alleles. *Diabetes* 1992; **41**: 914–19.
21 Jacobs KH, Jenkins D, Mijovic CH, et al. An investigation of Japanese subjects maps susceptibility to type I (insulin-dependent) diabetes mellitus close to the DQA1 gene. *Hum Immunol* 1992; **33**: 24–8.
22 Cavan DA, Jacobs KH, Penny MA, et al. Both DQA1 and DQB1 genes are

implicated in HLA-associated protection from type I (insulin-dependent) diabetes in a British Caucasian population. *Diabetologia* 1993; **36**: 252–7.

23 Todd JA, Mijovic C, Fletcher J, et al. Identification of susceptibility loci for insulin-dependent diabetes mellitus by trans-racial gene mapping. *Nature* 1989; **338**: 587–9.

24 Khalil I, d'Auriol L, Gobet M, et al. A combination of HLA-DQβ Asp57-negative and HLA DQα Arg 52 confers susceptibility to insulin-dependent diabetes mellitus. *J Clin Invest* 1990; **85**: 1315–19.

25 Jenkins D, Mijovic C, Jacobs KH, et al. Allele-specific gene probing supports the DQ molecule as a detemINant of inherited susceptibility to type I (insulin-dependent) diabetes mellitus. *Diabetologia* 1991; **34**: 109–13.

26 Mijovic CH, Jenkins D, Jacobs KH, et al. HLA-DQA1 and -DQB1 alleles associated with genetic susceptibility to IDDM in a black population. *Diabetes* 1991; **40**: 748–53.

27 Jacobs KH, Cavan DA, Penny MA, Barnett AH. DR4-associated susceptibility to Type I diabetes mellitus does not result from DQA1 promoter region polymorphism. *Diabetic Med* (in press).

28 Andersen CL, Beaty JS, Nettles JW, et al. Allelic polymorphism in transcriptional regulatory regions of HLA-DQB genes. *J Exp Med* 1991; **173**: 181–92.

29 Carrier C, Mollen N, Ginsberg-Fellner F, Rothman WC, Rubinstein P. A BglII fragment labels a subset of B8, DR3 haplotypes uniquely associated with insulin-dependent diabetes mellitus. *Hum Immunol* 1989; **26**: 344–52.

30 Easteal S, Kohonen-Corish MRJ, Zimmet P, Serjeantson SW. HLA-DP variation as additional risk factor in IDDM. *Diabetes* 1990; **39**: 855–7.

31 Jenkins D, Penny MA, Mijovic CH, et al. Tumour necrosis factor-beta polymorphism is unlikely to determine susceptibility to type I (insulin-dependent) diabetes mellitus. *Diabetologia* 1991; **34**: 576–8.

32 Louis EJ, Thomson G. Three-allele synergistic mixed model for insulin-dependent diabetes. *Diabetes* 1986; **35**: 958–63.

33 Deschamps I, Hors J, Clergot-Darpoux F, et al. Excess of maternal HLA-DR3 antigens in HLA DR3,4 positive type I (insulin-dependent) diabetic patients. *Diabetologia* 1990; **33**: 425–30.

34 Warram JH, Krolewski AS, Gottlieb MS, Kahn CR. Differences in risk of insulin-dependent diabetes in offspring of diabetic mothers and fathers. *N Engl J Med* 1984; **311**: 149–52.

35 Thomson G, Robinson WP, Kuhner MK, et al. Genetic heterogeneity: modes of inheritance and risk estimates for a joint study of Caucasians with insulin-dependent diabetes mellitus. *Am J Hum Genet* 1988; **43**: 799–816.

36 Kohonen-Corish MRJ, Serjeantson SW, Lee HK, Zimmet P. Insulin-dependent diabetes mellitus: HLA-DR and -DQ genotyping in three ethnic groups. *Dis Markers* 1987; **5**: 153–64.

37 Ronningen KS, Spurkland A, Iwe T, Vartdal F, Thorsby E. Distribution of HLA-DRB1, -DQA1 and -DQB1 genotypes among Norwegian patients with insulin-dependent diabetes mellitus. *Tissue Antigens* 1991; **37**: 105–11.

38 Awata T, Kuzuya T, Matsuda A, Iwamoto Y, Kanazawa Y. Genetic analysis of HLA class II alleles and susceptibility to type I (insulin-dependent) diabetes mellitus in Japanese subjects. *Diabetologia* 1992; **35**: 419–24.

39 Marsh SGE, Bodmer JG. HLA class II nucleotide sequences. *Tissue Antigens* 1991; **37**: 181–9.

40 Awata T, Kuzuya T, Matsuda A, et al. High frequency of aspartic acid at position

57 of HLA-DQ β-chain in Japanese IDDM patients and nondiabetic subjects. *Diabetes* 1990; **39**: 266–9.

41 Miyazaki T, Uno M, Uehira M. Direct evidence for the contribution of the unique I-A^{NOD} to the development of insulitis in non-obese diabetic mice. *Nature* 1990; **345**: 722–4.

42 Ronningen KS, Gjertsen HA, Iwe T, et al. Particular HLA-DQ α β heterodimer associated with IDDM susceptibility in both DR4-DQw4 Japanese and DR4-DQw8/DRw8-DQw4 whites. *Diabetes* 1991 **40**: 759–63.

43 Gutierrez-Lopez MD, Bertera S, Chantres MT, et al. Susceptibility to type I (insulin-dependent) diabetes mellitus in Spanish patients correlates quantitatively with expression of HLA-DQα Arg52 and HLA-DQβ non-Asp 57 alleles. *Diabetologia* 1992; **35**: 583–8.

44 Penny MA, Mijovic CH, Cavan DA, et al. An investigation into the role of HLA DQα Arg52–DQβ Non-Asp57 heterodimers in susceptibility to type I (insulin-dependent) diabetes mellitus: studies in five racial groups. *Human Immunol* (in press).

45 Jenkins D, Penny MA, Uchigata Y, et al. Investigation of the mode of inheritance of insulin-dependent diabetes mellitus in Japanese subjects. *Am J Hum Genet* 1992; **50**: 1018–21.

46 Onodera T, Ray UR, Melez KA, et al. Virus induced diabetes mellitus: autoimmunity and polyendocrine disease prevented by immunosuppression. *Nature* 1982; **297**: 66–8.

47 Bodansky HJ, Grant PJ, Dean BM, et al. Islet cell antibodies and insulin autoantibodies in association with common viral infections. *Lancet* 1986; **ii**: 1351–3.

48 Jenson AB, Rosenberg HS, Notkins AL. Pancreatic islet cell damage in children with fatal viral infections. *Lancet* 1980; **ii**: 354–8.

49 Yoon JW, Austin M, Onodera T, Notkins AL. Virus-induced diabetes mellitus: isolation of a virus from the pancreas of a child with diabetic ketoacidosis. *N Engl J Med* 1979; **300**: 1173–9.

50 Lo SSS, Tun RYM, Leslie RDG. Non-genetic factors causing type I diabetes. *Diabetic Med* 1991; **8**: 609–18.

51 Toniolo A, Onodera T, Yoon JW, Notkins AL. Induction of diabetes by cumulative environmental insults from viruses and chemicals. *Nature* 1980; **288**: 383–5.

52 Lund T, O'Reilly L, Hutchings P, et al. Prevention of insulin-dependent diabetes mellitus in non-obese diabetic mice transgenes encoding modified I-A β-chain or normal I-E α-chain. *Nature* 1990; **345**: 727–9.

53 Bill J, Kanagawa O, Woodland DL, Palmer E. The MHC molecule I-E is necessary but not sufficient for the clonal deletion of VβII-bearing T cells. *J Exp Med* 1989; **169**: 1405–19.

54 Bain SC, Todd JA, Barnett AH. The British Diabetic Association–Warren Repository. *Autoimmunity* 1990; **7**: 83–5.

55 Tuomilehto-Wolf E, Tuomilehto J, Cepaitis Z, et al. New susceptibility haplotype for type I diabetes. *Lancet* 1989; **ii**: 299–302.

56 Julier C, Hyer RN, Davies J, et al. Insulin-IGF2 region on chromosome 11p encodes a gene implicated in HLA-DR4 dependent diabetes susceptibility. *Nature* 1991; **354**: 155–9.

57 Bain SC, Prins J-B, Hearne CM, et al. Insulin gene region-encoded susceptibility to type I diabetes is not restricted to HLA-DR4-positive individuals. *Nature Genet* 1992; **2**: 213–15.

58 Millward BA, Welsh KI, Leslie RDG, Pyke DA, Demaine AG. T cell receptor

beta chain polymorphisms are associated with insulin-dependent diabetes. *Clin Exp Immunol* 1987; **70**: 152–7.

59 Field LL. Non-HLA region genes in insulin-dependent diabetes mellitus. *Baillière's Clin Endocrinol Metab* 1991; **5**: 413–37.

60 Field LL, Anderson CE, Neiswanger K, et al. Interaction of HLA and immunoglobulin antigens in type I (insulin-dependent) diabetes. *Diabetologia* 1984; **27**: 504–8.

61 Todd JA, Aitman TJ, Cornall RJ, et al. Genetic analysis of an autoimmune disease, murine type I (insulin-dependent) diabetes mellitus. *Nature* 1991; **351**: 542–7.

62 Cornall RJ, Pins J-B, Todd JA, et al. Type I diabetes in mice is linked to the interleukin-1 receptor and the Lsh/Ity/Bcg genes on chromosome 1. *Nature* 1991; **353**: 262–5.

Interaction of Genetic and Non-genetic Factors

Chapter Two

Population Studies

N. Tajima[a], M. Matsushima[b] and R. E. LaPorte[b]

[a]Third Department of Internal Medicine, Jikei University School of Medicine, Tokyo, Japan; [b]Department of Epidemiology, Graduate School of Public Health, Pittsburgh, USA

GEOGRAPHICAL VARIATION IN INSULIN-DEPENDENT DIABETES MELLITUS INCIDENCE

VARIATION BETWEEN COUNTRIES

Worldwide Incidence Data

Accumulated population-based data have demonstrated a marked diversity in the incidence of insulin-dependent diabetes mellitus (IDDM) worldwide. Rewers et al., as part of the Diabetes Epidemiology Research International (DERI) group, first mapped existing IDDM incidence data in subjects under age 15 years using the standardized incidence measures with the collaboration of 24 registries from ethnically and geographically diverse countries[1]. There were extraordinary large variations in incidence rates, from 1.7 per 100 000 for Hokkaido, Japan, to 29.5 per 100 000 in Finland during the years 1978–1980. This was subsequently updated as part of the World Health Organization (WHO) report, again demonstrating the enormous diversity across all countries[2].

Causes of Diabetes. Edited by R. D. G. Leslie

Standardized Prospective Surveillance for IDDM

Most recently, prospective monitoring based on a standard protocol on the newly diagnosed cases of IDDM in subjects up to 15 years was conducted by the Eurodiab Ace Study Group during 1989–1990 in 24 geographically well-defined regions in Europe and Israel[3]. It was demonstrated that the incidence ranged from 4.6 per 100 000 for northern Greece to 42.9 per 100 000 for two regions in Finland, with an almost ten-fold difference in Europe itself. The most striking new finding from this report was a very high rate in Sardinia (30.2 per 100 000). It has been speculated that the extremely high rates may be the result of a large proportion of susceptible gene in this island[4]. However, the rise in IDDM incidence over time in Sardinia would tend to argue against this. Detailed further analyses are warranted. Another large project to determine IDDM incidence worldwide for the year 2000, using the standardized procedure, was started by the WHO Diamond Project Group in 1990[5]. Approximately 110 centres from 64 countries agreed to participate. The preliminary data will be available in the next few years.

Geographical Mapping of the IDDM Incidence Rate for Age 0–14 years

Reported data basically followed a classical finding of a north–south gradient; however, it did not show a simple gradation (Figure 1). Sardinia, Italy, which is located in the Mediterranean region, had the second highest rate in the world. In contrast, a relatively low rate in Iceland (10.8 per 100 000, 1980–1989), with a similar latitude to Finland, was reported[6]. It was interesting that the genetic background in Iceland is from Norway, yet the incidence in Norway (20.8 per 100 000, 1989)[3] is approximately two times higher than that seen in Iceland. The north–south gradient in IDDM incidence, namely, the greater the distance from the equator, the higher the incidence rate, has been interpreted as evidence for the involvement of environmental factors, especially viruses, in the occurrence of this disorder[7]. The demonstration of outliers of 'hot spot' and 'cold spot' in IDDM incidence rate, emerging from the recent studies, suggests a complicated interaction of genetic and non-genetic factors associated with the aetiology of IDDM.

WITHIN-COUNTRY VARIATION

Finland

In Finland, earlier studies by Reunanen et al.[8] have shown that the IDDM incidence rate in the 1970s was lower in the northern than in the southern

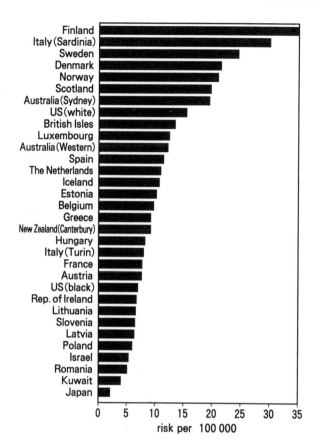

Figure 1 Geographical variation in age-adjusted IDDM incidence rate for 0–14 years after 1985. Estimated case ascertainment in each registry is more than 95%. (Data are cited from references 3, 6, 9, 10, 14, 18, 20–22, 25, 34, 47, 48, 53, 63 and 64)

part of the country. However, the most recent observation by Tuomilehto et al.[9] failed to detect within-country variation in IDDM incidence. In this chapter, the average annual incidence rate of cases under 15 years for 1987–1989 was reported to be 35 per 100 000, with 95% confidence interval (CI) of 33–38. Furthermore, comparative study of the incidence rate between Finland and Estonia has revealed that the incidence rate in Estonia was 10.3 per 100 000 for the year 1988[10], which is approximately one-third of that in Finland; it has been speculated that the large difference might be attributed to viral infection and diet[11]. Although different countries, their populations are genetically and linguistically similar, and are geographically close (Figure 2).

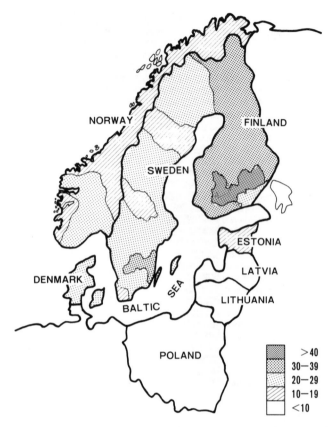

Figure 2 Intra-/inter-country variation in IDDM incidence rate per 100 000 per year for 0–14 years in the Baltic area. (Data are cited from references 9 (Finland, 1987–1989), 12 (Sweden, 1977–1983), 40 (Norway, 1973–1982), 3 (Denmark, 1990) and 34 (Poland, Lithuania, Latvia and Estonia, 1983–1988))

Sweden

The data from Sweden for the years 1977–1983[12] suggested that age- and sex-standardized IDDM incidence rate varied, but not systematically, among the 24 counties. It ranged from 17.1 per 100 000 to 32.8 per 100 000, including two geographically close counties which had significantly higher incidence rates in the south-eastern part of Sweden, which is closer to the Baltic Sea. Another two counties with significantly low incidence rates were located in mid- and northern Sweden. The reason for this geographical variation within the country has yet to be explained. Swedish people are considered to be a genetically homogeneous and static population; therefore, possible differences in non-genetic factors should be taken into account.

Norway

A considerable geographical variation in IDDM incidence in Norway has been reported[13]. The rate for the age group 0–14 years in 1973–1977 was 6.8 per 100 000 in Finnmark County in northernmost Norway and 24–28 per 100 000 in the southern part of the country. Cases were identified retrospectively by using two independent sources, and the degree of ascertainment was estimated as more than 90%. Authors argued that the lowest rates, seen in the county of Finnmark, may be related to the low prevalence of diabetes in Lapps.

British Isles

Nationwide surveillance of IDDM patients in the British Isles[14] also demonstrated a large within-country variation. Metcalfe et al. studied the incidence rate of IDDM in subjects under 15 years during 1988 using an active reporting system. The incidence rates varied from 6.8 per 100 000 in the Republic of Ireland to 19.8 per 100 000 in Scotland. The national incidence rate was 13.5 per 100 000.

The USA and Canada

The USA and Canada are areas where the importance of an accurate ongoing population-based IDDM registry was recognized from the early years. In 1986, the DERI study group sent a letter to all the centres within the USA and other countries where they have registries, asking them to provide details of the number of new IDDM cases. Using standardized data reporting, age-adjusted IDDM incidence data for 0–14 years by ethnic group within the USA were summarized (Table 1). The rates varied remarkably with place and in different ethnic groups. It ranged from 4.1 per 100 000 in Hispanics in San Diego[15], to 28.9 per 100 000 in whites in the US Virgin Islands[16]. A very high incidence rate is also observed in Prince Edward Island, Canada (25.5 per 100 000)[1,17].

Japan

In contrast to the finding in high and medium-risk countries, geographical variation in a low-risk country such as Japan is infinitesimal[18,19]. The overall incidence rates by area during the 1980s for age 0–14 years were reported to be approximately 2 per 100 000, with no north–south gradient (Hokkaido: 2.1 per 100 000, 1985–1989; Tokyo: 1.7 per 100 000, 1978–1989; Kagoshima: 1.8 per 100 000, 1980–1989). The age-specific incidence rates were amazingly similar across very different areas.

Table 1 Geographical and ethnic diversities in IDDM incidence within the USA
(cited from references 1 and 16)

Registry	Ethnic group			
	White	Black	Oriental	Hispanic
Rochester, MN, 1970–1979	20.6 (13.9–29.5)			
North Dakota, 1979–1983	20.3 (17.2–24.0)			
Colorado, 1978–1983	16.4 (15.0–17.8)			9.7 (7.4–12.4)
Allegheny Co., PA, 1978–1983	16.2 (14.1–18.4)	11.8 (7.9–17.2)		
Jefferson Co., Al, 1979–1983	16.9 (13.4–21.4)	4.4 (2.3–7.5)		
San Diego, CA, 1978–1980	13.8 (9.8–18.9)	3.3 (0.4–11.9)	6.4 (1.3–18.7)	4.1 (1.3–9.6)
US Virgin Islands, 1979–1988	28.9 (3.9–53.8)	5.9 (3.0–8.8)		7.2 (0–15.1)

What is most interesting is the extremely low variation in incidence rates in Japan in contrast to the British Isles and the USA. What information does the intra-/inter-country variation provide? The range, including semi-interquartile range, in incidence rates for various parts of the British Isles[14] and the USA[1] was much greater than that seen in Japan[18] (Table 2). The within-country variability due to a race/ethnic component, because the semi-interquartile range for US whites is much less than the US total population (3.00 versus 5.95). Furthermore, the 95% CI surrounding the variance estimates completely overlapped for the British Isles (variance: 10.16; 95% CI: 5.72–22.84) and the USA (variance: 17.53; 95% CI: 6.83–105.43), but noticeably did not overlap with the 'tight' CI seen in Japan (variance: 0.03; 95% CI: 0.01–0.27). It was not only the absolute variation which was much smaller in Japan, but also the relative variation. The ratio of the highest to the lowest incidence rates in the British Isles (2.90) and the USA (2.20) was almost twice as great as that in Japan (1.25). The coefficient of variation in Japan was also about half that seen in the British Isles and the USA. It was interesting also that when the incidence rates were examined for whites only in the USA, the variation in the incidence rates was still considerably lower in Japan, which likely reflects the large ethnic variation among Europeans in the USA, with Minnesota, for example, having as their parent population Scandinavia, a high-risk area of Europe, and Allegheny County, Pennsylvania, having as their parent population the low-risk area of Eastern

Table 2 Within-country difference in British Isles[14], the USA[1] and Japan[18]. Figures in the table are the incidence rate by the area in each country. Almost infinitesimal intra-Japan variation but large range and semi-interquartile range in incidence in the other two countries are observed

	British Isles	US (total)	USA (white)	Japan
	19.80	20.00	20.60	2.07
	17.70	17.80	20.30	1.93
	17.10	15.10	16.90	1.78
	15.80	13.40	16.40	1.66
	15.80	11.40	16.20	1.65
	15.20	9.40	13.80	
	14.90			
	14.60			
	13.50			
	13.40			
	13.30			
	13.10			
	12.80			
	12.40			
	11.80			
	10.90			
	8.00			
	6.80			
Mean	13.72	14.65	17.37	1.82
SD	3.11	4.19	2.62	0.16
Median	13.40	13.40	16.20	1.72
Range	13.00	11.40	6.80	0.42
Q3–Q1[a]	3.65	5.95	3.00	0.25

[a]Semi-interquartile range.

Europe. It is thus likely that much of the inter- and intra-country variation results from genetic factors.

Oceania

An IDDM incidence survey was conducted in Western Australia primarily by the school health services with external validation in 1983. An incidence rate of 12.3 per 100 000 for age 0–14 years was found with almost complete ascertainment[20]. In Sydney[21], a population-based IDDM register of IDDM cases in the 0–14-year age group was completed with high ascertainment in the Southern Metropolitan Health Region of Sydney. New cases were ascertained retrospectively for 1984 and prospectively for the years 1985–1987. Age-specific incidence rates were 13.6 per 100 000 for 1984 and 19.4 per

100 000 for 1987. However, the increase was not statistically significant. A prospective study based on a register started in 1982 was conducted by Canterbury Hospital Board with almost complete ascertainment. The average incidence rate for age less than 20 years was 11.7 per 100 000 for the period 1982–1986, with non-significant sex differences and temporal trends[22]. Data are also available from a small series of cases in Auckland[23]. The reported incidence of 9.3 per 100 000 for age 0–15 years is similar to that for Canterbury, since the age range is greater in the Canterbury registry than in that of Auckland. The procedures utilized in the different areas of Oceania were not standardized; therefore, direct comparisons cannot be made. However, overall there seems to be relatively little variability of incidence in Oceania.

TEMPORAL VARIATION

SECULAR TRENDS IN IDDM INCIDENCE

Importance of Data Selection

In assessing secular trends, one should consider possible undernumeration of cases in earlier years. If the degree of case ascertainment was not analysed in the text, the accuracy of the data presented may be questionable. Furthermore, low incidence rates observed in the earlier years may be attributed, in part, to a birth cohort effect. The major point is that we now have much better incidence data than before. There are few reliable data on the incidence of IDDM prior to 1940. The most reliable data come from 1965 onward.

Linear Increase in Scandinavian Countries

There have been many instances where European countries have shown an increase in IDDM incidence[24]. In Sweden, the incidence data of children aged 0–14 years for all 24 counties over 1977–1983 were reported[12] to be 23.6 per 100 000 and increased dramatically in the second 3-year period (22.7–25.1 per 100 000). This increase was consistent when the cohort was subdivided by age, sex and area. This cohort was followed for further analyses of temporal variation, and an increasing linear trend in IDDM for both sex and different age groups during 1978–1987 was found[25]. In Finland, all individuals with IDDM are included in the Central Drug Registry, by which these patients receive reimbursement for the cost of insulin. Therefore, this system provides the most accurate data. It has been demonstrated that the incidence rate showed a common linear trend of 20.4 per 100 000 in 1966 to 38.0 per

100000 in 1983 for the 0–14-year age group[26]. Among male birth cohorts in Denmark, there was evidence for a significant increase in incidence independent of age effects for the early 1950s to a maximum in the late 1970s[27].

Observations in Other Parts of Europe

The incidence of IDDM up to age 14 years inclusive in the three decades 1951–1980 using the register of Leicestershire was evaluated[28]. The rate was 5.34 per 10000 during 1961–1970, and increased to 10.6 per 100000 for 1971–1980, with a significant change in each age group for boys and girls The register started in the early 1940s dating back to the 1920s; however, authors eliminated the data before 1950 owing to the ascertainment problem. As was mentioned earlier in this chapter, an annual national IDDM incidence rate under age 15 years during 1988 in the British Isles of 13.5 per 100 000 was reported[14]. In this chapter, the incidence rate in Trent Regional Health Authority, where Leicestershire is included, is reported as the same as the national mean. This figure appears to be much higher than the incidence rate by registry data in Leicestershire, which was 7.7 per 100 000 for age 0–15 years in 1973–1974[14]. Owing to the different methodology utilized in the two surveys, it is impossible to make a direct comparison; however, it is very likely that the incidence of IDDM has increased in the past three decades in England. A rising incidence was also found using a retrospective study in Hungarian children under age 15 years[29]. During the period 1978–1987, the incidence rate increased very rapidly from 3.8 per 100 000 to 8.2 per 100 000. Following the procedures utilized in the Danish study, the IDDM incidence rate in male army conscripts was examined in the Netherlands[30]. A significant non-linear increase in the birth cohorts of 1960–1970 was observed.

IDDM 'EPIDEMIC': THE NATURE OF COMMUNICABLE DISEASE

Earliest Appearance of Epidemics

It has been reported that, unlike practically any other non-communicable diseases, IDDM exhibits epidemic patterns like that seen in infectious disease. Evidence of rapid fluctuations in incidence can only be ascribed to potent, non-genetic factors. The earliest observation was recognized in Oslo, Norway[31], where the incidence of IDDM increased from 10 per 100 000 in 1926 to approximately 20 per 100 000 in 1936 for both sexes. The rate declined again to 5–10 per 100 000 in 1940–1950. In Erie County, New York, USA[32], IDDM incidence rate increased from 9.9 per 100 000 to 12.5 per 100 000 during the period 1946–1961. The rates fluctuated, whereby the first peak of 9.2 per 100 000 was observed in 1953, 2 years after the earlier nadir year of 1951 (5.8 per 100 000). These data should be cited with caution because neither provided an estimate of the degree of case ascertainment. However, rapid year to year fluctuations of incidence are unlikely to be completely explained by ascertainment.

Suggestion of Peak Incidence in the Mid-1980s Worldwide

The first reliable data of IDDM epidemic come from midwestern Poland[33], where the incidence almost doubled from 3.5 per 100 000 in 1970–1981 to 6.6 per 100 000 in 1982–1984. A similar observation was detected in the Baltic populations geographically close to Poland. The IDDM incidence rate for age below 15 years among Finland, Estonia, Latvia, Lithuania and Poland for the years 1983–1988 varied remarkably within a small area (Finland: 36.9; Estonia: 10.7; Latvia: 6.4; Lithuania: 6.5; and Poland: 6.0), with a peak incidence around 1986 in all countries except for Poland[34,35]. Japan, known as an IDDM low-risk country, is one of the countries where accurate data on time trends are needed. Two population-based ongoing IDDM registries started from mid-1970s suggested a relatively constant incidence from 1980 to 1987, followed by a slight decline[18]. A preliminary report from Shanghai[36] demonstrated that there were 70 newly diagnosed IDDM cases identified during 1980–1991, which represents an IDDM incidence rate of 0.67 per 100 000. The striking finding was that not only a world record low incidence rate, but also a spiking incidence, was seen in the year 1986.

Apparent Epidemic of IDDM Following Virus Outbreak

A classic epidemic pattern was seen in Jefferson County, Alabama, immediately after an aseptic meningitis outbreak due to Coxsackie virus B5[37]. The rate increased from an average annual incidence of 12.8 per 100 000 in 1979–1983 to 23.3 per 100 000 in 1984. The rise was greatest in females and among all children aged 10–14 years. In Finland, the incidence rate reached a peak level in 1983 after a linear increase. After that, the rate declined somewhat during the two subsequent years, which was argued to be associated with a mumps outbreak that occurred during the years 1979–1980 throughout Finland[38]. In that paper, the authors suggested that the geographical variation in mumps within Finland, which paralleled the regional trends in the incidence of IDDM, supported their speculation. Although not confirmed, there are some reports which strongly suggest the association of viral epidemic and the occurrence of IDDM. Tull et al. investigated the epidemiology of IDDM in the US Virgin Islands[16] during the period 1979–1988. An average annual IDDM incidence rate from children below 15 years of age was 7.5 per 100 000, with a significant increase in incidence observed in 1984 (28.4 per 100 000). The doubling increase of IDDM incidence was seen in 15–17-year-old males from 1980 to 1982 in Colorado[39]. Similar changes were also reported from Pittsburgh[2] and Norway[40].

SEX DIFFERENCE, AGE AT ONSET, SEASONALITY AND ETHNICITY

SEX-SPECIFIC IDDM INCIDENCE RATE

Sex-specific IDDM incidence data from various parts of the world suggest that there is a slight excess for females in the non-Caucasian population, a mostly low-risk group, whereas an equal or slightly male predominance is observed in Caucasians (Figure 3). The relationship between incidence rate and sex ratio appears to follow the regression formula[41]. The reason for the female excess in a low-risk area remains to be elucidated. The influence of intrinsic factors such as sex hormones, height at onset[42,43] and growth spurt[44] on the aetiology of IDDM is very intriguing, yet has not been sufficiently explained.

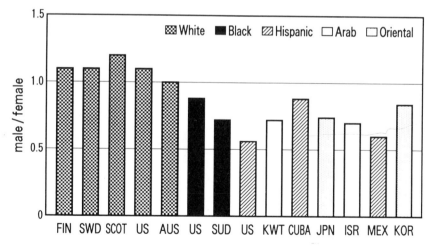

Figure 3 Sex ratio in IDDM incidence by race. The similar male/female ratio is seen in high-and medium-risk countries, but female predominance is observed in low-risk countries. (FIN, Finland; SWD, Sweden; SCOT, Scotland; US, Allegheny County, USA; AUS, Western Australia; SUD, Sudan; KWT, Kuwait; CUBA, Cuba; JPN, Japan; ISR, Israel; MEX, Mexico; KOR, Korea)

AGE AT ONSET

In both sexes, the incidence rates of IDDM were highest in the 10–14-year age group, followed by a sharp decline towards the end of adolescence. The peak age of onset is 1–2 years earlier in females than in males. These findings are consistent regardless of the ethnicity or the risk of disease incidence[2,45].

SEASONALITY

There have been many data available regarding the seasonality of the occurrence of IDDM. In the northern hemisphere, most cases are diagnosed during December to February, whereas in the southern hemisphere cases are identified mostly during June to August[45] (Figure 4). Little is known about the findings in countries close to the equator.

ETHNICITY

As was mentioned earlier, in Allegheny County, Jefferson County and San Diego, incidence rates are significantly higher in whites than in blacks[45]. The Colorado registry reveals that non-Hispanics have a 2.5-fold increased risk for IDDM compared to the Hispanic population within the same registry. These differences seem to be more related to ethnicity than geography, and

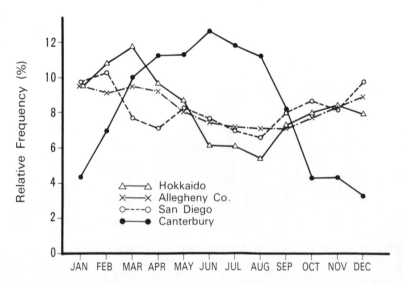

Figure 4 Seasonality of IDDM incidence in Hokkaido, Allegheny County (PA), San Diego (northern hemisphere) and Canterbury (southern hemisphere). Data are cited from reference 45. Reproduced by permission of Karger, Basel

this is discussed later in this chapter (Heritage studies). An ethnic difference in IDDM incidence is also clearly demonstrated in Israel. A retrospective survey of the entire population was performed for 1975–1980[46] and the data were recently updated[47]. The reported incidence rate for Jewish children of age 0–17 years in 1989 was 5.5 per 100 000, with an ethnic difference (Ashkenazi: 8.2; mixed: 4.6; Sephardi: 5.7; mid-East: 4.7; and Arab: 3.4 per 100 000). The incidence rate for Arabs in Israel is similar to that for Kuwait. Using the data provided by the free treatment system of the national health service, Taha et al. conducted an IDDM incidence study in Kuwait and reported[48] that the IDDM incidence rate for 0–14 years for 1980–1981 was 4.0 per 100 000.

HERITAGE STUDIES

Investigations to identify interactions of genetic and environmental factors associated with the occurrence of IDDM may be best examined with the development of heritage studies. A heritage study can be defined as the evaluation of changes in incidence of disease in populations that are constrained by a common gene pool, e.g. Spanish heritage, but with varying degree of admixture and environmental change. However, without having the well-documented and standardized incidence registries both in each parent country and in the host country, one cannot conduct in-depth comparative analyses for genetic and non-genetic risk factors. The rapid development of prospective IDDM incidence registries in the various parts of the world would soon provide valuable information on the epidemiology of heritage populations. These types of heritage studies can provide very valuable information concerning the aetiology of IDDM.

ITALIAN HERITAGE POPULATION

A considerable geographical variation in IDDM incidence within Italy itself gives a unique opportunity to examine non-genetic factors[49]. Northern Italy showed a relatively low incidence (4–13 per 100 000), whereas Sardinia, located in the south, had the highest incidence (30.2 per 100 000), which is approaching the rate in Finland. The magnitude of these differences has not been documented. On the other hand, the incidence in Italian children aged 0–14 years in Montreal was reported to be 10.7 per 100 000[50]. They came mainly from the southern and central parts of Italy, where the registries are not well established. Italian heritage research is to be conducted in a uniform way through collaboration with the Eurodiab Ace project[49].

IBERIAN HERITAGE POPULATION

DERI group evaluated the incidence of IDDM in the Spanish and Portuguese heritage population[51], and demonstrated at least a 10-fold difference in risk between people with Hispanic ancestry in Colorado and Mexicans in Mexico City. The Colorado Registry revealed[52] that the rate is 9.5 per 100 000 for the 0–17-year age group—significantly lower than that for non-Hispanics, which is about 15 per 100 000. In contrast, incidence rates were 4.1 per 100000 for San Diego and 2.6 per 100 000 for Cuba. New data from Mexico City and the surrounding metropolitan area indicate an even lower incidence, but which has not as yet been validated[52]. Overall, there is at least a three-fold or maybe as high as 15-fold difference in incidence among Hispanic populations, depending on where they live.

AFRICAN HERITAGE POPULATION

Reported IDDM incidence data in African–Americans aged below 15 years are limited but are available from the USA and the Caribbean[16]. It varies remarkably, ranging from 3.3 per 100 000 in San Diego to 11.8 per 100 000 in Allegheny County, PA, with a four-fold difference[45]. It was demonstrated also that whites had about a 1.5 greater risk of developing IDDM than blacks. Both in Jefferson County[53] and San Diego[15], African heritage populations have a significantly lower risk for IDDM than that seen in whites, even after controlling for socio-economic status. The comparison of incidence data between African heritage populations in the USA and African blacks is extremely important. The preliminary data indicate that the risk for African blacks in Tanzania[54] is extremely low (less than 1 per 100 000), but this figure may be underestimated because of children dying before the diagnosis of diabetes was made. New data for the African heritage population in the Caribbean have recently become available. It was reported that the rate of IDDM in children under 15 years of age was 5.6 per 100 000 for the 10-year period 1979–1988[16,55]. The massive differences seen among African heritage populations living in the same geographical area indicate that those groups are at markedly different risks of IDDM. Factors associated with ethnicity influencing IDDM incidence may be explained by differences in degree of racial admixture, diet, lifestyle or socio-economic status.

FUTURE DIRECTIONS

WHERE WOULD ONE MOST EFFECTIVELY USE POPULATION STUDIES TO IDENTIFY NON-GENETIC FACTORS?

Assessment of epidemics and geographical variation within low-risk countries appear to be the most effective means to identify non-genetic factors associated with IDDM. There may be two reasons. One is that identification of the factors responsible for an increase of 4 per 100 000 persons at risk per year in incidence in a population in which the incidence is 1 per 100 000 would be easier than in a population with a 20 per 100 000 incidence rate: a rise from 1 to 5 per 100 000 would be much more noticeable than from 20 to 24 per 100 000. The second reason is that people in a low-risk area may be less susceptible to IDDM, so that if one could identify a potential responsible agent it should be a very potent triggering factor for IDDM. However, it is very important to note that the target population should be genetically homogeneous and the genetic pool estimated to be constant. In this respect, Japan is a good example for testing this hypothesis[56,57]. Also, the population should be relatively 'static', with minimum rates of influx and efflux. Moreover, there should be an accurate ongoing registry system with almost 100% ascertainment. Otherwise a small number of missing cases would influence the incidence figure.

MIGRANT STUDIES

Migrant studies differ from heritage work as the former assume that there is little admixture between the migrant and host populations. Migrant studies are one of the best approaches for evaluating the 'pure' effect of environmental factors on the occurrence of IDDM. A recent report from England[58] indicates that England appears to be diabetogenic for its Asian minorities. We might expect a similar finding if we examined Asian migrants to the USA. It is, therefore, very important to establish a system to determine whether the IDDM incidence rate among the Asian heritage population is increased. The Han nationality in mainland China is a possibility for a study like this as the Han are the largest group among more than 50 ethnic groups in China, living in a geographically and culturally diverse area[59]. As part of the WHO DIAMOND project, a collaborative study on establishing IDDM registries from a population base of 30 000 000 children throughout China was recently started with the collaboration of the Chinese Academy of Preventive Medicine.

NEW REGISTRY SYSTEM: IDDM AS 'A REPORTABLE DISEASE'

Establishment of population-based IDDM registries is one of the most important occurrences in the field of diabetes epidemiology. From registry data very accurate descriptions of the epidemiology of past and future epidemics can be undertaken because of the high degree of ascertainment. However, it is not a panacea for monitoring the disease because typically one cannot detect an occurrence with sufficient time to find out what was causing the rise. Most registry systems have a lag of 1–5 years between case identification and registration. By the time the data are collected and analysed, the epidemic has passed and the diabetogenic stimuli may no longer be present in the community. Identification of the specific exposure factors would thus be difficult.

In order to overcome this problem, an alternative approach would be to use the existing surveillance systems for reportable diseases, using multiple sources of ascertainment. As IDDM has many features in common with communicable disease, this system should work very well. In the reporting system, health professionals at each hospital or clinic would be responsible for reporting new cases of 'notifiable' diseases. The nationwide IDDM surveillance in mainland China has started by adopting this strategy in some provinces.

One of the possible disadvantages may be that all voluntary reporting systems are subject to under-ascertainment. However, the problem of ascertainment for determining incidence rates actually need not be a major problem. Using multiple independent sources, one can apply a simple statistical method called capture–recapture, which was developed to count wildlife, to accurately estimate true IDDM incidence rate. The detailed mathematical background is discussed in the literature[60-62]. In this method, achieving 100% ascertainment is not crucial. The incidence study in Madrid[63] clearly demonstrated the advantage of this method. The capture–mark–recapture method has been also utilized in Italy[64], The Netherlands[30] and Colorado[39].

SUMMARY

Accumulated population-based data on the descriptive epidemiology of IDDM have enabled us to understand that the risk for individuals to develop IDDM differs remarkably according to place of residence and ethnicity. The geographical variation in incidence appears to be constrained by the genetic background of the population. It is likely that most of the 40–50-fold variation results from differences in host susceptibility. However, the environment clearly contributes to the geographical variation, with evidence for a three- to four-fold difference in incidence between countries having a similar genetic heritage, e.g. Iceland and Norway, Estonia and Finland.

The strongest evidence for non-genetic factors comes from temporal trends and epidemic data. There is little question that in many countries the incidence of disease is rapidly increasing. In addition, there are epidemic years seen in many registries. These temporal trends and epidemics can only be the result of non-genetic factors. Evaluation of these findings, especially in low-risk countries, where the people seem to be resistant to IDDM, may give us a major clue to identify the responsible non-genetic factors. However, unfortunately, accurate data from low-risk areas such as Asia, Africa and

South America are still very limited. If we knew what was causing the changing incidences of IDDM over time, we would know the non-genetic factors causing IDDM.

IDDM is unlike most non-communicable diseases in that we know much more about the contributing genetic factors than we do about non-genetic factors responsible for disease occurrence. The monitoring of IDDM through registries and the reportable disease system will greatly aid in our search for the environmental factors responsible for IDDM. We still have a major 'environmental challenge' in understanding the aetiology and prevention of IDDM[65].

REFERENCES

1 Diabetes Epidemiology Research International Group. Geographic patterns of childhood insulin-dependent diabetes mellitus. *Diabetes* 1988; **37**: 1113–19.
2 Rewers M, LaPorte RE, King H, Tuomilehto J. Trends in the prevalence and incidence of diabetes: insulin-dependent diabetes mellitus in childhood. *World Health Stat Q* 1988; **41**: 179–89.
3 Green A, Gale EAM, Patterson CC, for the Eurodiab Ace Study Group. Incidence of childhood-onset insulin-dependent diabetes mellitus: the Eurodiab Ace study. *Lancet* 1992; **339**: 905–9.
4 Nasa GLa, Carcassi C, Cirillo R, et al. Serological and molecular studies of HLA in insulin-dependent diabetes mellitus in Sardinia. *Dis Markers* 1990; **8**: 333–40.
5 WHO Diamond Project Group. WHO multinational project for childhood diabetes. *Diabetes Care* 1990; **13**: 1062–8.
6 Helgason T, Danielsen R, Thorsson AV. Incidence and prevalence of type 1 (insulin-dependent) diabetes mellitus in Icelandic children 1970–1989. *Diabetologia* 1991; **35**: 880–3.
7 LaPorte RE, Tajima N, Akerblom HK, et al. Geographic differences in the risk of insulin-dependent diabetes mellitus: the importance of registries. *Diabetes Care* 1985; **8** (Suppl 1): 101–7.
8 Reunanen A, Akerblom HK, Kaar ML. Prevalence and ten-year (1970–1979) incidence of insulin-dependent diabetes mellitus in children and adolescents in Finland. *Acta Paediatr Scand* 1982; **71**: 893–9.
9 Tuomilehto J, Lounamaa R, Tuomilehto-Wolf E, et al. Epidemiology of childhood diabetes mellitus in Finland: background of a nationwide study of type 1 (insulin-dependent) diabetes mellitus. *Diabetologia* 1992; **35**: 70–6.
10 Kalits I, Podar T. Incidence and prevalence of type 1 (insulin-dependent) diabetes in Estonia in 1988. *Diabetologia* 1990; **33**: 346–9.
11 Tuomilehto J, Podar T, Reunanen A, et al. Comparison of incidence of IDDM in childhood between Estonia and Finland, 1980–1988. *Diabetes Care* 1991; **14**: 982–8.
12 Dahlquist G, Blom L, Holmgren G, et al. The epidemiology of diabetes in Swedish children 0–14 years: a six year prospective study. *Diabetologia* 1985; **28**: 802–8.
13 Joner G, Sovik O. Incidence, age at onset and seasonal variation of diabetes mellitus in Norwegian children, 1973–1977. *Acta Paediatr Scand* 1981; **70**: 329–35.
14 Metcalfe MA, Baum JD. Incidence of insulin dependent diabetes in children aged under 15 years in the British Isles during 1988. *Br Med J* 1991; **302**: 442–6.

15 Lorenzi M, Cagliero E, Schmidt NJ. Racial differences in incidence of juvenile-onset type 1 diabetes: epidemiologic studies in southern California. *Diabetologia* 1985; **28**: 734–8.

16 Tull ES, Roseman JM, Christian CLE. Epidemiology of childhood IDDM in US Virgin Islands from 1979 to 1988: evidence of an epidemic in early 1980s and variation by degree of racial admixture. *Diabetes Care* 1991; **14**: 558–64.

17 Tan MH, Wornell MC, Beck AW. Epidemiology of diabetes mellitus in Prince Edward Island. *Diabetes Care* 1981; **4**: 519–24.

18 Japan IDDM Epidemiology Study Group. Lack of regional variation in IDDM risk in Japan. *Diabetes Care* 1993; **16**: 796–800.

19 Matsuura N, Fukushima N, Fujuta H, et al. Epidemiologic survey of juvenile onset insulin dependent diabetes mellitus (IDDM) in Hokkaido, Japan, 1973–1981. *Tohoku J Exp Med* 1983; **141** (Suppl): 181–9.

20 Glatthaar C, Whittall DE, Welborn TA, et al. Diabetes in Western Australian children: descriptive epidemiology, *Med J Aust* 1988; **148**: 117–23.

21 Sutton DL, Lyle DM, Pierce JP. Incidence and prevalence of insulin-dependent diabetes mellitus in the zero- to 19-years' age-group in Sydney. *Med J Aust* 1989; **151**: 140–6.

22 Mason DR, Scott RS, Darlow BA. Epidemiology of insulin-dependent diabetes mellitus in Canterbury, New Zealand. *Diabetes Res Clin Pract* 1987; **3**: 21–9.

23 Elliott RB, Pilcher CC. Childhood diabetes in the Auckland area. *NZ Med J* 1985; 23 October: 922–3.

24 Diabetes Epidemiology Research International Group. Secular trends in incidence of childhood IDDM in 10 countries. *Diabetes* 1990; **39**: 858–64.

25 Nystrom L, Dahlquist G, Rewers M, et al. The Swedish childhood diabetes study: an analysis of the temporal variation in diabetes incidence 1978–1987. *Int J Epidemiol* 1990; **19**: 141–6.

26 Tuomilehto J, Rewers M, Reunanen A, et al. Increasing trend in type 1 (insulin-dependent) diabetes mellitus in childhood in Finland: analysis of age, calendar time and birth cohort effects during 1965 to 1984. *Diabetologia* 1991; **34**: 287–7.

27 Green A, Andersen PK, Svendsen AJ, et al. Increasing incidence of early onset type 1 (insulin-dependent) diabetes mellitus: a study of Danish male birth cohorts. *Diabetologia* 1992; **35**: 178–82.

28 Burden AC, Hearnshaw JR, Swift PGF. Childhood diabetes mellitus: an increasing incidence. *Diabetic Med* 1989; **6**: 334–6.

29 Soltesz G, Madacsy L, Bekefi D, et al. Rising incidence of type 1 diabetes in Hungarian children (1978–1987). *Diabetic Med* 1989; **7**: 111–14.

30 Drykomingen CEM, Mulder ALM, Vaandrager GJ, et al. The incidence of male childhood type 1 (insulin-dependent) diabetes mellitus is rising rapidly in The Netherlands. *Diabetologia* 1992; **35**: 139–42.

31 Westlund K. Incidence of diabetes mellitus in Oslo, Norway 1925–1954. *Br J Prev Med* 1966; **20**: 105–16.

32 Sultz HA, Schlesinger ER, Mosher WE, et al. Childhood diabetes mellitus, In: *Long-term Childhood Illness*. University of Pittsburgh Press, Pittsburgh, 1972, pp 223–48.

33 Rewers M, LaPorte RE, Walczak M et al. Apparent epidemic of insulin-dependent diabetes mellitus in Midwestern Poland. *Diabetes* 1987; **36**: 106–13.

34 Tuomilehto J, Podar T, Brigis G, et al. Comparison of the incidence of insulin-dependent diabetes mellitus in childhood among five Baltic populations during 1983–1988. *Int J Epidemiol* 1992; **21**: 518–27.

35 Grabauskas V, Urbonaite B, Padaiga Z. Incidence of childhood insulin-dependent diabetes mellitus in Lithuania 1983–1988. *Acta Paediatr Scand* 1991; **80**: 718–19.
36 Unpublished data. Fu H, Shen SX, Chen ZW, et al. The lowest confirmed incidence of childhood diabetes in the world, Shanghai, China (submitted for publication).
37 Wagenknecht LE, Roseman JM, Herman WH. Increased incidence of insulin-dependent diabetes mellitus following an epidemic of Coxsackie virus B5. *Am J Epidemiol* 1991; **133**: 1024–31.
38 Hyoty H, Leinikki P, Reunanen A, et al. Mumps infections in the etiology of type 1 (insulin-dependent) diabetes. *Diabetes Res* 1988; **9**: 111–16.
39 Hamman RF, Gay, EC, Cruikshanks KJ, et al. Colorado IDDM registry: incidence and validation of IDDM in children aged 0–17 yr. *Diabetes Care* 1990; **13**: 499–506.
40 Joner G, Sovik O. Increasing incidence of diabetes mellitus in Norwegian children 0–14 years of age 1973–1982. *Diabetologia* 1989; **32**: 79–83.
41 Tuomilehto J, Podar T, Tuomilehto-Wolf E. Variation in insulin-dependent diabetes mellitus (IDDM) in Finland and in the Baltic region: a case of genetic–environmental interaction? In: *Diabetes* 1991 (eds JA Rifkin, SL Taylor) Elsevier, Amsterdam, pp 995–1001.
42 Songer TJ, LaPorte RE, Tajima N, et al. Height at diagnosis of insulin dependent diabetes in patients and their non-diabetic family members. *Br Med J* 1986; **292**: 1419–22.
43 Japan and Pittsburgh Childhood Diabetes Research Groups. Height at onset of insulin-dependent diabetes mellitus in high- and low-risk countries. *Diabetes Res Clin Pract* 1989; **6**: 173–6.
44 Blom L, Persoon LA, Dahlquist G. A high linear growth is associated with an increased risk of childhood diabetes mellitus. *Diabetologia* 1992; **35**: 528–33.
45 Tajima N, LaPorte RE. Incidence of IDDM outside Europe. In: *Epidemiology and Etiology of Insulin-dependent Diabetes in the Young* (eds C Levy-Marchal, P Czernichow) Karger, Basel, 1992, pp 31–41.
46 Laron Z, Karp M, Modan M. The incidence of insulin-dependent diabetes mellitus in Israeli children and adolescents 0–20 years of age: a retrospective study, 1975–1980. *Diabetes Care* 1985; **8** (Suppl 1): 24–8.
47 Laron Z, Mansour T, Karp M, et al. The incidence of childhood IDDM in various ethinic groups in Israel: a populations-based study—1989. In: *Epidemiology and Etiology of Insulin-dependent Diabetes in the Young* (eds C Levy-Marchal, P Czernichow) Karger, Basel, 1992, pp 42–7.
48 Taha TH, Moussa MAA, Rashid AR, et al. Diabetes mellitus in Kuwait: incidence in the first 29 years of life. *Diabetologia* 1983; **25**: 306–8.
49 Diabetes Epidemiology Research International (DERI) Study Group. The epidemiology and immunogenetics of IDDM in Italian-heritage populations. *Diabetes Metab Rev* 1990; **6**: 63–9.
50 Siemiatycki J, Colle E, Campbell S, et al. Incidence of IDDM in Montreal by ethnic groups and by social class and comparisons with ethnic groups living elsewhere. *Diabetes* 1988; **37**: 1096–102.
51 Diabetes Epidemiology Research International Group. Evaluation of epidemiology and immunogenetics of IDDM in Spanish- and Portuguese-heritage registries: a key to understanding the etiology of IDDM? *Diabetes Care* 1989; **12**: 487–93.
52 Gay EC, Hamman RF, Carosone-Link PJ, et al. Colorado IDDM registry: lower incidence of IDDM in Hispanics. Comparison of disease characteristics and care patterns in biethnic population. *Diabetes Care* 1989; **12**: 701–8.

53 Wagenknecht LE, Roseman JM, Alexander WJ. Epidemiology of IDDM in black and white children in Jefferson County, Alabama, 1979–1985. *Diabetes* 1989; **38**: 629–33.

54 Swai ABM, Lutale J, McLarty DG. Diabetes in tropical Africa: a prospective study, 1981–7. 1. Characteristics of newly presenting patients in Dar es Salaam, Tanzania, 1981–7. *Br Med J* 1990; **300**: 1103–6.

55 Tull ES, Makame MH for the Diabetes Epidemiology Research International Group. Evaluation of type 1 diabetes in black African-heritage populations: no time for further neglect. *Diabetic Med* 1992; **9**: 513–21.

56 Matsumoto H. Characteristics of Mongoloid and neighboring populations based on the genetic markers of human immunoglobulins. *Hum Genet* 1988; **80**: 207–18.

57 Matsumoto H. On the origin of the Japanese race: studies of genetic markers of the immunoglobulins. *Proc Jpn Acad* 1984; **60**: 211–16.

58 Bodansky HJ, Staines A, Stephenson C, et al. Evidence for an environmental effect in the aetiology of insulin dependent diabetes in a transmigratory population. *Br Med J* 1992; **304**: 1020–2.

59 Zhao T, Lee TD. Gm and Km allotypes in 74 Chinese populations: a hypothesis of the origin of the Chinese nation. *Hum Genet* 1989; **83**: 101–10.

60 Petersen CGJ. The yearly immigration of young plaice into the Limfjord from the German sea. *Report of the Danish Biological Station to the Ministry of Fisheries* 1896; **6**: 1–48.

61 Robles SC, Marrett LD, Clarke EA, et al. An application of capture–recapture methods to the estimation of completeness of cancer registration. *J Clin Epidemiol* 1988; **41**: 495–501.

62 LaPorte RE, McCarty DJ, Tull ES, Tajima N. Counting birds, bees, and NCDs. *Lancet* 1992; **339**: 494–5.

63 Serrano-Rios M, Moy CS, Serrano RM, et al. Incidence of type 1 (insulin-dependent) diabetes mellitus in subjects 0–14 years of age in the comunidad of Madrid, Spain. *Diabetologia* 1990; **33**: 422–4.

64 Bruno G, Merletti F, Pisu E, et al. Incidence of IDDM during 1984–1986 in population aged less than 30 yr. Residents of Turin, Italy. *Diabetes Care* 1990; **13**: 1051–6.

65 Diabetes Epidemiology Research International. Preventing insulin dependent diabetes mellitus: the environmental challenge. *Br Med J* 1987; **295**: 479–81.

Chapter Three

Family Studies and the Causes of Insulin-dependent Diabetes Mellitus

Polly J. Bingley and Edwin A. M. Gale

Department of Diabetes and Metabolism, St Bartholomew's Hospital, London, UK

INTRODUCTION

The 1970s brought final confirmation that idiopathic diabetes mellitus is a heterogeneous disease. Lines of evidence pointing to this conclusion included epidemiological differences between insulin-dependent diabetes mellitus (IDDM) and non-insulin-dependent diabetes mellitus (NIDDM), recognition of the human leucocyte antigen (HLA) associations with IDDM but not NIDDM, and the discovery of islet cell antibodies (ICA) in the circulation of most patients presenting with clinical features of IDDM but only a small fraction of those with NIDDM. The growing realization that autoimmune processes are involved in the pathogenesis of IDDM resulted within 10 years or so in controlled (or uncontrolled) clinical trials of immunosuppression in newly diagnosed patients.

Causes of Diabetes. Edited by R. D. G. Leslie
© 1993 John Wiley & Sons Ltd.

The prospective family study represented a logical step forward in this climate of thought—a step that will be lastingly associated with the name of Andrew Cudworth—and has provided much of the basis of our current understanding of the genetics and natural history of the disease process. It has allowed increasingly useful predictive models to be developed, and family studies provide the basis for the controlled trials of intervention in high-risk relatives that are now getting under way in many countries.

What are the advantages of the family study approach? In the first place, it allows genetic analysis to be undertaken, and should in time allow genes conferring susceptibility or protection to be identified in the major histocompatitility complex (MHC) region and other parts of the genome. Second, it allows prospective observation of the natural history of the disease process. Third, it allows risk assessment to be tested and refined on the basis of experience. Fourth, it permits interventions designed to delay or prevent the onset of IDDM to be tested in those relatives at highest risk.

There are practical advantages to this approach. Children with diabetes are easy to identify, and their parents are are already well aware that their siblings are at increased risk of the disease, and in consequence highly motivated to help with research which might eventually lead to its prevention. There are corresponding disadvantages. Only some 10% of newly diagnosed children already have a first-degree relative with IDDM[1,2]. The presence of two affected family members might imply a heavy load of diabetes susceptibility genes—but might equally be due to shared environmental influences. Genes and environment are notoriously difficult to disentangle, and in any case families with multiple cases may in some way be 'special'. Is it reasonable to extrapolate lessons learned in this setting to the population at large?

In this chapter we shall consider the contribution of the family study approach to our understanding of the causes of IDDM, and its potential value for the future.

TYPES OF FAMILY STUDY

There are currently 30 or more prospective family studies in progress around the world, and study groups are also recruited from family members for other purposes. For example, repositories of cells from families with multiple cases of IDDM (multiplex families) have been established in the USA, UK and elsewhere for genetic analysis. These families have usually been recruited by advertising among physicians or through patient organizations. Other family studies (usually based around large diabetic clinic populations) simply set out to screen as many family members as possible in order to identify the maximum number of high-risk individuals. This approach has yielded a lot of valuable information, but has potential limitations. It may lead to a distorted selection of patients since highly motivated families, or families with multiple cases of diabetes, may be drawn to the screening centre from elsewhere. Equally, concentration on the subpopulation at highest risk will tend to give a false impression of the power of predictive models because false negatives and individuals at lower degrees of risk have been excluded. A few groups, notably the Pittsburgh group in the USA, the DiMe study group in Finland, and our own Bart's–Oxford group, have attempted to overcome these problems by setting up population-based family studies. The main disadvantage of this approach is that it is labour-intensive and unlikely to identify such large numbers of high-risk individuals as 'one-off' screening programmes. On the other hand, it allows the issue of false negative prediction to be tackled, and permits results to be handled using an epidemiological approach. It is important to recognize these differences in sample selection. Each may be appropriate for the question it seeks to answer, but important differences in emphasis may emerge as attempts are made to generalize results generated in different ways.

ENVIRONMENTAL INFLUENCES AND THE PATHOGENESIS OF IDDM

IDDM is presumed to arise on a basis of genetic susceptibility, but the majority of those with genetic susceptibility will never develop the disease. There is considerable evidence to support this inference, which originally arose from the classic observation that only about a third of monozygotic twin pairs are concordant for IDDM[3]. Equally, there is good evidence that autoimmune processes play a role in the disease. Evidence for this includes the strong HLA associations with IDDM, and its overlap with other organ-specific autoimmune disease, while the appearance of autoantibodies and lymphocytes directed towards antigens present on or within islet cells points to the same conclusion. Most conclusively, β cell survival is prolonged in newly diagnosed patients treated with immunotherapy[4]. Circulating immune markers such as ICA may in appropriate circumstances be highly predictive of the development of diabetes[5]. The observation that their detection may herald disease many years in advance of the clinical onset suggests a slow, smouldering disease prodrome, and the patchy nature of islet infiltration observed in the pancreata of young patients who died shortly after diagnosis would be consistent with this interpretation[6].

While it is increasingly possible to identify those at genetic risk of IDDM, and to pick up those in whom a slow subclinical disease process is under way, the link between the diathesis and the disease is missing. It has for many years been assumed that environmental influences supply this link, and more recently it has come to be believed (at least by some) that the decisive contact is made very early in life, most probably in the neonatal period. The importance of environmental factors is well established in animal models of spontaneous diabetes, and many papers have reported differences in the rate of diabetes produced by variations in diet[7], exposure to infection, or even differences in air temperature[8]. Human populations are inevitably more difficult to analyse, but evidence for the existence of a major environmental influence(s) includes study of migrant populations in whom the rate of IDDM appears to have increased[9,10], and other data from stable populations indicating a sudden surge ('epidemic') in incidence of IDDM[11]. Despite difficulties with the interpretation of both types of study, there is probably some basis for these claims, although perhaps less solid than has sometimes been maintained. In contrast, there is no doubt that the incidence of IDDM has risen and continues to rise in Europe and other parts of the world, while no report has as yet described a falling incidence. The change in Europe represents a two- to three-fold increase over the past 20–40 years (in most cases linear rather than abrupt), and seems to provide conclusive evidence that non-genetic influences are at work[12].

Before considering candidate environmental influences, we should pause to consider the likely time at which these might interact with the growing child. IDDM has a well-marked peak in incidence around the time of puberty in almost all reported studies, and an equally marked decline thereafter— even though the disease may present as late as extreme old age. A population-based study from Finland found that some 60% of all clinically defined negative cases of IDDM had presented before the age of 22[13]. About a quarter of childhood cases present before the age of 5, and prospective studies suggest that a child who presents at the age of 13 will typically (but not always) have had detectable circulating levels of ICA 5 years or more before onset of the disease. There is therefore a strong presumption that the disease process is most commonly initiated in early childhood.

Other evidence supports this. Insulitis appears early in the neonatal period in the non-obese diabetic (NOD) mouse[14]. In man, high titres of insulin autoantibodies (IAA) appear early in childhood and decline rapidly with age[15]. Initial seroconversion to ICA positivity usually develops before the age of 5 (Elliott, personal observations; see Chapter 8), and our own experience with a sensitive ICA assay suggests that conversion from ICA negativity to ICA positivity is a rare event over the age of 10[5]. If these inferences are correct, the majority of cases of IDDM developing in adolescence or even well into adult life are nonetheless the end result of a process initiated in infancy. The observation that progression to IDDM slows with increasing age[16] would be consistent with this view. Taken together, these observations suggest that the immune process is initiated either *in utero* or in the early stages of neonatal life, and that the *time* at which such agent (or agents) are presented to the developing immune system plays a crucial role in determining loss of self-tolerance.

Possible environmental causes of IDDM need to be considered from this point of view. Arguments for a viral aetiology seem quite plausible, for example, with cytomegalovirus perhaps the most intriguing candidate at present[17]. Even so, it is hard to explain the steady rise in incidence in so many countries on this basis, especially with the added assumption that contact with the virus would need to occur either *in utero* or within the early neonatal period.

The nutritional hypothesis of causation performs rather better in this respect. In 1984 Borch-Johnsen and colleagues[18] suggested that the incidence of IDDM was inversely related to the prevalence of breast-feeding. Despite some conflicting reports[19,20] a protective effect for breast-feeding as an independent risk determinant has been supported by subsequent studies[21-24]. These observations are consistent with the animal data. In the BB rat—another animal model of spontaneous diabetes—progression to diabetes is markedly reduced if L-amino acids are substituted for protein in their diet[25], while spontaneous diabetes can be totally prevented in the NOD mouse by hydrolysing the protein content of the diet[26]. These experiments suggest that intact foreign protein is a requirement for the expression of diabetes in these genetically susceptible animals.

Further, analysis of the bovine albumin molecule has identified a 17-amino acid sequence, known as ABBOS, which differs markedly from the equivalent sequence in man and other species, including the mouse and rat. Antibodies to bovine serum albumin (BSA) are more common in recently diagnosed diabetes than in controls, and cross-react with a β cell peptide referred to as p69 (see Chapter 7). This is not presented at the β cell membrane and therefore—according to this argument—does not enter the repertoire of self-antigens tolerated by the immune system. However, p69 does appear on the cell surface when the cells are exposed *in vitro* to interferon-γ, as might occur *in vivo* in response to infection. The 'cow's milk' theory would therefore postulate that individuals with genetic susceptibility to IDDM are capable of generating antibodies against the ABBOS sequence, and that these are capable of cross-reacting with p69, but only when this is expressed on the surface of β cells, as during intercurrent infection[27]. This sequence of events might explain an indolent relapsing and remitting immune attack directed against the β cell. In many this may prove abortive, but in others it results, even after many years, in the development of diabetes. This hypothesis fits well with the evidence that the imune response leading to IDDM is generated very early in life, but does not explain the rapid rise in incidence of the condition since the 1950s—except on the (not implausible) assumption that commercial processing of cow's milk, or of milk-based food products, has in some way increased its antigenicity.

GENETICS OF IDDM

A major advantage of family studies is that genotypes rather than phenotypes can be defined. Investigation can therefore be taken beyond single marker studies, and the role of combinations of markers in determining genetic susceptibilty for IDDM can be examined, allowing the role played by specific haplotypes in determining susceptibility to IDDM to be defined. Various approaches have been used to distinguish 'affected' and 'unaffected' haplotypes within families. The relative risk associated with a given haplotype can be calculated by comparing the haplotypes of the diabetic child with the remaining two parental haplotypes not present in the affected child. An alternative method is to identify the four parental haplotypes and then designate them 'affected' or 'non-affected' according to the disease status of each family member. Parental haplotypes present only in unaffected family members are defined as 'unaffected' while those present in family members with diabetes are 'affected'.

Four principal 'high-risk haplotypes' for IDDM were described in the Ninth International Histocompatibility Workshop:

1. A1, Cw7, B8, w6 (C4-AQ0, C4-B1, C2-1, Bf-S), DR3, DQw2.
2. A2, Cw3, Bw62, w6 (C4-A3, C4-B3, C2-2, Bf-S) DR4, DQw8.
3. A2, Cw3, Bw60, w6 (C4-A3, C4-B3, C2-1, Bf-S) DR4, DQw8.
4. A30, Cw5, B18, w6 (C4-A3, C4-BQ0, C2-1, Bf-F1) DR3, DQw2.

The first three are found in European and American Caucasoid families and the fourth in IDDM patients in southern Europe[28]. A recently described haplotype (A2, Cw1, Bw56, w6, DR4) may explain—although only in part—the very high incidence of IDDM in Finland[29].

Further examination of the data from the Finnish DiMe study has shown that extended haplotypes identical at the DQB1 loci are associated with very different risks of IDDM, implying that MHC genes outside the DQ region also play an important role in determining genetic susceptibility[30]. This approach also demonstrates the advantage of a population-based family study, since it has allowed absolute risks for developing IDDM to be estimated for the first time, albeit with relatively wide confidence intervals; these risks for identical DQB1 alleles ranged from 35 (corresponding to the overall risk in Finland) to as high as 218 per 100 000 per year.

The risk of diabetes developing in a family member is modulated by two other factors: HLA haplotype sharing and transmission ratio distortion.

HLA HAPLOTYPE SHARING

HLA genotyping in 120 diabetic sibling pairs recruited to the British Diabetic Association register established that the risk of developing diabetes was concentrated among siblings who were HLA identical with the proband. Fifty-seven per cent of the affected siblings were HLA identical and 6% non-identical, compared with the 25% expected by Mendelian laws[31]. In the Bart's–Windsor study HLA non-identical siblings had a risk of diabetes which could not be distinguished from that in the background population. Haploidentical siblings (those with one haplotype in common with the proband) had an estimated risk of 9%, whereas HLA identical siblings (both haplotypes in common) had a risk of 16%[32]. HLA testing can therefore be used to stratify risk within a family setting.

TRANSMISSION RATIO DISTORTION

The observation that children of fathers with IDDM appear to be at higher risk of developing the disease than children of affected mothers[2,33] has provoked interest in the issue of preferential transmission of diabetic alleles within the HLA complex. Sixty-eight per cent of the children of DR3 fathers inherited the DR3 allele, and 65.1% of children of DR3 mothers, compared with the expected 50% ($p < 0.0005$ and $p < 0.002$ respectively); 72.1% of offspring of DR4 fathers but only 55.6% of those of DR4 mothers inherited this allele ($p < 0.001$)[34]. Distortion of transmission of the diabetic haplotypes A1-B8-Dw3-DR3 and A2-B15-Cw3-Dw4-DR4 has also previously been described in 150 families in the Bart's–Windsor family study. The prevalence of the paternal A1-B8 haplotype was increased significantly (1.7 : 1), while the maternal haplotype followed the expected segregation pattern. In contrast, the maternal A2-B15-CW3 haplotype was transmitted preferentially (76%) while showing the expected distribution as a paternal haplotype[35]. It was suggested that this might be the result of natural selection at the gamete or post-zygotic stage of development or that genes outside the HLA region might influence the transmission rate of haplotypes.

NON-MHC GENES

Concordance for IDDM in monozygotic twins has been estimated at 30–55%[3] and in HLA identical siblings is 15–20%. This difference implies that genes outside the MHC complex must also contribute to genetic susceptibility. These include the insulin gene on chromosome 11 and immunoglobulin heavy chain haplotypes[36,37]. Further progress may be achieved by linkage analysis of DNA markers in large numbers of families with two or more affected siblings.

PREDICTION OF IDDM IN FAMILIES

OVERALL RISK

Tillil and Kobberling studied the families of 554 subjects with IDDM and calculated the lifetime risk for first-degree relatives in three consecutive generations. The overall risk (± 1 SE) was $6.6 \pm 1.1\%$ for siblings and $4.8 \pm 1.7\%$ for children[38]. Other studies have also found a risk for siblings between 4% and 8%[32,39-41]. The Pittsburgh group found a higher overall risk of 11% in 442 siblings in 132 families but this may have been due to selection bias resulting in recruitment of a higher proportion of multiplex families[42].

IMMUNE MARKERS AND PREDICTION

ICA are detectable in 70–80% of new cases of childhood IDDM[43], and in 5–8% of first-degree relatives, provided a sensitive assay is used. Within the group of relatives, the majority of future cases of IDDM will come from the ICA-positive subgroup, and risk will be roughly proportional to ICA titre. This means that some 5% of those with ICA in the range 4–19 JDF units, and 35% of those with ICA $\geqslant$ 20 JDF units, will develop insulin-requiring diabetes within 5 years. Those non-diabetic after 5 years will still have a high risk of progression[5,16], even though diabetes is not inevitable even after 10 years of persistent ICA positivity[44]. Despite technical difficulties with its measurement, ICA thus continue to provide the basis of prediction of IDDM. Recent research efforts have been directed mainly towards refinement of prediction based on this single marker, and we have recently described a decision tree approach which can allow a complex and evolving body of data to be integrated and analysed within a relatively simple format[45].

IMPROVING RISK PREDICTION BASED ON ICA

Family members have an increased baseline risk, together with a high dose of genes conferring susceptibility to IDDM, and genetic markers appear relatively uninformative in this context, although they do improve specificity to some extent[46]. Age also correlates inversely with risk[16]. ICA appear to carry widely differing predictive value according to the population in which they are measured, and risks ascertained within a population of, for example, first-degree relatives should not be extrapolated to the population at large.

Heterogeneity within ICA-positive individuals has also been recognized. Some ICA stain β cells predominantly (β *cell-selective* or *restricted* pattern) and are associated with a much lower risk of progression than ICA that stain all types of islet cells (*whole islet* or *non-restricted* pattern)[47-49]. These β cell-selective antibodies may account for the pattern of staining in about 25% of all ICA positive first-degree relatives[48].

The two other autoantibodies of major importance in diabetes prediction[50] are autoantibodies to insulin (IAA)[51] and to the islet 64 000 M_r antigen identified as the enzyme glutamic acid decarboxylase (GAD)[52]. IAA probably have little predictive value in the absence of ICA provided a sensitive ICA assay is used, but the combination, present in around 50% of those who develop IDDM, is highly predictive[53,54]. IAA are inversely related to age[15], as is risk of progression to IDDM in ICA-positive individuals, so these variables might not be truly independent. Antibodies to GAD appear in some 80% of high-risk relatives prior to diagnosis, but their prognostic value currently appears limited; it has been suggested that they may overlap with β cell-selective ICA. In contrast, tryptic fragments of 64 000 M_r antigen, notably the 37 kDa moiety, correlate well with whole islet ICA, appear in only 2% of discordant twins and are absent in ICA-positive polyendocrine patients who have not developed diabetes[55,56].

We have recently undertaken a combined analysis of risk in 101 ICA-positive first-degree relatives, using ICA titre and staining pattern in addition to IAA, GAD, 37 kDa and 40 kDa tryptic fragments. No single 'marker of choice' emerged from this analysis. Instead, risk mounted according to the number of antibody species present, from 6% for ICA alone ($\geq$ 10 JDF units) to 86% for cases with three or more antibodies. This approach promises to enhance prediction of diabetes without loss of sensitivity; it suggested additionally that anti-37 kDa might be of value as a marker of impending onset[57].

METABOLIC MARKERS

A logical extension of the approach outlined above would be to assess the extent of target organ damage. Since pancreatic biopsy is impracticable, tests of β cell function have been used as an indirect measure of β cell survival. The obvious limitation of this approach is the difficulty of extrapolating from β cell function to β cell mass. Further, differences in method and poor reproducibility of insulin responses have limited comparisons between centres and between or within individuals, although a new international standard for performance of the intravenous glucose tolerance test (IVGTT) has recently been agreed[58]. It is, however, clear that the first-phase insulin response to intravenous glucose falls well in advance of onset of diabetes in most individuals, although this is only really useful as a predictive measure when absolute secretory failure (i.e. below the first centile) can be defined. ICA-positive relatives in this category developed diabetes at the rate of 0.48 per subject-year of follow-up in one study, compared with only 0.05 per subject-year in those with first-phase insulin release above this level[59]. A predictive model based on combined analysis of IAA and first-phase insulin response has been proposed by the group at the Joslin Clinic, and has been claimed to give highly specific prediction in 'end-stage prediabetes', with progression within 3–4 years in some 90% of those identified, although prediction beyond 3 years is less certain[60]. This model has yet to be independently validated, however, and may prove to be less specific than originally thought.

SUMMARY: PREDICTION IN FIRST-DEGREE RELATIVES

Highly specific prediction is becoming increasingly feasible in relatives, based on the approach outlined above. Certain limitations should, however, be recognized. One is that prediction works best close to the onset of diabetes, and therefore by definition at a time when there is least scope for β cell salvage. Moreover, increased specificity implies reduced sensitivity. In other words, we must pass over many individuals at lower degrees of risk to arrive at a subset in whom early onset of diabetes appears almost inevitable. For example, if you consider all future cases of IDDM from a population of first-degree relatives, we estimate that no more than 20–30% of these could be identified by the dual-parameter model at a single screening point. The remainder would be excluded by virtue of absence of IAA, persistence of insulin secretory responses, low titre or undetectable ICA. If we then go on to reflect that only around 10% of new cases of childhood diabetes have an affected first-degree relative, it becomes apparent that this strategy would only have the potential to detect 2–3% of all future cases. Even highly effective treatment of this group would have little impact upon the future incidence of IDDM; this could only be reduced by screening and intervention in the population at large.

FROM FAMILY STUDIES TO POPULATION STUDIES

Only about one in 10 children who develop diabetes have an affected first-degree relative[1,2], which means that for intervention strategies to have a significant impact on the overall incidence of IDDM, the disease must be predicted and prevented in the general population. We must first ask if familial and non-familial IDDM is the same disease. In fact there is no direct evidence that familial cases of IDDM differ from sporadic cases. Anderson and colleagues found no differences in HLA associations, family history of diabetes or thyroid disease, or antibody positivity between simplex, multiplex and multigenerational families[61]. At the same time genetic and immune markers of susceptibility are likely to prove to have a different significance within families than in the general population, and we shall summarize this argument below.

Since genetic markers of susceptibility have relatively low specificity, their principal value in prediction of IDDM within the general population is likely to be in identification of high-risk groups for more intensive screening with immune and metabolic markers. Oligonucleotide probes to HLA-DR and DQ alleles have the potential to identify individuals in a Caucasian population with a 6–8% risk of IDDM[62,63], a risk similar to that for siblings of a child with IDDM. A Finnish study has reported experience using a panel of four sequence-specific oligonucleotide probes to identify alleles conferring susceptibility to and protection against IDDM. DQw8 in the absence of a protective DQ allele, was found in 82% of patients as against 3% of controls, giving a lifetime absolute risk (for a Finnish population) of 13.7%— considerably greater than the risk of an unselected sibling[64].

There is still some controversy concerning the predictive value of ICA within the general population, although it is clear that ICA are associated with increased risk of IDDM in children with no family history of diabetes. Studies of ICA in school children have found a prevalence varying between 0.3% and 4%[65–68]. In a study in the Netherlands, at least 10 years' follow-up was available on 2805 children with no family history of diabetes who had blood taken as part of a population health screening exercise. Eight of 2805 (0.3%) were found to have detectable ICA, and four (50%) of these had developed IDDM 10 years later, compared with three of 2797 (0.1%) who did not have detectable ICA on the first sample[69].

These findings suggest that ICA should constitute a useful predictor of IDDM in the general population. In our own study in the Oxford region we have obtained an indirect estimate of the positive predictive value of ICA by combining data from an incidence study and a prospective population-based family study with the results of screening 2925 school children. The prevalence of ICA $\geq$ 4 JDF units in the school children was 2.8% compared with 6.6% in 274 age-matched siblings of children with IDDM living in the same area. Life table analysis showed that the siblings' risk of developing IDDM between the ages of 10 and 20 was 2.8%, while the cumulative incidence of IDDM in the general population was only 0.21%. These data imply that ICA would be expected to have positive predictive value some six to seven times lower in the general population than that observed in family studies[45].

THE EFFECT OF DIFFERENCES IN OVERALL RISK

First-degree relatives have a cumulative risk of IDDM of about 3%, whereas that in the general population is about 0.3%. This difference alone can have a major effect on the positive predictive value of a test (the proportion of those who have a positive test who have disease), which is perhaps the most useful determinant of its clinical usefulness. This is a function of its sensitivity and specificity, but is also influenced by the prevalence of disease in the population being studied. General population screening for ICA alone is therefore likely always to be associated with an unacceptable proportion of false positives.

This problem can possibly be overcome by using a two-test strategy whereby an initial test of high sensitivity (e.g. selecting genetically susceptible individuals) is followed by ICA testing. If, as outlined above, initial screening with oligonucleotide probes for HLA-DR and DQ allelles in a Caucasian population might identify a population with an 8% risk of developing IDDM, then the positive predictive value of ICA >20 JDF units would rise to levels greater than those seen in first-degree relatives[62,63].

The practical value of screening healthy populations for markers of susceptibility could, however, be enormously enhanced by changes in intervention strategy. For example, vaccination aimed at preventing the autoimmune process would need to be given to all those who are genetically susceptible. If very safe preventive measures become available, use of sensitive but nonspecific screening tests would then become equally appropriate, since these could also be given to large numbers of children who may not otherwise develop diabetes.

ETHICAL CONSIDERATIONS

A family study is a form of screening, carried out within a population that is by definition already at high risk, well informed and highly motivated. What happens when the screening process is extended to a low-risk, relatively ill-informed population? Screening within families, for example with ICA, usually brings reassurance since only about one relative in 40 will be identified as at very high risk. In contrast, a major consequence of screening within the wider population must be to generate anxiety where none existed. Worse still, much of this anxiety will be unfounded if the screening test results in a large number of false positive predictions. In the longer term, increased public awareness of the possibility of predicting IDDM would awaken the possibility that predictive tests—however inaccurate—might be used to the disadvantage of the individual with regard to employment, health insurance and so forth. These troubled waters will need to be navigated over the next few years. In the interim screening should not be undertaken lightly, and should always be carried out with appropriate counselling and possibilities for follow-up[70,71].

CONCLUSIONS

The family study approach is unlikely in itself to contribute directly to our understanding of the environmental causes of IDDM. These are more likely to be resolved by standard epidemiological techniques, such as case-control studies, or by direct testing of hypotheses generated in animal models. On the other hand, family studies are indispensable to an understanding of the genetics of the disease, and of the natural history of the prodromal events leading up to a diagnosis of diabetes. These clinical studies complement the work of the epidemiologist by directing attention to high-risk situations and pinpointing the period during which crucial interactions with the environment are likely to occur. Family studies also provide the basis for current ability to predict the disease, and to design and assess interventions designed to delay its onset. In this context sample size becomes paramount, since clinical onset is the endpoint for both prediction and prevention, and very large numbers of high-risk individuals must be studied to enable adequate statistical power to be achieved. For this reason large-scale, almost inevitably international, collaborative studies, with standardization and pooling of data, represent an essential step on the road to prevention of IDDM.

REFERENCES

1 Bloom A, Hayes TM, Gamble DR. Register of newly diagnosed diabetic children. *Br Med J* 1975; **ii**: 580–3.
2 Dahlquist G, Blom L, Holmgren G, et al. The epidemiology of diabetes in Swedish children 0–14 years: a six-year prospective study. *Diabetologia* 1985; **28**: 802–8.
3 Barnett AH, Eff C, Leslie RDG, Pyke DA. Diabetes in identical twins: a study of 200 pairs. *Diabetologia* 1981; **20**: 87–93.
4 Canadian–European Randomized Control Trial Group. Cyclosporin-induced remission of IDDM after early intervention: association with enhanced insulin secretion. *Diabetes* 1988; **37**: 1574–82.
5 Bonifacio E, Bingley PJ, Dean BM, et al. Quantification of islet-cell antibodies and prediction of insulin-dependent diabetes. *Lancet* 1990; **335**: 147–9.
6 Foulis AK, Stewart JA. The pancreas in recent-onset type 1 (insulin-dependent) diabetes mellitus: insulin content of islets, insulitis and associated changes in the exocrine acinar tissue. *Diabetologia* 1984; **26**: 456–61.
7 Scott FW, Daneman D, Martin JM. Evidence for a critical role of diet in the development of insulin-dependent diabetes mellitus. *Diabetes Res* 1988; **7**: 153–7.
8 Williams AJK, Krug Ji P, Lampeter EF, et al. Raised temperature reduces the incidence of diabetes in the NOD mouse. *Diabetologia* 1990; **33**: 635–7.
9 Siemiatycki J, Colle E, Campbell S, et al. Incidence of IDDM in Montreal by ethnic group and by social class and comparisons with ethnic groups living elsewhere. *Diabetes* 1988; **37**: 1096–102.
10 Bodansky HJ, Staines A, Stephenson C, et al. Evidence for an environmental effect in the aetiology of insulin-dependent diabetes in a transmigratory population. *Br Med J* 1992; **304**: 1020–22.
11 Rewers M, La Porte RE, Walczak M, Dmochowski, K, Bogaczynska E. Apparent epiolemic of insulin-dependent diabetes in Poland. *Diabetes* 1987; **36**: 106–13.
12 Bingley PJ, Gale EAM. Rising incidence of IDDM in Europe. *Diabetes Care* 1989; **12**: 289–95.
13 Laakso M, Pyorala K. Age of onset and type of diabetes. *Diabetes Care* 1985; **8**: 114–17.

14 Fujita T, Yui R, Kusumoto Y, et al. Lymphocytic insulitis in a 'non-obese diabetic (NOD)' strain of mice: an immunohistochemical and electron microscope investigation. *Biomed Res* 1982; **3**: 429.

15 Vardi P, Ziegler AG, Mathews JH, et al. Concentration of insulin autoantibodies at onset of type 1 diabetes: inverse log-linear correlation with age. *Diabetes Care* 1988; **11**: 736–9.

16 Riley WJ, Maclaren NK, Krischer J, et al. A prospective study of the development of diabetes in relatives of patients with insulin-dependent diabetes. *N Engl J Med* 1990; **323**: 1167–72.

17 Pak CY, Eun HM, McArthur RG, Yoon J-W. Association of cytomegalovirus infection with autoimmune type 1 diabetes. *Lancet* 1988; **ii**: 1–5.

18 Borch-Johnsen K, Joner G, Mandrup-Poulsen T, et al. Relation between breast-feeding and incidence rates of insulin-dependent diabetes mellitus. *Lancet* 1984; **ii**: 1083–6.

19 Nigro G. Breast-feeding and insulin-dependent diabetes mellitus in children (Letter). *Lancet* 1985; **i**: 467.

20 Fort P, Lanes R, Dahlem S, et al. Breast feeding and insulin-dependent diabetes mellitus in children. *Am J Coll Nutr* 1986; **5**: 439–41.

21 Mayer EJ, Hamman RF, Gay EC, et al. Reduced risk of IDDM among breast-fed children. *Diabetes* 1988; **37**: 1625–32.

22 Siemiatycki J, Colle E, Campbell S, Dewar RAD, Belmonte MM. Case-control study of IDDM. *Diabetes Care* 1989; **12**: 209–16.

23 Blom L, Dahlquist G, Nystrom L, Sandstrom A, Wall S. The Swedish Childhood Diabetes Study: social and perinatal determinants for diabetes in childhood. *Diabetologia* 1989; **32**: 7–13.

24 Virtanen SM, Rasanen L, Aro A, et al. Infant feeding in Finish children <7 yr of age with newly diagnosed IDDM. *Diabetes Care* 1991; **14**: 415–17.

25 Elliott RB, Martin JM. Dietary protein: a trigger of insulin-dependent diabetes in the BB rat? *Diabetologia* 1984; **26**: 297–9.

26 Coleman DL, Kuzava JE, Leiter EH. Effect of diet on incidence of diabetes in nonobese diabetic mice. *Diabetes* 1990; **39**: 432–6.

27 Karjalainen J, Martin JM, Knip M, et al. A bovine serum albumin peptide as a possible trigger of insulin-dependent diabetes mellitus. *N Engl J Med* 1992; **327**: 302–7.

28 Bertrams J, Baur MP. Insulin dependent diabetes mellitus. In: *Histocompatibility Testing 1984* (eds ED Albert, WR Mayr) Springer-Verlag, Berlin, 1984, pp 348–58.

29 Tuomilehto-Wolf E, Tuomilehto J, Cepaitis Z, Lounnama R. The DIME study. New susceptibility haplotype for type 1 diabetes. *Lancet* 1989; **ii**: 299–302.

30 Tienari PJ, Tuomilehto-Wolf E, Tuomilehto J, Peltonen L. The DIME Study Group. HLA haplotypes in type 1 (insulin-dependent) diabetes mellitus: molecular analysis of the HLA-DQ locus. *Diabetologia* 1992; **35**: 254–60.

31 Walker A, Cudworth AG. Type 1 (insulin-dependent) diabetic multiplex families: mode of genetic transmission. *Diabetes* 1980; **29**: 1036–9.

32 Tarn AC, Thomas JM, Dean BM, et al. Predicting insulin-dependent diabetes. *Lancet* 1988; **i**: 845–60.

33 Warram JH, Krolewski AS, Gottlieb MS, Kahn CR. Differences in risk of insulin dependent diabetes in offspring of diabetic mothers and diabetic fathers. *N Engl J Med* 1984; **ii**: 299–302.

34 Vadheim CM, Rotter JI, Maclaren NK, Riley WJ, Anderson CE. Preferential transmission of diabetic alleles within the HLA gene complex. *N Engl J Med* 1986; **315**: 1314–18.

35 Cudworth AG, Wolf E, Gorsuch AN, Festenstein H. A new look at HLA genetics with particular reference to type 1 diabetes. *Lancet* 1979; **ii**: 389–91.
36 Bell GI, Horita S, Karam JH. A polymorphic locus near the insulin gene is associated with insulin-dependent diabetes mellitus. *Diabetes* 1984; **33**: 176–83.
37 Rich SS, Weitkamp LR, Guttormsen S, Barbosa J. Gm, Km, and HLA in insulin-dependent type 1 diabetes mellitus: a log-linear analysis of association. *Diabetes* 1986; **35**: 927–32.
38 Tillil H, Kobberling J. Age-corrected empirical genetic risk estimates for first degree relatives of IDDM patients. *Diabetes* 1987; **36**: 93–9.
39 Simpson NE. The genetics of diabetes: a study of 223 families of juvenile diabetics. *Ann Hum Genet* 1962; **26**: 1–21.
40 Gottlieb MS. Diabetes in offspring and siblings of juvenile and maturity-onset-type diabetics. *J Chronic Dis* 1979; **33**: 331–9.
41 Gamble DR. An epidemiological study of childhood diabetes affecting two or more siblings. *Diabetologia* 1980; **19**: 341–4.
42 Cavender DE, Wagener DK, Rabin BS, et al. The Pittsburg insulin-dependent diabetes mellitus (IDDM) study: HLA antigens and haplotypes as risk factors for the development of IDDM in IDDM patients and their siblings. *J Chronic Dis* 1984; **37**: 555–68.
43 Lendrum R, Walker G, Gamble DR. Islet-cell antibodies in juvenile diabetes mellitus of recent onset. *Lancet* 1975; **i**: 880–3.
44 McCulloch DK, Klaff LJ, Kahn SE, et al. Nonprogression of subclinical β-cell dysfunction among first-degree relatives of IDDM patients: 5-yr follow-up of the Seattle Family Study. *Diabetes* 1990; **39**: 549–56.
45 Bingley PJ, Bonifacio E, Gale EAM. Can we really predict IDDM? *Diabetes* 1993; **42**: 213–20.
46 Deschamps I, Boitard C, Hors J, et al. Life table analysis of the risk of type 1 (insulin-dependent) diabetes in siblings according to islet cell antibodies and HLA markers. *Diabetologia* 1992; **35**: 951–7.
47 Genovese S, Bonifacio E, Dean BM, et al. Distinct cytoplasmic islet cell antibodies with different risks for type 1 (insulin-dependent) diabetes mellitus. *Diabetologia* 1992; **35**: 385–8.
48 Gianini R, Pugliese A, Bonner-Weir S, et al. Prognostically significant heterogeneity of cytoplasmic islet cell antibodies in relatives of patients with type 1 diabetes. *Diabetes* 1992; **41**: 347–53.
49 Timsit J, Caillat-Zucman S, Blondel H, et al. Islet cell antibody heterogeneity among type 1 (insulin-dependent) diabetic patients. *Diabetologia* 1992; **35**: 792–5.
50 Harrison LC. Islet cell antigens in insulin-dependent diabetes: Pandora's box revisited. *Immunol Today* 1992; **13**: 348–52.
51 Palmer JP, Asplin CM, Clemons P, et al. Insulin antibodies in insulin-dependent diabetes before insulin treatment. *Science* 1983; **222**: 1337–9.
52 Baekkeskov S, Aanstoot HJ, Christgau S, et al. Identification of the 64K auto-antigen in insulin-dependent diabetes as GABA-synthesizing enzyme glutamic acid decarboxylase. *Nature (Lond)* 1990; **347**: 151–6.
53 Ziegler AG, Ziegler R, Vardi P, et al. Life-table analysis of progression to diabetes of anti-insulin autoantibody-positive relatives of individuals with type 1 diabetes. *Diabetes* 1989; **38**: 1320–5.
54 Atkinson MA, Maclaren NK, Riley WJ, et al. Are insulin autoantibodies markers for insulin-dependent diabetes mellitus? *Diabetes* 1986; **35**: 894–8.
55 Christie MR, Tun RYM, Lo SSS, et al. Antibodies to GAD and trypic fragments

of the islet 64K antigen as distinct markers for development of IDDM: studies with identical twins. *Diabetes* 1992; **41**: 782–7.

56 Genovese S, Cassidy D, Bonifacio E, Bottazzo GF, Christie MR. Antibodies to 37/40kD tryptic fragments of 64kD antigen are markers of rapid progression to type 1 insulin-dependent diabetes (Abstract). *Diabetes Res Clin Pract* 1991; **14** (Suppl 1): S11.

57 Bingley PJ, Christie MR, Bonfanti R, et al. Combined analysis of autoantibodies enhances prediction of IDDM in islet cell antibody (ICA) positive relatives. *Diabetic Med* 1993 (in press).

58 Bingley PJ, Colman PG, Eisenbarth GS, et al. Standardization of IVGTT to predict IDDM. *Diabetes Care* 1992; **15**: 93–102.

59 Vardi P, Crisa L, Jackson RA. Predictive value of intravenous glucose tolerance test insulin secretion less than or greater than the first percentile in islet cell antibody positive relatives of type 1 (insulin-dependent) diabetic patients. *Diabetologia* 1991; **34**: 93–102.

60 Colman PG, Eisenbarth GS. Immunology of type 1 diabetes: 1987. In: *Diabetes Annual 4* (eds. KGGM Alberti, LP Krall) Elsevier, Amsterdam, 1988, pp 17–45.

61 Anderson CE, Hodge SE, Rubin R, et al. A search for heterogeneity in insulin dependent diabetes mellitus (IDDM): HLA and autoimmune studies in simplex, multiplex and multigenerational families. *Metabolism* 1983; **32**: 471–7.

62 Sheehy MJ, Scharf SJ, Rowe JR, et al. A diabetes-susceptibility HLA haplotype is best defined by a combination of HLA-DR and -DQ alleles. *J Clin Invest* 1989; **83**: 830–5.

63 Owerbach D, Gunn S, Gabbay KH. Primary associations of HLA-DQw8 with type 1 diabetes in DR4 patients. *Diabetes* 1989; **38**: 942–5.

64 Reijonen H, Ilonen J, Knip M, Akerblom HK. HLA-DQBI alleles and absence of Asp 57 as susceptibility factors of IDDM in Finland. *Diabetes* 1991; **40**: 1640–4.

65 Maclaren NK, Horne G, Spillar RP, et al. Islet cell antibodies (ICA) in US school children. *Diabetes* 1985; **34** (Suppl 1): 84A.

66 Bergua M, Sole J, Marion G, et al. Prevalence of islet cell antibodies, insulin antibodies and hyperglycaemia in 2291 schoolchildren. *Diabetologia* 1987; **30**: 724–6.

67 Landin-Olsson M, Karlsson A, Dahlquist G, et al. Islet cell and other organ specific autoantibodies in all children developing type 1 (insulin-dependent) diabetes in Sweden during one year and in matched control children. *Diabetologia* 1989; **32**: 387–95.

68 Karjalainen J. Islet cell antibodies as predictive markers for IDDM in children with high background incidence of disease. *Diabetes* 1990; **39**: 1144–50.

69 Bruining GJ, Molenaar JL, Grobbee DE, et al. Ten-year follow-up study of islet cell antibodies and childhood diabetes mellitus. *Lancet* 1989; **i**: 1100–3.

70 Lee JM. Screening and informed consent. *N Engl J Med* 1993; **328**: 438–40.

71 Siegler A, Amiel SA, Lantos J. Scientific and ethical consequences of disease prediction. *Diabetologia* 1992; **35** (Suppl 2): S60–S68.

Chapter Four

Diabetic Twin Studies

R. D. G. Leslie
St Bartholomew's Hospital, London, UK

INTRODUCTION

Diabetic twin studies have provided important information about the causes of diabetes, including the cause of insulin-dependent diabetes mellitus (IDDM). IDDM is due to non-genetically determined factors, probably environmental agents, operating in genetically susceptible individuals. The environmental event operates over a brief period in early childhood to induce an immune process which destroys the islet β cell. β cell destruction in some is chronic and progressive, leading to IDDM, but it others it can remit without diabetes developing. In the months or years before the onset of IDDM, clinical, immune and metabolic changes can be detected and these changes are predictive of diabetes. The nature, intensity, extent and persistence of these immune changes distinguish twins who develop IDDM from those who do not.

Two major types of diabetes are recognized: IDDM and non-insulin-dependent diabetes mellitus (NIDDM). In this review I discuss how the study of diabetic twins has contributed to our understanding of events leading to IDDM.

Causes of Diabetes. Edited by R. D. G. Leslie.
© 1993 John Wiley & Sons Ltd.

RATIONALE FOR STUDYING TWINS

In the method of analysing twins proposed by Sir Francis Galton, the rates of concordance of a disease for identical and non-identical twins are compared. Both identical and non-identical twins share the same environment in childhood but only identical twins share the same genes. Therefore identical and non-identical twins will be concordant to the same degree for factors determined by the environment. In contrast, the concordance rates in identical and non-identical twins will differ for genetically determined features. The greater the difference between identical and non-identical twins, the more powerful the genetic influence causing a particular feature. In this twin method the difference between the concordance rates for identical and non-identical twins reared together is doubled to give an index of heritability[1].

Heritability reflects gene expression or penetrance in a given environment. Perhaps the best estimate of heritability can be obtained by determining the concordance rate of identical twins reared apart, although one cannot, even then, exclude the potentially important influence of a shared environment *in utero*. Concordance rates are usually expressed as the pairwise concordance, i.e. $C / C + D$ (where C is the number of pairs concordant and D the number of pairs discordant for the disease). When ascertainment is complete it is possible to calculate the proband concordance, i.e. $2C / 2C + D$.

There are five reasons for studying identical twins with a disease:

1. To define heritability: this is defined by the Galton method and requires the study of identical and non-identical twins.
2. As a control group: to define the effect of diabetes, appropriate control subjects should be matched for factors including genetic susceptibility to diabetes. Only the non-diabetic identical co-twins of diabetic patients are known to be genetically susceptible to diabetes, as the nature of all the disease genes is unclear. Thus the ideal control is a non-diabetic identical twin who has been reared with the index diabetic co-twin in childhood.
3. To define non-genetic factors: differences between identical twins must be due to non-genetically determined factors, while similarities could be due to shared genetic or non-genetic factors.
4. To define genetic factors: if a factor is inherited then identical twins will be concordant for it and levels of that factor between twins of a pair will be correlated irrespective of whether they have diabetes or not. Finally, if altered levels of that factor are found in IDDM twins they will also be abnormal in the non-diabetic identical co-twin as compared with a normal control subject.
5. To define groups at high and low disease risk: the concordance rates for IDDM between identical twins (36%) means that we can study twins at high disease risk to identify changes which do or do not lead on to

diabetes; twins who remain non-diabetic more than 6 years from the diagnosis of their index twin have a low disease risk $(<2\%)$[2].

Most studies of twins with diabetes have not used this panoply of techniques. Until recently, our own study has been concerned only with identical twins.

OUR PRESENT SERIES

We have been studying identical twins with diabetes for 26 years. The twins have been referred by colleagues from throughout Britain[3]. They were referred because the index twin had diabetes, not because they were twins. Our ascertainment of twins is therefore biased. This is the largest, longest-running and most comprehensive twin study in the world. The study was started by Dr David Pyke and has been based at King's College Hospital, Westminster Hospital and, more recently, at St Bartholemew's Hospital, London. As of 1st December 1992 the total number of twins was 332 pairs. Of 211 pairs in which the index twin has IDDM, 113 are concordant and 98 pairs are discordant for diabetes. Of the remainder 115 pairs have an index twin with NIDDM and in six pairs the type of diabetes is uncertain. We also have 21 pairs of non-identical twins all of whom to date are discordant for IDDM and eight pairs of non-identical twins discordant for NIDDM.

OTHER TWIN SERIES

Of the reported studies of diabetic twins, in only three has diabetes been categorized by disease type, monozygosity confirmed and the unaffected twins examined by glucose tolerance testing. Only five twin studies have ascertained index twins who were either young at diagnosis or had IDDM. In all but two of these studies ascertainment was incomplete, twins either being referred because they were diabetic or ascertained from a clinic population. The two exceptions are the study from the Danish Twin Register by Harvald and Hauge and a more recent study using the Finnish Twin Register[4,5]. In the Danish study, of 36 'younger onset' pairs 24 were discordant, but the unaffected twins were not tested[4]. The Finnish study made use of a Central Population Registry, a national registry for hospital discharges and a registry for patients provided with free-of-charge medication. In this study three of 23 pairs of identical twins and two of 81 pairs of non-identical twins were concordant for IDDM; the concordance rates were therefore higher among identical (23% probandwise and 13% pairwise) than non-identical twins (5% probandwise and 3% pairwise)[5]. The unaffected twins were not tested for zygosity or glucose tolerance, nor have they been followed for a long period as the study has only recently been initiated. Nevertheless the results suggest that many identical twin pairs can be discordant for IDDM. Then Berg reported discordance in six of 12 identical twin pairs in which the index twin was diagnosed under 43 years of age[6]. Gottlieb and Root, from the Joslin Clinic, found discordance in 18 of 20 co-twins of patients diagnosed under the age of 40 years[7]. Soeldner and Eisenbarth, also from the Joslin Clinic, reported detailed prospective studies on 24 co-twins of diabetic twins with IDDM, of whom 20 remain discordant[8]. The University of Southern California used national advertising and a postal questionnaire to identify twins; of 130 identical twin pairs 95 were discordant for IDDM but the unaffected twins were not tested[9]. Finally, the Japan Diabetes Society collected twins by correspondence with their members and identified 21 twins with IDDM, 11 of them identical twins and 10 non-identical twins[10]. The twins were not tested for zygosity but the non-diabetic twins had oral glucose tolerance tests. Of 11 identical twin pairs five were concordant for diabetes, as compared with none of the 10 non-identical twin pairs. In summary, the majority of identical twins with IDDM have a non-diabetic co-twin irrespective of their country of origin. In all studies the concordance rate for IDDM in identical twins is higher than that for non-identical twins.

PATHOGENESIS OF IDDM

There are two types of diabetes which must be treated with insulin, i.e. the patients are insulin-dependent. One type is associated with diabetes insipidus, optic atrophy and high-tone deafness (DIDMOAD or Wolfram's syndrome) and is due to malformation of islet β cells. The other is type 1 or insulin-dependent diabetes (IDDM) and is due to destruction of the β cells. At diagnosis of IDDM about 80% of islets contain no β cells and the islets may be heavily infiltrated with lymphocytes[11]. Not all the insulin-secreting β cells will be destroyed, and even in long-standing diabetic patients about 10% of the islets have insulin-containing cells. There is no evidence that the exocrine pancreatic cells or the other islet cells secreting glucagon, somatostatin or pancreatic polypeptide are involved in this destructive process. Those residual islets which contain β cells hyperexpress class I human leucocyte antigen (HLA) but only the β cells express class II HLA and contain immunoreactive interferon α[11]. At diagnosis, cellular and humoral immune changes are present in peripheral blood. Cellular changes include increased numbers of activated T lymphocytes expressing the HLA-DR antigen on their cell surface[12], and alterations in both the number and function of immuno-regulatory T lymphocytes[13] and natural killer cells[14]. Autoantibodies can be detected in up to 100% of patients. These antibodies recognize antigens in the islet cell cytoplasm (islet cell antibodies or ICA), in β cell glucose

Table 1 Antibodies associated with IDDM recognize a variety of structural and functional elements in the islet β cell

Cytoplasmic islet cell antigens	Carboxypeptidase H
Islet cell surface antigens	Glutamic acid decarboxylase
Tubulin	Insulin
Albumin	Proinsulin
37/40 kDa islet fragments	?Glucose transporter

recognition systems (possibly the glucose transporter) and in β cell hormone secretion systems including enzymes (carboxypeptidase H and glutamic acid decarboxylase or GAD) and hormones (insulin and proinsulin)[15-18] (Table 1).

LIMITED ROLE OF GENETIC FACTORS IN IDDM

Genetic influences are important in IDDM but are not paramount. In our twin series only about 36% of identical twins of diabetic patients develop the disease[2]. From the University of Southern California Diabetes Twin Registry the concordance rates in twin pairs in which the index twin was diagnosed under 10 years of age were 48% in identical twins and 15% in non-identical twins at 15 years follow-up[9]. Thus the estimated heritability is no more than 66%; even this figure is likely to be exaggerated as the method of ascertainment preferentially identified concordant pairs. This genetic influence declines with increasing age at diagnosis. Heritability falls from 66% to 2% according to whether the index twin is diagnosed under 10 years of age or between 15 and 30 years of age respectively[9].

Genes in the class II region of the HLA system on chromosome 6 are associated with IDDM. Current evidence suggests that the HLA DQ region of chromosome 6 is more important than the HLA DR region[19]. In particular, genes which code for an amino acid other than aspartate at position 57 of the DQ β chains and for arginine in position 52 of DQ α chains are associated with disease susceptibility[19,20]. Other DQB1 genes, including a gene which codes for aspartate at position 57 of the DQ β chain, confer disease protection[19-21]. The overall structure of the HLA molecule is probably more important than any single amino acid residue alone. It is possible that genes outside the HLA region play a role in this disease but they have not yet been clearly identified in man. One candidate gene for such an association is the insulin gene hypervariable region on chromosome 11[22].

HLA genes are important if IDDM is to develop. Thus, in families with several affected members, about 95% of the diabetic siblings are HLA identical or haploidentical[23]. Even in identical twin pairs discordant for diabetes non-genetic factors are not entirely responsible for their diabetes, since they also have the HLA disease susceptibility genes[24]. The concordance rate for diabetes between identical twins is greater if they are heterozygous for HLA DR3 and HLA DR4 than either one alone[2,24]. This observation suggests that HLA DR3 and HLA DR4 genes confer greater predisposition to IDDM than either alone; i.e. genetic susceptibility to IDDM is polygenic.

Nevertheless the role of these HLA genes as disease susceptibility alleles is limited. Thus two of the most important genes, HLA DR3 and DR4, are found in 60% of the normal population yet only 0.25% of the population will develop IDDM. The chances of an HLA identical sibling developing IDDM is about 10%—44 times greater than the normal risk. Such risks are very small when compared with the relative risk of 230 for an identical twin of a diabetic developing IDDM, even though only one-third will do so[2]. Since the main candidate for genetic susceptibility to IDDM is in the HLA region which codes for proteins involved in antigen presentation and recognition, the immune response is probably important in the aetiology of IDDM.

GENETIC SUSCEPTIBILITY TO NON-GENETIC FACTORS

Non-human somatic studies of the HLA DQ β region suggests that this region has been in balanced polymorphism for 10 or more million years. To maintain the extraordinary diversity of HLA types over this time selection pressures must have been operating; otherwise most alleles would have been lost through genetic drift. It has been proposed that infectious pathogens are the major cause of HLA diversity. HLA associations with IDDM may therefore operate through susceptibility to certain undefined infections. Other factors may be genetically determined and associated with susceptibility to infections. Both cellular and humoral immune changes associated with IDDM can be detected in the non-diabetic co-twins of patients with IDDM; they include a reduction in natural killer cells, complement function and suppressor/cytotoxic cells (expressing the CD8 antigen)[14,25,26]. These changes have poor predictive power and may be inherited. Natural killer cells are primary effectors of antiviral defence, the complement component C4 plays a key role in virus neutralization and CD8$^+$ lymphocytes are important in clearing viruses. The reduction in these immune parameters suggests an inherited predisposition to viral infections, which may explain why diabetic patients are less likely to mount a protective antibody response following vaccination against hepatitis[27]. There is no evidence that these immune changes would predispose to damage by a toxin—another environmental agent which could cause diabetes. Finally, patients with IDDM have an increased red blood cell sodium–lithium countertransport activity[28]. We have recently shown that this change is not due to the disease but is probably inherited, since the non-diabetic identical co-twins of IDDM patients also have an increased countertransport activity which correlates with that of their diabetic twin[28]. It is likely, therefore, that increased activity of a cell membrane ion transporter is inherited as part of the genetic susceptibility to IDDM, though how such a change could influence susceptibility to IDDM remains unclear.

IMPORTANCE OF NON-GENETICALLY DETERMINED FACTORS

The most powerful evidence that IDDM is due to non-genetically determined factors comes from the study of identical twins. As identical twins usually live together in childhood, similarities (concordance) between twins might be due to shared genetic or non-genetic factors. Differences or discordance between identical twins, on the other hand, must be due to non-genetically determined factors.

In view of the major ascertainment biases in all previous diabetic twin studies, including our own, it was not possible to reach a firm conclusion that

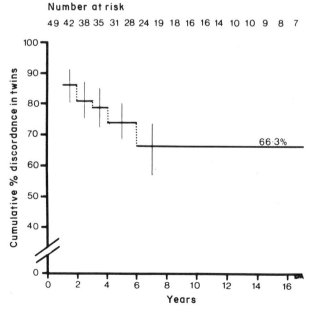

Figure 1 Life table showing percentage (±SE) of identical twins of IDDM patients who remain non-diabetic

twin pairs would remain discordant for diabetes irrespective of the period of follow-up. We therefore studied prospectively a cohort of 49 non-diabetic identical twins of recently diagnosed patients with IDDM for up to 24 years (median 9 years)[2]. During this time 15 twins developed diabetes. Actuarial analysis indicated that by 12 years 34% of the twins would have developed diabetes and that thereafter only another 2% could be expected to do so (Figure 1). The striking degree of discordance between identical twins for this disease suggests that non-genetically determined factors must play a major role in its aetiology. Estimates of heritability based on the American postal questionnaire suggest that heritability falls with increasing age of diagnosis, indicating an increasing non-genetic influence[9].

NON-GENETIC FACTOR LIKELY TO BE ENVIRONMENTAL, NOT SOMATIC MUTATION

Differences between identical twins for IDDM must be due to causes other than the germline genes. However, even identical twins could be genetically different for certain genes. For example, genes could undergo random and ordered rearrangement or mutation and may differ between identical twins[29]. In contrast to antibody genes, genes of the T cell receptor do not appear to undergo somatic hypermutation. If, as is widely believed, T cells are responsible for the immune destruction of islet β cells then it is unlikely that somatic mutations give rise to IDDM. Several other observations argue against somatic mutations causing the disease. It is unlikely that random somatic mutations could explain the almost constant year-on-year disease incidence within different populations without epidemicity[30]. In addition, there is no evidence of randomness in either the clinical syndrome or the antigens recognized by antibodies in patients with the disease[31,32]. If a somatic mutation of the immune system caused IDDM, the aberrant immune response would probably be monoclonal and not polyclonal as is the case in IDDM[33]. In fact, the evidence is that the immune antibody response is antigen-driven given that the antibodies associated with IDDM show polyclonality, isotype switching, recognition of diverse antigens, persistence in the prediabetic period and disappearance after the clinical onset of diabetes as the antigen source (the islet β cell) is destroyed[34]. We therefore believe, though we cannot be certain, that the disease is not due to a random genetic mutation but is caused by an environmental agent acting in a genetically susceptible individual.

NATURE OF ENVIRONMENTAL FACTOR UNKNOWN

What is the environmental agent which causes IDDM? Attention has focused on viruses and toxins[35]. While both these factors have been shown in some cases to cause diabetes in man, it remains unclear whether either is the environmental agent responsible for the generality of IDDM. Several environmental factors may precipitate the clinical onset of IDDM, including the seasons (the disease is more common in warmer months), peripuberty and stressful life events[36]. However, as discussed below, the disease process is likely to have been initiated many months earlier. Twin studies have been singularly unhelpful to date in identifying important environmental factors.

ENVIRONMENTAL FACTOR PROBABLY OPERATES OVER A BRIEF PERIOD

The age-specific pattern of incidence of IDDM is similar worldwide. The disease is extremely rare before 9 months of age, the peak incidence is between 5 and 15 years of age; and there is a sharp decline in the incidence after 15 years of age[30] (Figure 2). The decline in disease incidence is a consistent and striking feature. This decline in incidence could be due to either a loss of the genetically susceptible pool in a population or a limited period of effect of the environmental agent. We know from twin studies that the majority of genetically susceptible individuals do not develop the disease[2]. Therefore the decreasing disease incidence with age must be due to a decreased effect of the environmental factor. We have already seen that the decrease in concordance rates in twins with increasing age is due to a reduced

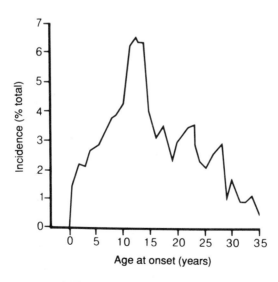

Figure 2 Age at onset of IDDM compiled from several sources to estimate age-specific incidence

heritability. It is likely, therefore, that the decline in disease rates with age is due to a decline in both genetic and environmental influences.

If the environmental factor operated over a prolonged period to cause IDDM the disease rate would rise with time, as the incidence of lung cancer rises with increasing duration of smoking. The fall in disease incidence with time in populations and in identical co-twins of patients with IDDM favours a brief critical period in which the process leading to β cell destruction is initiated[2,30].

EXPOSURE OR SUSCEPTIBILITY TO EXPOSURE

It is not possible at present to determine whether the decreasing environmental effect is due to a lack of exposure to the environmental factor or a change in susceptibility to such a factor. It is difficult to envisage an environmental agent to which only children are exposed. On the other hand, the pattern of disease incidence does resemble that for common viral infections which cause less illness with age as immunity develops. Current evidence favours the latter as twins can have immune changes (see below), consistent with exposure to an environmental agent, yet not develop IDDM, possibly because exposure induces tolerance to developing diabetes[36].

MULTIPLE HIT OR SINGLE HIT

It is not known whether the disease is initiated by single or multiple exposures during the brief critical period. Diabetes can be produced in animal models using viruses and chemical toxins in combination[35]. Cumulative damage, if it were to occur, would have to occur within a brief time frame.

AGE OF EXPOSURE

It is not possible from these twin studies to suggest the likely age of exposure other than to suggest that it is probably in early childhood, since immune changes can be detected in many young prediabetic individuals at the earliest time of ascertainment[32]. Some evidence points to the peripartum or even the *in utero* period being important[35].

DESTRUCTIVE PROCESS IS PROBABLY IMMUNE-MEDIATED

While the destruction of the β cell could result from the direct effect of an environmental agent, the destructive process must also involve the immune system. The most striking evidence supporting involvement of the immune system comes from a study of identical twins in Minneapolis[37]. Three insulin-dependent diabetic twins received a segmental pancreas transplantation (without immunosuppression) from their non-diabetic co-twins, who were themselves unlikely to develop IDDM because they had been discordant for diabetes for more that 17 years[37]. Diabetes was temporarily cured but then relapsed as the graft stopped functioning. Examination of the pancreatic graft showed that, unlike a graft rejection response, only the β cells were destroyed. The destructive process could not have been inherited since the pancreas came from one of the twins who was not himself diabetic. The rapid destruction of apparently normal β cells when transplanted from one twin to their co-twin suggests that the destructive process must:(1) be outside the islet; (2) be β cell-specific; and (3) have retained its cytotoxic memory for at least 17 years. The immune system is the most likely candidate for such an extra-islet cell effect. In line with this argument the islets showed an inflammatory infiltrate in which cytotoxic/suppressor T cells were predominant. It remains possible that the non-diabetic twins β cells had previously been transformed so that this immune attack need not necessarily be autoimmune.

EXPOSURE NEED NOT LEAD TO IDDM

The immune changes associated with IDDM do not always lead on to the disease[36]. Increased levels of activated T lymphocytes have been detected in the majority of non-diabetic identical twins of recently diagnosed diabetic patients who were then followed for up to 10 years without developing diabetes themselves[38,39]. Autoantibodies to islet cells, insulin, GAD and tryptic fragments of the 64 kDa islet antigen have also been detected in non-diabetic twins and siblings of diabetic patients who, we calculate, are unlikely now to develop diabetes[31,32,34,39]. In both twin- and population-based studies islet cell antibodies can remit without progression to diabetes[39,40]. As identical twins can be discordant for these immune changes, namely the production of ICA, GAD antibodies and activation of T lymphocytes, the changes probably reflect exposure to an environmental event[39]. By implication, then, exposure to the critical environmental event which causes these immune changes need not lead on to IDDM.

Evidence now suggests that the islet β cells can be damaged without progression to IDDM. Impaired glucose tolerance was observed in five of 41 identical twins of patients with IDDM, none of whom developed diabetes themselves, and all of whom now have normal glucose tolerance[41]. Some of these non-diabetic twins also had a decreased insulin response to intravenous glucose and an altered insulin-to-glucose dose–response relationship[42]. Finally, increased peripheral blood levels of proinsulin, the precursor of insulin, have been found in twins and siblings of diabetic patients many years after the diagnosis of the index case, and when they themselves are unlikely to develop IDDM[43-45]. It should be noted that the changes in proinsulin secretion were detected in non-HLA identical siblings; this observation raises the possibility that β cell damage, in contrast to β cell destruction, is not HLA-restricted.

We have known for some years that immune charges in organ-orientated diseases such as thyroiditis can occur without necessarily leading to destruction of the target cells. It now looks as if the disease process associated with IDDM also encompasses a wide spectrum, including immune and metabolic changes which do not lead on to diabetes.

CHRONIC PROGRESSIVE β CELL DESTRUCTION LEADING TO IDDM

The evidence suggests that a destructive immune process, once initiated, pursues in some a chronic progressive course of β cell destruction, while in others the process remits spontaneously. We have detected immune changes up to 14 years before the onset of diabetes[32]. During this prediabetic period we have detected immune, metabolic and clinical changes which herald the onset of clinical diabetes[32,42,46].

CLINICAL CHANGES BEFORE IDDM

Diabetes can retard growth. In a group of young non-diabetic twins of patients with IDDM, there was a significant tendency for growth to fall below the third percentile compared with their diabetic twins[46]. These changes were only detected in twins who subsequently developed IDDM, and not in twins who remain non-diabetic. Growth delay occurred many months before the diagnosis of diabetes. Subtle changes in glucose tolerance and sex hormones at growth nadir raises the possibility that either metabolic or hormonal disturbances account for the growth delay[46]. Twins usually grow at the same rate and to the same final height. However, at diagnosis of diabetes the index twin is often shorter than his unaffected co-twin, consistent with growth delay being prevalent in the prediabetic period[47].

IMMUNE PROCESS LEADING TO IDDM

CELLULAR CHANGES

Twins studied before they developed IDDM already show activation of T lymphocytes when first ascertained, irrespective of the time before they develop diabetes[26,38,39]. These changes persist until the diagnosis of diabetes months, even years, later without any consistent alteration in their level[38].

CYTOKINE CHANGES

Lymphocytes and macrophages which are activated and involved in an immune response should produce cytokines. The detection of interferon-α in islet β cells at diagnosis of IDDM suggests that cytokines are involved in the immune response associated with disease and is important evidence that β cells have been exposed to a virus[11]. Cytokines may be responsible for the aberrant expression of class II glycoproteins on islet β cells and may themselves cause islet β cell destruction. In preliminary studies we have studied circulating levels of tumour necrosis factor (TNF)-α, interleukin 1α and interferon-γ using sensitive immunoassays[48]. During the prediabetic period TNF and interleukin 1 levels were elevated above the normal range in about 70% of samples, in contrast to twins who remain non-diabetic who had elevated levels in less than 15% of samples.

HUMORAL CHANGES

Antigens recognized by serum antibodies in twins tested in the prediabetic period include: islet cell cytoplasmic antigens (ICA); insulin; GAD; a 64 kDa antigen which incorporates GAD; and trypsin-derived fragments of this 64 kDa antigen, including 37 kDa, 40 kDa and 50 kDa fragments[32] (see Table 1). There is evidence that the 64 kDa antigen is associated with two antibody specificities which are distinct; one specificity is associated with the 50 kDa fragment, which retains GAD activity, and the other with both the 37 kDa and 40 kDa fragments, which tend to be associated and neither of which have GAD activity[32]. It is proposed therefore that 37 kDa and 40 kDa antigens are part of the 64 kDa antigen complex but they may not be fragments of

Table 2 Frequency of antibodies in 58 non-diabetic identical twins of diabetic patients who later developed IDDM ($n = 12$) or remain non-diabetic ($n = 46$). 37/40 kDa antibodies had the highest positive predictive value

	Prediabetic twins	Non-diabetic twins
GAD	67%	13%
50 kDA	75%	15%
37/40 kDa	67%	2%
ICA (>4 JDF units)	75%	11%
IAA	25%	4%

GAD. Antibodies to all these islet antigens have been found in the non-diabetic twins of patients with IDDM[32]: of 58 non-diabetic twins tested 12 developed IDDM subsequently and the remainder are unlikely now to develop diabetes. Islet cell antibodies and antibodies to GAD and its tryptic fragments were detected at similar frequencies in prediabetic twins (67–75%), but only 25% had insulin autoantibodies. In contrast, twins who remain non-diabetic had a lower frequency of these antibodies (11–13%) except for insulin autoantibodies (4%) and most notably 37 kDa antibodies (2%) (see Table 2). Eight of nine twins with 37/40 kDa antibodies and all six twins with ICA >20 JDF units developed diabetes. Thus antibodies to 37/40 kDa fragments or high-titre ICA were the best markers for diabetes development in these twins.

CELLULAR AND HUMORAL CHANGES

Previous family studies have indicated that both cellular and humoral immune changes can be detected together in the prediabetic period, but there are no prospective studies to assess the predictive value of these changes. In a 10-year prospective study of a cohort of 20 non-diabetic twins, 10 of whom developed IDDM, we found that increased levels of activated T lymphocytes and either ICA or insulin autoantibodies were strongly predictive of diabetes[38]. In contrast to the prediabetic twins, the 10 twins who remain non-diabetic showed the combination of T cell activation and ICA in only one of 40 samples taken during the study period (unpublished observations). Thus the presence of both cellular and humoral immune changes emerged as one feature which distinguished twins who went on to develop IDDM from those who did not. The second important feature which distinguished twins who develop diabetes was the persistence of both cellular and humoral immune changes in the prediabetic period. Since the levels of both ICA and activated T lymphocytes persist up to the onset of the disease in those twins who develop diabetes mellitus but decrease thereafter with the destruction of the target (the β cell), it is likely that these immune changes are antigen-dependent and antigen-driven. In summary, the immune response during the prediabetic period involves both cellular and humoral changes, probably initiated by an environmental factor and maintained by specific islet cell antigens. This response persists over a prolonged period up to diagnosis, indicating that the process associated with it is not intermittent but continuous.

METABOLIC CHANGES BEFORE IDDM

Metabolic changes can precede the onset of IDDM by many months. Many metabolic changes have been described, including changes in both glucose metabolism and β cell function.

QUALITATIVE CHANGES IN β CELL FUNCTION

Possibly the earliest abnormality is an increase in the fasting proinsulin level even when the fasting glucose and insulin levels are normal[44]. The nature of the increased proinsulin is unclear; it could be due to an excess release of the precursors, including partially processed forms of proinsulin from the secretory pathway, or to release of the intact hormone from the non-secretory pathway. The proinsulin assays which have been used do not distinguish between intact proinsulin and proinsulin intermediates[44]. The increased proinsulin secretion could result from an inherited susceptibility to IDDM or, alternatively, it could be secondary to β cell damage. Studies of baboons confirm that β cell damage which leads to IDDM can cause an increase in fasting proinsulin levels[49].

The β cell normally secretes insulin as regular oscillatory pulses which can be detected in the peripheral circulation as basal insulin oscillations with a mean period of 13 minutes. A group of siblings of patients with IDDM who also had ICA were tested to establish whether they showed oscillatory insulin secretion[50]. They did, though regular oscillatory activity was generally absent even when the insulin response to intravenous glucose was in the normal range.

Insulin secretion responds to increasing intravenous glucose loads in a stepwise fashion[42]. The increasing response to glucose provides a dose–response relationship which shows a high degree of fit in a non-linear logarithmic curve-fitting programme. We found that twins tested up to 10 months before the onset of IDDM did not demonstrate such a stepwise increase in their insulin responses[42]. The loss of normal glucose to insulin relationship in prediabetic twins is consistent with a qualitative β cell defect before the onset of IDDM.

Sites on the cell membrane that could provide specific targets for β cell destruction include the glucose recognition system and those systems responsible for insulin secretion. If the glucose recognition system is involved early in the disease, then it should be possible to demonstrate differential sensitivity of the β cell to glucose as compared to other insulin secretagogues. Both ourselves and others have demonstrated in prediabetic patients an absent response to intravenous glucose when the response to glucagon or arginine is present but greatly reduced[51,52]. One reason for the rapid disappearance of the insulin response to glucose could be the attendant hyperglycaemia. A number of studies have shown the deleterious effect of hyperglycaemia on the islet's ability to recognize glucose, resulting in differential responses to various secretagogues[53]. A group of non-diabetic twins with ICA were studied, all of whom have developed IDDM; they showed a similar decrease in their insulin response to both intravenous glucose and glucagon as compared with controls[51]. It appears, therefore, that glucose and glucagon recognition may decline in parallel before the onset of clinical diabetes. The differential response, while it can occur, is not a characteristic feature of the prediabetic period.

QUANTITATIVE CHANGES IN β CELL FUNCTION

During the prediabetic period the insulin response to intravenous glucose may be decreased[8,42]. The insulin response can decline over a number of years even when it is the normal range[8]. This decreased insulin response could be due either to decreased sensitivity to glucose or decreased islet β cell secretory capacity. To define the glucose–insulin dose–response relationship we studied a group of 22 non-diabetic twins who were followed until seven developed IDDM and the remainder were considered unlikely to develop diabetes[42]. In contrast to the twins who remain non-diabetic, who had similar insulin responses to their control group, the prediabetic twins had a decreased maximum insulin secretory response to the intravenous glucose.

CHANGES IN GLUCOSE METABOLISM

Impairment of glucose tolerance and glucose clearance has been observed many months before the onset of diabetes and before changes in fasting glucose[41]. Impaired glucose tolerance can occur without changes in either other intermediary metabolites or insulin. However, glucose tolerance can improve with time in some twins who do not develop diabetes[41]. In our experience the 2-hour glucose level after an oral glucose load starts to increase above the control range as early as 3 years before the diagnosis of diabetes, while the fasting glucose remains normal[41]. In the final stage glucose tolerance deteriorates rapidly[41]. Fasting glucose increases gradually over the last 18 months before the clinical onset of IDDM but only increases dramatically at the time of diagnosis (unpublished observations).

PREDICTING IDDM

The predictive values of immune changes can be calculated by studying twins who subsequently developed IDDM as compared with those who are now unlikely to develop the disease, as calculated by actuarial analysis. The positive predictive value is determined by calculating the number of twins with an abnormality who develop IDDM as a percentage of the overall number of twins with that abnormality. Predictive values for immune or metabolic changes will be different in twins as compared with family or population studies, as twins have a greater genetic susceptibility to IDDM. As the HLA and non-HLA genetic susceptibility is defined this discrepancy will be less apparent; already family studies are using genetic data to enhance the predictive value of immune changes.

IDENTICAL TWINS

The risk of developing IDDM if you are the identical co-twin of an IDDM patient is about 36%[2]. If the index twin was diagnosed under the age of 15 years this risk is then 42%, but it is only 13% if the the index twin was over 15 years of age[9].

IMMUNE CHANGES:

The immune changes with the highest predictive value were those induced by environmental events in that identical twins were discordant for them. Antibodies to the 37 kDa islet protein fragment or ICA with a titre greater than 20 JDF units had the highest positive predictive value (89% and 90% respectively), while GAD antibodies had a positive predictive value of 62%[32]. Antibodies with the highest sensitivity as predictors were to the 50 kDa fragment and ICA (both 75%). Increased levels of activated T lymphocytes had a positive predictive value of only 60% but a sensitivity of 100%[38]. Since all the prediabetic twins tested had antibodies to at least one islet tryptic fragment but some had neither ICA nor GAD antibodies, antibodies to proteolytic fragments of the 64 kDa antigen could be used to provide more sensitive and specific predictors of IDDM. Therefore, population screening could use different sets of antibodies to provide maximum sensitivity or maximum specificity for disease prediction. In a preliminary study the presence of two or more antibodies was more predictive of subsequent diabetes than of one antibody alone[32]. The extent and persistence of immune changes are also important in that activation of T cells with ICA gave a positive predictive value of 90% and their persistence in two consecutive samples a predictive value of 100% (reference 37 and unpublished observations).

METABOLIC CHANGES

A decrease in the first-phase insulin response to intravenous glucose in a group of non-diabetic co-twins of patients with IDDM gave a positive predictive value of 58%[42]. In the same group of twins an altered glucose–insulin dose–response relationship as represented by a decreased coefficient of determination (R^2) gave a positive predictive value of 67%[42]. The only other metabolic change of any predictive value is impaired glucose tolerance, which gave a value of 33% in a small group of twins[41]. That these predictive values do not reach 100% is testament to the fact that metabolic changes can be detected in twins who are now unlikely to develop IDDM.

DIFFERENCES DETERMINING IDDM

The question arises as to how individuals who develop diabetes differ from those who do not. A critical role may be played by the molecular complex comprising the HLA molecule, the antigen and the T cell receptor, which is central to the development of an immune response. The HLA molecules comprise an α and a β chain of amino acids which probably form a 'pocket' in which the antigen sits[54]. The nature of the amino acids lining this 'pocket', or peptide binding site, could determine the ability of antigen to bind and, by implication, to be presented to the peptide receptor on T lymphocytes. However, identical twins with the same HLA genes are usually discordant for IDDM, suggesting that factors other than HLA genetic susceptibility must be important. A second essential factor is the nature of the antigen; for example, antibodies to the islet cell are more predictive of IDDM than antibodies to insulin[54], and high-titre antibodies are more predictive than low-titre antibodies[32,55]. Little is known of the third component of the molecular complex—the T cell receptor. The presence of both cellular and humoral immune changes and their persistence in two or more consecutive samples distinguish twins who develop IDDM from those who do not. Thus it is the nature, intensity, extent and persistence of changes which determine whether diabetes will develop.

ACKNOWLEDGEMENTS

The British Diabetic Twin Study has been supported by the Diabetic Twin Research Trust, the Juvenile Diabetes Foundation, the Medical Research Council, the Wellcome Trust, the Charing Cross and Westminster Medical School Joint Research Committee, the King's College Hospital Joint Research Committee and the Nuffield Foundation. I acknowledge the support of many research fellows and collaborators in these studies and, in particular, of Dr David Pyke.

REFERENCES

1 Falconer DS. *Introduction to Quantitative Genetics*, 2nd edn. Longman, New York, 1981, pp 148–69.
2 Olmos P, A'Hern R, Heaton DA, et al. The significance of the concordance rate for type 1 (insulin-dependent) diabetes in identical twins. *Diabetologia* 1988; **31**: 747–50.
3 Barnett AH, Eff C, Leslie RDG, Pyke DA. Diabetes in identical twins: a study of 200 pairs. *Diabetologia* 1981; **20**: 87–93.
4 Harvald B, Hauge M. Selection in diabetes in modern society. *Acta Med Scand* 1963; **173**: 459–65.
5 Kaprio J, Tuomilehto J, Koskenvuo M, Romanov K, et al. Concordance for type

1 (insulin-dependent) diabetes mellitus in a population-based cohort of twins in Finland. *Diabetologia* 1992 **35**: 1060–7.

6 Then Berg H. Zur frage der psychischen und neurologischen ercheinungen bei diabeteskranken und deren verwandten. *Z. Gesamte Neurol Psychiatrie Referate Ergebrisse* 1939; **165**: 278–83.

7 Gottlieb MS, Root HF. Diabetes mellitus in twins. *Diabetes* 1968; **17**: 693–704.

8 Srikanta S, Ganda OP, Jackson RA, et al. Type 1 diabetes mellitus in monozygotic twins: chronic progressive β cell dysfunction. *Ann Int Med* 1983; **99**: 320–6.

9 Kumar D, Gemayel NS, Mack TM. Significance of age at onset of insulin-dependent diabetes mellitus and disease concordance in monozygotic and dizygotic twins. *Diabetes* 1992 **41** (Suppl 1): 129A.

10 Committee of Diabetic Twins, Japan Diabetes Society. Diabetes mellitus in twins: a cooperative study in Japan. *Diabetes Res Clin Pract* 1988; **5**: 271–80.

11 Foulis AK, Farquharson MA, Meager A. Immunoreactive alpha-interferon in insulin-secreting beta cells on type 1 diabetes mellitus. *Lancet* 1987; **ii**: 423–7.

12 Alviggi L, Johnston C, Hoskins PJ, et al. Pathogenesis of insulin-dependent diabetes: a role for activated T lymphocytes. *Lancet* 1984; **ii**: 4–6.

13 Vergani D. Cell mediated immunity. In: *Immunogenetics of Insulin-dependent Diabetes* (ed AH Barnett) MTP Press, Lancaster, 1987, pp 80–90.

14 Hussain MJ, Alviggi L, Millward BA, et al. Evidence that the reduced number of natural killer cells in type 1 (insulin dependent) diabetes may be genetically determined. *Diabetes* 1987; **30**: 907–11.

15 Bottazzo GF, Dean B, Gorsuch AN, Cudworth AG, Doniach D. Complement-fixing islet cell antibodies in type 1 diabetes: possible monitors of active beta cell damage. *Lancet* 1980; **i**: 668–72.

16 Wilkin T, Hoskins PJ, Armitage M, et al. Value of insulin autoantibodies as serum makers for insulin dependent diabetes mellitus. *Lancet* 1985; **i**: 480–2.

17 Palmer JP, Asplin CM, Clemens P, et al. Insulin antibodies in insulin dependent diabetes before insulin treatment. *Science* 1983; **222**: 1337–9.

18 Baekkeskov S, Aanstoot H-J, Christgau S, et al. Identification of 64K autoantigen in insulin-dependent diabetes as the GABA-synthesizing enzyme glutamic acid decarboxylase. *Nature* 1990; **347**: 151–6.

19 Todd JA, Bell JI, McDevitt HO. HLA DQ beta gene contributes to susceptibility and resistance to insulin-dependent diabetes mellitus. *Nature* 1987; **329**: 599–604.

20 Khalil I, d'Auriol L, Gobet M, et al. A combination of HLA-DQB Asp 57-negative and HLA DQA Arg 52 confers susceptibility to Insulin-dependent diabetes mellitus. *J Clin Invest* 1990; **85**: 1315–19.

21 Todd JA, Mijovic C, Fletcher J, et al. Identification of susceptibility loci for insulin dependent diabetes mellitus by transracial gene mapping. *Nature* 1989; **338**: 587–9.

22 Julier C, Hyer RN, Davies J, et al. Insulin-IGF2 region on chromosome 11p encodes a gene implicated in HLA-DR4 dependent diabetes susceptibility. *Nature* 1991 **354**: 155–9.

23 Tarn AC, Thomas JM, Dean BM, et al. Predicting insulin-dependent diabetes. *Lancet* 1988; **i**: 845–50.

24 Johnston C, Pyke DA, Cudworth AG, Wolf E. HLA-DR typing in identical twins with insulin-dependent diabetes: difference between concordant and discordant pairs. *Br Med J* 1983; **286**: 253–5.

25 Senaldi G, Millward BA, Hussain MJ, et al. Low serum haemolytic function of the fourth complement component (C4) in insulin dependent diabetes. *J Clin Pathol* 1988; **41**: 1114–16.

26 Johnston C, Alviggi L, Millward BA, et al. Alterations in T-lymphocyte

subpopulations in type 1 diabetes: exploration of genetic influence in identical twins. *Diabetes* 1988; **37**: 1484–8.

27 Pozzilli P, Arduini P, Visalli N, et al. Reduced protection against hepatitis B virus following vaccination in patients with type 1 (insulin-dependent) diabetes. *Diabetologia* 1987; **30**: 817–19.

28 Hardman TC, Dubrey SW, Leslie RDG et al. Erythrocyte sodium–lithium countertransport and blood pressure in identical twin pairs discordant for insulindependent diabetes. *Br Med J* 1992; **305**: 215–19.

29 Cains J, Overbaugh J, Miller S. The origins of mutants. *Nature* 1988; **335**: 142–5.

30 Gamble DR. The epidemiology of insulin-dependent diabetes with particular reference to the relationship of virus infection to its aetiology. *Epidemiol Rev* 1980; **2**: 49–70.

31 Johnston C, Millward BA, Hoskins P, Leslie RDG, Bottazzo GF. Islet cell antibodies as predictors of the later development of type 1 (insulin-dependent) diabetes. *Diabetologia* 1989; **32**: 382–6.

32 Christie MR, Tun RYM, Lo SSS, et al. Antibodies to glutamate acid decarboxylase as markers for the development of insulin-dependent diabetes: studies with identical twins. *Diabetes* 1992; **41**: 782–7.

33 Millward BA, Hussain MJ, Peakman M, et al. Characterization of islet cell antibody in insulin-dependent diabetes: evidence for IgG1 subclass restriction and polyclonality. *J Clin Exp Immunol* 1988; **71**: 353–6.

34 Riley WJ, Maclaren NK, Krischer J, et al. A prospective study of the development of diabetes in relatives of patients with insulin-dependent diabetes. *N Engl J Med* 1990; **323**: 1167–72.

35 Lo SSS, Tun RYM, Leslie RDG. Non-genetic factors causing type 1 diabetes. *Diabetic Med* 1991; **8**: 609–18.

36 Leslie RDG, Pyke DA. Escaping insulin dependent diabetes. *Br Med J* 1991; **302**: 1103–4.

37 Sutherland DE, Sibley R, Yu X-Z et al. Twin-to-twin pancreas transplantation: reversal and reenactment of the pathogenesis of type 1 diabetes. *Trans Assoc Am Physicians* 1984; **97**: 80–87.

38 Peakman M, Alviggi L, Hussain MJ, et al. Persistent T cell activation predicts diabetes in unaffected identical co-twins of type 1 diabetics. *Diabetologia* 1991; **34** (Suppl 2): A56 P222.

39 Millward BA, Alviggi L, Hoskins PJ, et al. Immune changes associated with insulin dependent diabetes may remit without causing diabetes: a study in identical twins. *Br Med J* 1986; **292**: 793–6.

40 Notsu K, Oka N, Note S, et al. Islet cell antibodies in the Japanese population and subjects with type 1 (insulin-dependent) diabetes. *Diabetologia* 1985; **28**: 660–2.

41 Beer SF, Heaton DA, Alberti KGMM, Pyke DA, Leslie RDG. Impaired glucose tolerance precedes but does not predict insulin-dependent diabetes mellitus: a study of identical twins. *Diabetolgia* 1990; **33**: 497–502.

42 Lo SSS, Hawa M, Beer SF, Pyke DA, Leslie RDG. Altered islet beta-cell function before the onset of type 1 (insulin-dependent) diabetes mellitus. *Diabetologia* 1992; **35**: 277–82.

43 Heaton DA, Millward BA, Gray IP, et al. Evidence of beta cell dysfunction which does not lead on to diabetes: a study of identical twins of insulin dependent diabetics. *Br Med J* 1987; **294**: 145–6.

44 Heaton DA, Millward BA, Gray IP, et al. Increased proinsulin levels as an early indicator of beta cell dysfunction in non-diabetic twins of type 1 (insulindependent) diabetic patients. *Diabetologia* 1988; **31**: 182–4.

45 Hartling SG, Lindgren F, Dahlqvist G, Persson B, Binder C. Elevated proinsulin in healthy siblings of IDDM patients independent of HLA identity. *Diabetes* 1989; **38**: 1271–4.
46 Leslie RDG, Lo S, Millward BA, Honour J, Pyke DA. Decreased growth velocity before IDDM onset. *Diabetes* 1991; **40**: 211–16.
47 Hoskins PJ, Leslie RDG, Pyke DA. Height at diagnosis of diabetes in children: a study in identical twins. *Br Med J* 1985; **290**: 278–80.
48 Hussain MJ, Peakman M, Lo SSS, Leslie RDG, Vergani D. Elevated levels of tumour necrosis factor-alpha and interleukin-1alpha presage the onset of type 1 (insulin-dependent) diabetes. *Diabetologia* 1991; **34** (Suppl 2): A191 P760.
49 Kahn SE, McCulloch DK, Schwartz W, Palmer JP, Porte D Jr. Effect of insulin resistance and hyperglycaemia on proinsulin release in a primate model of diabetes mellitus. J Clin Endocrin Metab 1992; **74**: 192–7.
50 Bingley PJ, Matthews DR, Williams AJK, Bottazzo GF, Gale EAM. Loss of regular oscillatory insulin secretion in islet cell antibody positive non-diabetic subjects. *Diabetologia* 1992; **35**: 32–8.
51 Heaton DA, Lazarus NR, Pyke DA, Leslie RDG. B-cell responses to IV glucose and glucagon in non-diabetic twins of patients with type 1 (insulin-dependent) diabetes mellitus. *Diabetologia* 1989; **32**: 814–17.
52 Ganda OP, Srikanta S, Brink SJ, et al. Differential sensitivity to beta cell secretogogues in 'early' type 1 diabetes mellitus. *Diabetes* 1984; **33**: 516–21.
53 Leahy JL, Cooper HE, Deal DA, Weir GG. Chronic hyperglycaemia is associated with impaired glucose influence on insulin secretion. *J Clin Invest* 1986; **77**: 908–15.
54 Bjorkman PJ, Saper MA, Samraoui B, et al. Structure of the human class 1 histocompatibility antigen, HLA-A2. *Nature* 1987; **329**: 506–12.
55 Bonifacio E, Bingley P, Shattock M, et al. Quantification of islet-cell antibodies and prediction of insulin-dependent diabetes. *Lancet* 1990; **335**: 147–9.

Chapter Five

Viruses as Triggering Agents of Insulin-dependent Diabetes Mellitus

J. W. Yoon and Y. H. Park

Laboratory of Viral and Immunopathogenesis of Diabetes, Julia McFarlane Diabetes Research Centre, and Department of Microbiology and Infectious Diseases, Faculty of Medicine, University of Calgary, Calgary, Alberta, Canada

INTRODUCTION

Insulin-dependent diabetes mellitus (IDDM), also known as type 1 diabetes, is the consequence of progressive β cell destruction during an asymptomatic period often extending over many years[1-4]. It is believed that a variety of aetiological factors, genetic and environmental, lead to the destruction of β cells. The familial occurrence of diabetes, or at least the tendency to develop the disease, has been observed and described for so long that it is considered to be factual. However, the concordance for IDDM between identical twins approaches 50%, suggesting that non-genetic factors are also involved in the expression of the disease[1-5]. Studies on viruses as an environmental factor go back to the turn of the century, when Dr Harris observed that one of his

Causes of Diabetes. Edited by R. D. G. Leslie
© 1993 John Wiley & Sons Ltd.

patients developed diabetes after having had mumps[6]. Since that time, there have been continual reports documenting a temporal relationship between the onset of certain viral infections and the subsequent development of diabetes[7]. In contrast to the induction of diabetes by viruses, there is also evidence that viruses protect against the development of autoimmune IDDM in animals such as BB rats and non-obese diabetic (NOD) mice[8,9]. In this review I will discuss candidate viruses that might be involved in the initial stages of triggering β cell-specific autoimmunity, leading to the development of IDDM. In addition, I will briefly discuss cytolytic infection of β cells as well as the involvement of viruses in the prevention of IDDM.

VIRUSES AS TRIGGERING AGENTS FOR β CELL-SPECIFIC AUTOIMMUNITY

RETROVIRUS

The endogenous retroviruses exist as a provirus (viral DNA) integrated into the genome of every cell of the host's body and are transmitted vertically to the next generation of animal species or humans via germ-line DNA. Such endogenous retroviruses do not usually cause disease, indeed are rarely expressed, but may be activated under certain conditions, e.g. in some strains of inbred mice. The virion of retrovirus has a unique three-layered structure. The genome–nucleoprotein complex, incorporating the enzyme reverse transcriptase, is thought to have helical symmetry, and is enclosed within an icosahedral capsid, which in turn is surrounded by a host-derived envelope from which project typical virus-coded glycoprotein peplomers. The various morphological forms of the virion observed in sections of infected cells by electron microscopy in earlier days reflected differences in the morphogenesis of particular retroviruses. The genome is also unique among mammalian viruses in that it is diploid. Two identical molecules of single-stranded RNA of positive polarity are linked together by hydrogen bonds at their 5' termini. Another unusual feature is that of terminal redundancy—an identical sequence of about 20 nucleotides occurs at both the 3' and the 5' end of each haploid unit. Uniquely also, a molecule of cellular tRNA is hydrogen-bonded to a particular site near the 5' end of the genome; this tRNA serves as a primer for the initiation of DNA synthesis. The 5' terminus of each haploid unit is capped, and the 3' terminus is polyadenylated. The genome of the typical non-defective leukaemia virus contains two copies of each three genes, known as gag (encoding the core proteins), pol (encoding the unique viral polymerase, reverse transcriptase), and env (encoding the two envelope glycoproteins). A fourth gene, onc (the oncogene responsible for oncogenesis) occurs only in certain exogenous retroviruses, the acutely transforming retroviruses, which are capable of transforming cells *in vitro* and inducing cancer *in vivo* with high efficiency. Because the oncogene has usually been incorporated into the viral RNA in place of one or more normal viral genes, the genome of most of these highly oncogenic retroviruses is defective and, therefore, is dependent on a non-defective helper retrovirus for its replication.

NOD mice develop a diabetic syndrome which, in many respects, resembles human IDDM[10]. Diabetes in NOD mice is characterized first by insulitis; β cell destruction follows and culminates in hypoinsulinaemia and hyperglycaemia. The precise events which trigger the onset of the disease remain largely unknown. Various effector systems, including macrophages, T lymphocytes and/or humoral mediators, have been implicated as possible effectors of immune responses. Recent studies from our laboratory and others reveal that the administration of cyclophosphamide to NOD mice produces a rapid progression to overt diabetes with severe insulitis within 2–3 weeks[11–13]. Cyclophosphamide significantly increases the incidence of diabetes in NOD mice, either by inhibiting suppressor T cells or by activating cytotoxic T cells. The depletion of macrophages by silica treatment, however, results in the prevention of insulitis and diabetes in cyclophosphamide-treated NOD mice. These findings suggest that (a) macrophages play a major role in the initiation of organ-specific autoimmunities in NOD mice and (b) the presentation of autoantigen(s) on specific target cells, such as β cells, by the macrophages may result in initiation of the immune process[11].

A recent investigation in our laboratory was initiated to determine whether there are any specific changes on the β cells that may lead to the attraction of macrophages for the initiation of β cell-specific autoimmune disease in cyclophosphamide-treated NOD male mice. Administration of cyclophosphamide to NOD male mice produced a rapid progression to overt diabetes (over 70%) with severe insulitis in 2–3 weeks; none of the untreated, control NOD male mice became diabetic. When thin sections of islets from NOD male mice, which had first received silica for the inhibition of insulitis and subsequently received cyclophosphamide, were examined under the electron microscope, clusters of endogenous retrovirus particles were frequently found in the β cells[14]. In contrast, retrovirus particles were rarely found in the β cells from NOD male mice which had received silica only. Other endocrine cells, including α cells, δ cells, pancreatic polypeptide producing (pp) cells, and exocrine acinar cells, did not contain such virus particles. These virus particles were not found in spleen, liver or kidney in either cyclophosphamide-treated or untreated NOD male mice. Earlier studies revealed that C-type-like retrovirus particles were found in pancreatic β cells from both C3H-db/db[15] and NOD mice[16]. In addition, intracisternal A-type particles (IAP) were also found in β cells from genetically diabetic mice, including C57BL/KSJ (db/db), DBA/2J (db/db) and CHeB/FeJ (db/db) mice[17]. There was a clear correlation between the presence of retrovirus particles in the β cells and insulitis lesions[14].

The role of β cell-specific expressed retrovirus in the pathogenesis of autoimmune IDDM in NOD mice has not been defined. Work in several laboratories has indicated that retrovirus (e.g. MuLV) gp 70 may be present on the cell surface without the production of detectable infectious virus[18-20]. Using immunofluorescent techniques, Lerner and his coworkers found that a protein similar or identical to the retrovirus (MuLV) gp 70 major envelope glycoprotein is present on the surface of mouse (SJL/J) thymocytes, in lymphoid tissues and in murine epithelial lining cells[20]. Since retroviruses (xenotropic viruses) were regularly recovered from the mouse tissues, it was believed that these immunofluorescent tests could be detecting a viral antigen

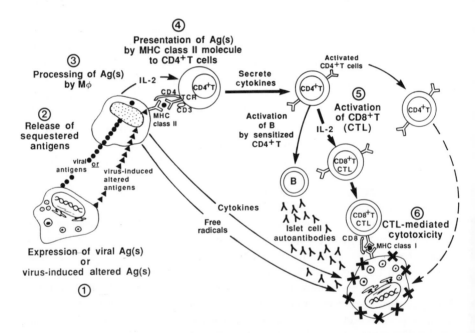

Figure 1 Certain viruses, e.g. retrovirus and rubella virus, may change a normally existing β cell antigen into an immunogenic form or induce new antigen or the expression of viral antigens. The viral antigens and/or virus-induced altered host antigens may be released from damaged β cells resulting from normal β cell turnover. The antigens are then processed by macrophages and presented to helper T cells in association with a class II MHC molecule. Helper T cells secrete interleukins that activate other helper T cells, B lymphocytes and cytotoxic T cells. The activated cytotoxic T cells recognize autoantigen on the β cells, where it is bound by class I MHC molecules. Macrophages, helper T cells and cytotoxic T cells act synergistically to destroy β cells, leading to the clinical onset of autoimmune IDDM

on the cell surface. Our recent studies revealed that the group-specific retroviral antigen translated from gag mRNA was found only in pancreatic β cells from diabetic NOD mice, but not from their parental strain, non-diabetic ICR mice. The precise role of retroviral gene expression and/or the gene product in β cells in the pathogenesis of autoimmune IDDM in NOD mice is not known. There is a possibility that the presentation of retrovirus antigen on the β cells by antigen-presenting cells may be the initial step in the autoimmune destruction of β cells. An immune response to the specific antigen on the target cell involves the activation of CD4$^+$ T cells, which are activated only when they interact with antigen presented on the surface of a macrophage or another antigen-presenting cell (Figure 1). Our previous experimental results support this possibility, since the elimination of antigen-presenting cells resulted in the prevention of a β cell-specific autoimmune process in NOD mice[11]. Another possible involvement of retrovirus in the initiation of autoimmune IDDM in NOD mice is that retroviral genomes (e.g. IAP) in the β cells can alter the expression of cellular genes, which may result in a β cell-specific altered antigen(s). This altered antigen(s) may act as foreign to immunocytes, leading to β cell-specific autoimmunity. Either β cell-specific expression of retrovirus group-specific antigen or retrovirus-induced β cell-specific altered antigens may eventually result in the generation of cytotoxic effector T lymphocytes that recognize specific determinants of 'self-proteins' on β cells, leading to β cell-specific autoimmune IDDM in NOD mice.

RUBELLA VIRUS

Congenital rubella syndrome (CRS) provides one of the best demonstrations in humans that a viral infection is associated with the subsequent development of autoimmune IDDM. We developed an animal model—neonatal golden Syrian hamsters, infected with rubella virus passaged in β cells—that closely parallels the diabetes observed with congenital rubella[21]. Seven- to ten-day-old Syrian hamsters developed hyperglycaemia, hypoinsulinaemia, a mononuclear cell infiltrate of the islets and positive immunofluorescence for rubella virus antigen in β cells following inoculation with β cell-passaged rubella virus. In addition, weak cytoplasmic islet cell antibodies were present in eight of the 20 infected animals. The mechanism of rubella virus-induced diabetes, however, is not known. Our preliminary data, showing insulitis in 34.5% of hamster islets and measurable circulating islet cell antibodies, is compatible with an autoimmune process. Rubella virus belongs to the togavirus family. This enveloped virus is surrounded by a lipoprotein coat derived from the host cell membrane when the virus buds through it. Thus rubella virus might insert, expose or alter antigens in the plasma membrane of the host cell during infection. Alternatively, the virus might induce an autoimmune syndrome by disturbing T cell subpopulations (helper or suppressor T cells) that regulate the host's immune response or the generation of viral antigen-specific cytotoxic (Tc) cells which recognize β cell-specific antigen(s) by molecular mimicry.

The CRS has emerged as an important human model for virus-induced IDDM. In CRS, diabetes takes 5–20 years to develop[22]. Although diabetes is the most common of the delayed manifestations of CRS, autoimmune thyroid disease[23], Addison's disease[23] and growth hormone deficiency[24] have also been reported. Patients with CRS and diabetes have a significantly increased frequency of human leucocyte antigen (HLA) DR3 and a significantly decreased frequency of HLA DR2[25]. There have been clues that endocrine abnormalities in CRS might have an autoimmune basis: an increased prevalence of islet cell surface antibody (21% of CRS patients, 50–80% of patients with abnormal carbohydrate metabolism)[26,27], an increased prevalence of antithyroid microsomal and/or antithyroglobulin antibody (26% of CRS patients) and an increased prevalence of anti-insulin autoantibody (13% of CRS patients compared with fewer than 1% of controls).

CYTOMEGALOVIRUS

Cytomegalovirus (CMV) infection is acquired subclinically during childhood, but in some of the more affluent communities it tends to be delayed until an age when it is capable of doing considerably more damage. Once infected with CMV, an individual carries the virus for life and sheds it intermittently in saliva, urine, semen, cervical discretions and/or breast milk. It is not known for certain which cells harbour the virus nor what form it is in. The B lymphocyte is the most likely candidate, but there is some evidence incriminating monocytes, polymorphs and epithelial cells. The genome of CMV has been recovered from oropharyngeal epithelium *in vivo*. Cell-mediated immunity (CMI) appears to be responsible for controlling CMV and for limiting exacerbations. Natural killer (NK) and cytotoxic T cells may both be involved. On the other hand, CMV itself is immunosuppressive, causing a general depression of CMI and an increase in suppressor T cells[28].

There was a case report that a child with congenital CMV infection developed diabetes mellitus at the age of 13 months[29]. At that time, he presented with a 2-week history of polydipsia, vomiting and weight loss, and was found to be severely dehydrated and ketoacidotic, with a blood glucose level of 50 mmol/l (900 mg/dl). In other reports, characteristic inclusion bodies have been found in the β cells of infants and children who died with disseminated CMV infections[30]. Insulitis and CMV-like particles have been observed in the pancreas of a particular rodent (*Octodon degu*) that manifests spontaneous diabetes[31].

Human CMV infection is ubiquitous and largely subclinical. In many persistent viral infections, the initial infection takes place before birth or very early in life, although the disease may not appear until later. The infection can be passed through the sperm or ovum if viruses integrate their genomes into the host DNA. Viral infections can also be transmitted transplacentally, perinatally or postnatally through close contact or breast milk. The immaturity of the immune systems of infants favours the establishment of persistent viral infections. Our finding, with both dot and *in situ* hybridization techniques, that about 15% of newly diagnosed IDDM patients had human CMV-specific viral genome in their lymphocytes and islet cell autoantibodies in their sera, suggests that autoimmune IDDM is sometimes associated with persistent CMV infections[32].

What might be the link between persistent CMV infection and autoimmune IDDM? Autoimmune disease could result from an immune response to viral antigens in the host cells, or to host cell-specific antigens that are exposed as a result of infection. If CMV infection persists in the β cells—in certain circumstances such as a particular genetic background and the presence of environmental factors (e.g. drugs, diet)—viral antigens may be expressed, or β cell-specific autoantigens may be induced, which may trigger β cell-specific autoimmunity. Alternatively, CMV may generate viral antigen-specific T cells which recognize β cell-specific autoantigen by molecular mimicry leading to β cell-specific autoimmune IDDM. Our recent study showed that human CMV can induce an islet cell antibody that a reacts with a 38 kDa autoantigen isolated from human pancreatic islets[33]. This is probably due to similar epitopes shared by islet cell-specific proteins and antigenic determinants of CMV.

PARVOVIRUS: KILHAM'S RAT VIRUS

Parvovirus consists of a simple icosahedral shell surrounding a single-stranded DNA molecule of very limited coding potential. The capsid is constructed from three species of polypeptide. The survival of parvovirus in nature is aided by persistent infections in which their genome becomes integrated with that of the cell. A striking feature of the parvoviruses is their selective replication in dividing cells. This requirement accounts for their evident predilection for bone marrow, gut and the developing embryo. Kilham's rat virus (KRV) is a member of the parvovirus family. KRV was originally isolated from a rat sarcoma[34] and has been found to cause a fatal neonatal disease, physical deformities and mental retardation in newborn rats. Recently, Guberski et al. found that KRV can cause autoimmune IDDM in diabetes-resistant (DR) BioBreeding (BB) rats[35].

BB rats spontaneously develop a diabetic syndrome that, in many respects, resembles human IDDM[36-38]. Diabetes-prone (DP) BB rats are lymphopenic and about 70–80% of the animals become diabetic at about 120 days of age. In contrast, DR BB rats, which were derived from DP progenitors, have normal lymphocyte numbers and phenotypes and do not develop diabetes. When these DR BB rats (21–25 days old) were infected with KRV, about 30% of the animals developed autoimmune diabetes within 2–4 weeks after KRV injection[35]. An additional 48% showed evidence of lymphocytic insulitis without diabetes. Guberski et al. analysed peripheral blood and lymph node cells from KRV-injected DR rats by flow cytometry[35]. When compared with vehicle controls, there were no significant changes in the percentages of peripheral blood CD4+ and CD8+T cells or NK cells 3, 6 and 10 days after infection, in diabetic rats. RT6.1+lymph node cells were also unchanged. The precise role of KRV in the induction of diabetes in DR BB rats is not known. It is speculated that KRV may generate viral antigen-specific effector T cells which can attack β cells. Whether KRV can generate viral antigen-specific T effector cells which recognize β cells remains to be determined.

MUMPS VIRUS

It has been hypothesized that a preceding infection with mumps virus may also trigger at least some cases of IDDM. Recent reports suggested that some children may develop islet cell antibody during parotitis[39]. Gamble[40] showed that mumps infection apparently precedes the development of diabetes in some newly diagnosed diabetic children. Other epidemiological studies do not support the hypothesis that mumps infection is associated with the onset of IDDM[41].

REOVIRUS

Since reoviruses produce a variety of lesions in newborn mice, we passaged reovirus type 3 in cultured pancreatic β cells to see whether the virus can be adapted to the β cells. When the β cell-passaged virus was infected into suckling SJL/J male mice, some of the infected animals showed an abnormal response in glucose tolerance tests 10 days after infection[42]. By immunofluorescence, specific viral antigens were found in some β cells as well as in acinar cells. By electron microscopy, viral particles were detected in the cytoplasm of some β cells. Surviving animals remained mildly hyperglycaemic for about 3 weeks, and then returned to normal.

In addition, mice infected with reovirus type 1, which was passaged in pancreatic β cell cultures, developed transient diabetes and a runting syndrome[43]. The runting syndrome consisted of retarded growth, oily hair, alopecia and steatorrhoea. Inflammatory cells and viral antigens, as well as virus particles, were found in the islets of Langerhans (α, β and δ cells) as well as in the anterior pituitary (growth hormone-producing cells). Examination of sera from infected mice revealed autoantibodies that reacted with cytoplasmic antigens in the islets of Langerhans, anterior pituitary and gastric mucosa of uninfected mice. To rule out a possible role for these autoantibodies in the pathogenesis of reovirus-induced diabetes, infected SJL and NFS mice were treated with different immunosuppressive drugs. The administration of antilymphocyte serum, antithymocyte serum or cyclophosphamide reduced or prevented the development of reovirus-induced diabetes[44]. In addition, virus-infected immunosuppressed mice gained weight at almost the same rate as uninfected controls, and mortality was greatly decreased. Thus Onodera et al. concluded that autoimmunity does play a role in the pathogenesis of reovirus-induced diabetes[43].

Precisely how reovirus infection triggers the development of autoantibodies is still unclear, but viruses have often been suspected as a cause of autoimmune disease. In contrast to reovirus type 1, reovirus type 3 does not induce autoantibodies in mice and does not infect the pituitary. The critical difference between reovirus type 1 and type 3 seems to reside at the level of the σ_1 polypeptide responsible for virus tropism. Therefore it is speculated that a single viral molecule appears to control pituitary infection and autoantibody production. In view of the histopathological changes seen in lymphoid organs of reovirus-infected mice, it may be that specific subsets of lymphocytes have receptors for the virus. Thus both infection of hormone-producing cells and infection of virus with cells of the immune system may be required to initiate the production of autoantibody[43]. The precise relationship between infection of reovirus type 1, the induction of autoantibodies and development of the diabetic syndrome remains to be determined.

CYTOLYTIC INFECTION OF PANCREATIC β CELLS AND DEVELOPMENT OF IDDM

PICORNAVIRUS

Encephalomyocarditis Virus

Picornavirus is the smallest RNA virus, which is a naked icosahedron. The capsid, appearing smooth and round in outline, is comprised of a single molecule of each of four polypeptides (VP1, 2, 3 and 4). The genome is a single linear molecule of single-stranded RNA of positive polarity. Encephalomyocarditis (EMC) virus belongs to the picornavirus family.

The best experimental evidence indicating that viruses have an aetiological role in the pathogenesis of IDDM comes from mice infected with EMC virus[45-47]. In genetically susceptible mice, the M variant of EMC (EMC-M) virus induces a diabetes-like syndrome, characterized by hypoinsulinaemia, hyperglycaemia, glycosuria, polydipsia and polyphagia. However, the development of diabetes after infection with EMC-M virus is not consistent. Statistically significant differences were consistently found upon repetition of the same experiment and between cages within experimental groups[48,49]. Plaque purification of EMC-M virus resulted in the isolation of two stable variants—one highly diabetogenic (EMC-D) and the other non-diabetogenic (EMC-B)[46]

The destruction of β cells in EMC virus-infected mice is dependent upon the genetic make-up of the virus and the genetic background of the host. With regard to the genetic make-up of the virus, two different variants (D and B) isolated from the M variant of EMC virus[46] showed biological and biochemical differences.[49,50,51]. The EMC-D virus produced diabetes in over 90% of infected animals, while none of the mice inoculated with the EMC-B virus developed diabetes. However, the D and B variants could not be distinguished antigenically by a sensitive plaque neutralization assay or a competitive radioimmunoassay. The complete nucleotide sequences of both diabetogenic EMC-D virus and non-diabetogenic EMC-B virus revealed 14 nucleotide differences between these two viral genomes[52]. Our most recent experimental results from the genomic sequence comparisons of several diabetogenic and non-diabetogenic variants isolated from EMC-D and EMC-B indicate that one amino acid, Ala776, on the capsid protein VP1, is responsible for the diabetogenicity of EMC virus[53].

With regard to the genetic background of the host, when mice were infected with diabetogenic EMC-D virus, only certain inbred strains (SJL/J, SWR/J, DBA/1J and DBA/2J) developed diabetes, while other strains (C57/BL/6J, CBA/J and AKR/J) did not[46]. The F1 hybrids resulting from the cross between susceptible SJL/J and resistant C57BL/6J mice were resistant to the development of EMC-D virus-induced diabetes. When the F1 hybrids were crossed with the resistant C57BL/6J parents, the backcross mice were found to be resistant to the development of EMC-D virus-induced diabetes. When the F1 hybrids were crossed with the susceptible SJL/J parents, about half (48%) of the backcross mice were found to be susceptible to the development of EMC-D virus-induced diabetes. When F1 hybrids were crossed with each other, 24% of the F2 mice (male) became diabetic. These experimental results show that susceptibility to EMC-D virus-induced diabetes is determined by an autosomal recessive gene and is inherited in a Mendelian mode[53]. The recent experiments, combined with earlier data, revealed that a single gene controlling susceptibility to EMC-D virus-induced diabetes in mice may operate by modulating the expression of viral receptors on the β cells[54–56].

Regarding the pathogenic mechanism for EMC-D virus-induced diabetes, earlier studies suggested that T lymphocytes may be involved in the destruction of β cells in EMC-M virus-induced diabetic mice[57]. However, later studies showed that depletion of lymphocytes failed to alter the incidence of diabetes[58]. Furthermore, athymic nude mice infected with EMC-D virus showed a response nearly identical to the diabetogenic response of hetero-zygous littermates. In addition, treatment of EMC virus-infected mice with cyclosporin A enhanced both the incidence and severity of diabetes rather than preventing the disease[59]. Our recent data showed that Mac-2 positive macrophages are predominant at an early stage of viral infection, whereas mixed immunocytes, including macrophages, helper/inducer T cells and cytotoxic/suppressor T cells, are present at the intermediate and late stages of viral infection[60]. Furthermore, the depletion of macrophages resulted in the prevention of diabetes when mice were inoculated with a low dose of EMC virus. In contrast, activation of macrophages in mice prior to viral infection clearly enhanced the incidence of diabetes. A low dose of virus infection is not enough to destroy a sufficient number of β cells for the development of clinical diabetes, and the involvement of activated macro-phages at the early stages of viral infection clearly contributes to the destruc-tion of the residual β cells[61].

Mengovirus

Antigenically, EMC-D virus and the 2T variant of mengovirus cannot be distinguished by hyperimmune sera; however, these two viruses are quite different in their tissue tropisms and mortality in mice[62]. The EMC-D virus induces diabetes mellitus in strains of susceptible mice, but does not produce neuropathology in or kill the mice[63]. In contrast, mengovirus 2T produces severe brain cell damage and high mortality[62,63]. By nucleic acid hybridiza-tion, these two viruses differ by about 20%; moreover, binding studies suggest that they recognize different viral receptors on the same cell[62].

The plaque-purified mengovirus 2T infects and destroys pancreatic β cells as demonstrated by immunofluorescence and histopathological examination. However, it has been difficult to study the tropism of the virus for β cells because of the rapid onset of paralysis and death after infection. Therefore, the capacity of this virus to infect the β cells and produce diabetes has to be studied early in the course of infection. It is interesting to note that the spectrum of host susceptibility to mengovirus-induced diabetes is strikingly different from that produced by the D variant of EMC virus. Both viruses produced diabetes in SJL/J mice, but only mengovirus produced abnormal glucose tolerance tests in the strains of mice which are resistant to EMC-induced diabetes, such as C57BL/6J, CBA/J, C3H/J, CE/J and AKR/J[63].

Immunofluorescent studies revealed that mengovirus infects pancreatic β cells from those mice, but EMC virus did not. Moreover, examination of islets of Langerhans from mengovirus-infected mice revealed marked necro-sis, severe inflammatory infiltration, and a decrease in the insulin content of the pancreas. To determine whether destruction of islet cells correlated with viral replication, islets from C3H/J mice infected with either mengovirus or EMC virus were assayed for infectious virus. At 1 and 2 days after infection, a significantly higher titre (10- to 100-fold) of the virus was observed in the mice infected with mengovirus. These studies showed that strain differences in the induction of diabetes by EMC virus and mengovirus could be due to the degree of virus replication in pancreatic β cells[63].

The precise mechanism by which mengovirus infects pancreatic β cells in the strains of mice resistant to EMC virus is not known. One of the many possibilities is that mengovirus and EMC virus are distinct viruses that bind to different receptors on the β cell surface. In different mouse strains, there may be quantitative differences in the expression of those receptors. Evidence in support of such a mechanism has been reported by Morishima et al., who found that the rate of binding of mengovirus to neuronal cell lines was 5–10 times greater than the rate of EMC virus binding[62]. Furthermore, receptor saturation experiments showed that unlabelled mengovirus and EMC virus effectively blocked the binding of labelled homologous but not heterologous virus, suggesting that these two viruses have different receptors on the cell surface. Thus receptors specific for mengovirus may be broadly expressed on the β cells of mice, while those for EMC virus may be restricted to a few strains.

In terms of a pathogenic mechanism, mengovirus can also infect, replicate and directly destroy pancreatic β cells independently of autoimmune responses. We have not found evidence of disturbances in T cell subpopulations nor have we seen the production of autoantibodies against pancreatic islet cells in mengovirus-induced diabetic animals. However, it is difficult to exclude the possibility that neurologically regulated hormones may contribute to some extent to the abnormalities in glucose homeostasis.

Coxsackie B Viruses

Earlier studies showed that Coxsackie B4 virus did not produce diabetes when inoculated into mice[64]. However, by repeatedly passaging Coxsackie B4 virus in murine-enriched pancreatic β cell cultures, it has been possible to enhance the diabetogenic capacity of this virus[65]. Nevertheless, it is very difficult to obtain a pure β cell tropic virus since the cells in primary cultures are a mixture of several different cell types[65,66]. Coxsackie B4 virus that had been passaged 14 times in cultures enriched for pancreatic β cells prepared from SJL/J mice can infect and destroy the pancreatic β cells in certain strains of mice. The destruction of β cells resulted in a decrease in the insulin content of the pancreas. This in turn led to hypoinsulinaemia and the subsequent development of hyperglycaemia. The reduction in immunoreactive insulin correlated inversely with the elevation in blood glucose. Thus the destruction of β cells by Coxsackie B4 virus appears to be responsible for the development of diabetes[65,66]. As in the case of the M variant of EMC virus, the degree of β cell damage is, in all probability, responsible for the observed difference in the metabolic response of individual animals. In the majority of animals, hyperglycaemia is transient. This may very well be due to the fact that a sufficient number of β cells are left intact after the infection so that proliferation and/or hypertrophy of these cells results in metabolic compensation. During the acute phase of the infection, viral antigens were found in the islets of Langerhans. The capacity of Coxsackie B4 virus to induce diabetes is influenced by the genetic background of the host. As in the case of EMC virus, only certain inbred strains of mice developed diabetes when exposed to Coxsackie B4 virus, and male mice developed more severe diabetes than female mice. Moreover, the strains of mice known to be susceptible to EMC-induced diabetes were also found to be susceptible to Coxsackie B4 virus-induced diabetes. Similarly, the strains of mice that were resistant to EMC-induced diabetes did not develop diabetes when exposed to Coxsackie B4 virus. The only exception thus far appears to be DBA/1J and DBA/2J mice, which developed diabetes when infected with EMC virus but were resistant to the disease when exposed to Coxsackie B4 virus.

In mice, EMC virus, mengovirus and Coxsackie B4 virus infect β cells and cause diabetes. In humans, there is evidence that Coxsackie B viruses may either cause or serve as the final insult in triggering some cases of IDDM[7,67]. The number of well-documented cases is small, however, and a non-human primate model would be of value. Several years ago, glucose and insulin levels were determined in several species of monkeys, including cynomolgus, rhesus, cebus and patas, after infection with EMC virus[68]. The glucose and insulin levels of the EMC-D virus-infected monkeys were within the normal range. Similarly, cynomoglus, rhesus and cebus monkeys had normal glucose tolerance and insulin secretion curves after infection with Coxsackie B4 virus. In the patas monkey, however, the glucose tolerance curves were clearly elevated, and the insulin secretion curves were markedly depressed[68]. These results clearly show that genetic factors are critical for the development of diabetes in monkeys infected with Coxsackie B4 virus.

The possibility that viruses might cause some cases of human IDDM by infecting and destroying pancreatic β cells has received considerable attention. However, it is difficult to demonstrate *in vivo* that viruses replicate in human β cells and produce diabetes. Therefore, an *in vitro* system has been developed to determine whether viruses are capable of infecting and destroying human β cells in culture. Several studies showed that some common human viruses, including mumps virus, Coxsackie B3 virus, Coxsackie B4 virus and reovirus type 3, could infect human β cells[67-71]. In addition, it was shown by radioimmunoassay that the infection markedly decreased the insulin content of β cells. Thus, at least under *in vitro* conditions, human β cells are not inherently resistant to viral infection. However, there is no way to prove that these viruses actually infect and destroy human pancreatic β cells and cause diabetes in man.

A more relevant approach is the isolation of viruses from the pancreata of children with acute-onset IDDM. A little over 10 years ago we obtained material from such a case[67]. A healthy 10-year-old boy was admitted to the hospital in diabetic ketoacidosis less than 3 days after the onset of a flu-like illness. Despite intensive therapy, the child's condition deteriorated and he died 7 days later. At autopsy, lymphocytic infiltration of the islets of Langerhans and necrosis of the β cells were observed. The picture was very similar to that seen in the islets of Langerhans of mice that developed diabetes after infection with EMC or Coxsackie B4 virus. When several inbred strains of mice were inoculated with the Coxsackie B4 variant isolated from the diabetic patient, SJL/J male mice developed diabetes, while CBA/J, C57BL/ 6J and BALB/c mice did not. Support for the idea that viruses can trigger some cases of diabetes in man has been strengthened by two additional case reports[72,73]. Recent careful epidemiological studies showed that some cases of IDDM are associated with Coxsackie B viral infection[74-76]. One recent interesting report showed that chronic Coxsackie B viral infection of the β cells could result in the synthesis and release of interferon-α, which in turn induces class I MHC hyperexpression on adjacent endocrine cells[77]. Recently, it was found that there was homology between the enzyme glutamic acid decarboxylase (GAD), formerly known as islet-specific 64 kDa protein[78], and Coxsackie B4 viral proteins[79]. It is speculated that Coxsackie B4 virus may generate viral antigen-specific cytotoxic T lymphocytes. The antigen-specific cytotoxic T cells may recognize GAD on the pancreatic β cells. This may be the initial step for T cell-mediated destruction of β cells under certain circumstances.

Whatever the mechanism, evidence from studies in mice, humans and non-human primates indicates that Coxsackie viruses can affect glucose homeostasis. Recent studies on Coxsackie B4 virus[80,81] have demonstrated that antigenic changes at the epitope level occur at a frequency greater than 10^{-2}. This suggests that even within the same virus pool there may be many antigenic variants, and that these variants may have different tissue tropism and different physiological properties. This could account for the wide spectrum of clinical disease produced by the Coxsackie viruses. A rare variant may be diabetogenic, which might explain why IDDM appears to be associated with a Coxsackie B virus infection under certain circumstances[82,83].

PROTECTIVE EFFECT OF VIRUSES AGAINST THE DEVELOPMENT OF DIABETES

EMC or Coxsackie B4 virus-induced diabetes can be prevented by vaccination using a live attenuated, killed or subunit vaccine. Our earlier studies have shown that EMC-D virus-induced diabetes can be prevented by a live attenuated vaccine[84]. SJL/J mice were immunized with the non-diabetogenic EMC-B virus and challenged 30, 43 or 90 days later with the diabetogenic EMC-D virus. Diabetes did not develop in any of the immunized mice, but it did develop in approximately 80% of the unimmunized control mice. The prevention of EMC-D virus-induced diabetes could be due to the neutralizing antibody, induced by a non-diabetogenic EMC-B virus.

Our recent experimental data revealed that retroviral proteins, such as the major envelope glycoprotein of C-type retrovirus (gp 70) and group-specific antigen of A-type retrovirus (p73), can prevent the development of diabetes in NOD mice when they have been immunized weekly with these viral proteins from the age of 2 days to 42 days[85]. We have screened the mice up to the age of 6 months. In the control group, the incidence of diabetes is 50%. In contrast, none of the NOD mice treated with p73 or gp 70 have developed diabetes. It is too early to draw a definite conclusion about the prevention of diabetes in NOD mice by immunization with retroviral proteins since the number of tested animals is small and the duration of the experiment is not sufficient.

In addition, inoculation of NOD mice (newborn or 6-week-old) with lymphocytic choriomeningitis virus (LCMV) also prevented or decreased the incidence of diabetes (0–6%)[8,86]. LCMV may infect and deplete the subpopulation of $CD4^+T$ cells. Selective suppression of $CD4^+T$ cell subsets was observed during virus infection[86]. Similarly, the inoculation of BB rats, another animal model of autoimmune diabetes, with LCMV (Armstrong strain, clone) reduced the incidence of diabetes and prevented mononuclear cell infiltration in the islets of Langerhans by somehow disordering particular lymphocyte subsets[9]. Oldstone suggested that LCMV, by directly aborting autoimmune-producing T lymphocytes, may prevent insulitis and diabetes. Furthermore, viral antibody-free BB rats show an increased frequency and accelerated onset of diabetes, suggesting that infection may be protective against the development of diabetes[87]. Thus, we speculate that infection or immune stimulation in humans may also reduce the penetrance of susceptibility genes. This could account for the low concordance rate for the development of diabetes between identical twins.

CONCLUSIONS

IDDM is known to run in families, but the hereditary factor(s) is not a sufficient explanation, since concordance in monozygous twins is 50% or less. Therefore, non-genetic factors must be involved in triggering IDDM. Viruses, as one of the non-genetic factors, may act as triggering agents for autoimmunity or as primary injurious agents to β cells. Certain viruses, such as retrovirus and rubella virus, may alter a normally existing β cell antigen into an immunogenic form or might induce a new antigen leading to β cell-specific autoimmune IDDM (Figure 1). For example, viral antigens or virus-induced autoantigens may be released from the β cells when β cells are destroyed due to the normal course of cell turnover; macrophages ingest this antigen (antigen processing) and present it, in asociation with a class II MHC molecule, to $CD4^+$ T cells (T_H cells) (antigen presentation). $CD4^+$ T cells secrete cytokines that activate other helper T cells, B lymphocytes and cytotoxic T cells. The activated cytotoxic T cells recognize autoantigen on the β cells where it is bound by class I MHC molecules, leading to the autoimmune destruction of β cells.

In addition, other viruses such as KRV may generate viral antigen-specific T effector cells. The viral antigen, which generates antigen-specific T effector cells, may have homology in the proteins of β cell-specific autoantigen. In this way, antigen-specific T cells can recognize β cell-specific autoantigen by mistake; this leads to the autoimmune destruction of β cells.

Some other viruses such as EMC-D virus, Mengo-2T virus, and Coxsackie B4 virus can induce IDDM by infecting and destroying β cells in genetically susceptible hosts. Certain species of monkey, such as patas, show elevated blood glucose levels and depressed insulin secretion after infection with Coxsackie B4 virus. Furthermore, an occasional case of IDDM in humans appears to be associated with infection of the β cells by Coxsackie B viruses. Viruses cannot only cause diabetes but they can prevent the development of IDDM. For example, inoculation of DP BB rats or NOD mice with lympho-cytic choriomeningitis virus can reduce the incidence of diabetes or prevent the disease by disordering particular subsets of lymphocytes.

In conclusion, viruses can induce diabetes by the induction of β cell-specific autoimmunity or the cytolytic infection of β cells. In addition, viruses can prevent the development of the disease by disordering particular lympho-cyte subsets. These factors may account for the low concordance rate for IDDM between identical twins.

ACKNOWLEDGEMENTS

This work was supported by the Medical Research Council of Canada and the Canadian Diabetes Association. The author is a Heritage Medical Scientist Awardee of the Alberta Heritage Foundation for Medical Research. We gratefully acknowledge the secretarial assistance of Ms Lorraine Pearson and editorial help of Dr Naomi Anderson.

REFERENCES

1 Gorusch AN, Spencer KN, Lister J, et al. Evidence for a long prediabetic period in type 1 (insulin-dependent) diabetes. *Lancet* 1981; **ii**: 1363–5.

2 Yoon JW. Viral pathogenesis of insulin-dependent diabetes mellitus. In: *Autoimmunity and the Pathogenesis of Diabetes* (eds F Ginsberg-Fellner, RC McEvoy) Springer-Verlag, Berlin 1990, 206–55.

3 Rossini AA, Mordes JP, Like AA. Immunology of insulin-dependent diabetes mellitus. *Ann Rev Immunol* 1985; **3** 289–320.

4 Drell, DW, Notkins AL. Multiple immunological abnormalities in patients with type 1 (insulin-dependent) diabetes mellitus. *Diabetologia* 1987; **30**: 132–43.

5 Pyke DA. The genetic perspective: putting research into practice. In: *Diabetes 1988* (eds RG Larkins, PZ Zimmet, DJ Chisolm) Excerpta Medical, Amsterdam, 1989, pp 1227–30.

6 Harris HF. A case of diabetes mellitus quickly following mumps on the pathological alterations of salivary glands, closely resembling those found in pancreas, in a case of diabetes mellitus. *Boston Med Surg J* 1989; **CXL**: 465.

7 Yoon JW. Role of viruses and environmental factors in induction of diabetes. *Curr Top Microbiol Immunol* 1990; **164**: 95–123.

8 Oldstone MBA. Prevention of type 1 diabetes in nonobese diabetic mice by virus infection. *Science* 1988; **239**: 500–2.

9 Dryberg T, Schwimmbeck PL, Oldstone MBA. Inhibition of diabetes in BB rats by virus infection. *J Clin Invest* 1988; **81**: 928–31.

10 Katoka S, Satoh J, Fujiya H, et al. Immunologic aspects of the nonobese diabetic (NOD) mouse: abnormalities of cellular immunity. *Diabetes* 1983; **32**: 247–53.

11 Lee KU, Amano K, Yoon JW. Evidence for initial involvement of macrophages in development of insulitis in NOD mice. *Diabetes* 1988; **37**: 1989–91.

12 Harada M, Makino S. Promotion of spontaneous diabetes in nonobese diabetes-prone mice by cyclophosphamide. *Diabetologia* 1982; **27**: 604–6.

13 Yasunami R, Bach JF. Anti-suppressor effect of cyclophosphamide on the development of spontaneous diabetes in NOD mice. *Eur J Immunol* 1988; **18**: 481–4.

14 Suenaga K, Yoon JW. Association of beta cell-specific expression of endogeneous retrovirus with the development of insulitis and diabetes in NOD mice. *Diabetes* 1988; **37**: 1722–6.

15 Leiter EH. Type C retrovirus production by pancreatic beta cells: association with accelerated pathogenesis in C3H-db/db ('diabetes') mice. *Am J Pathol* 1985; **119**: 22–32.

16 Fukino-Kurihara H, Fujita H, Hakura A, Nonaka K, Tarui S. Morphological aspects on pancreatic islets of non-obese diabetic (NOD) mice. *Virchows Arch* 1985; **49**: 107–20.

17 Leiter EH, Kuff EL. Intracisternal type A particles in murine pancreatic β cells: immunocytochemical demonstration of increased antigen (p73) in genetically diabetic mice. *Am J Pathol* 1984; **114**: 46–55.

18 Ikeda H, Pincus T, Yoshiki T, et al. Biological expression of antigenic determinants of murine leukemia virus proteins gp69/71 and p30. *J Virol* 1974; **14**: 1274–80.

19 Kennel SJ, Feldman JD. Distribution of viral glycoprotein gp 69/71 on cell surfaces of producer and nonproducer cells. *Cancer Res* 1976; **36**: 200–8.

20 Lerner RA, Wilson CB, Del Villano BC, McCohahey PJ, Dixon FJ. Endogenous oncornaviral gene expression in adult and fetal mice: quantitative, histologic, and physiologic studies of the major viral glycoprotein, gp 70. *J Exp Med* 1976; **143**: 151–66.

21 Rayfield EJ, Kelly KJ, Yoon JW. Rubella virus-induced diabetes in hamsters. *Diabetes* 1986; **35**: 1278–81.

22 Menser MA, Forrest JM, Bransby RD. Rubella infection and diabetes mellitus. *Lancet* 1978; **i**: 57–60.

23 Schopfer K, Matter L, Flueler U, Werder E. Diabetes mellitus, endocrine auto-antibodies and prenatal rubella infection. *Lancet* 1982; **ii**: 159.
24 Preece MA, Kearney PJ Marshall WC. Growth-hormone deficiency in congenital rubella. *Lancet* 1977; **ii**: 842–4.
25 Ginsberg-Fellner F, Fedun B, Cooper Z, et al. Interrelationships of congenital rubella and type 1 insulin-dependent diabetes mellitus. In: *The Immunology of Diabetes Mellitus* (eds MA Jaworski, GD Molnar, RV Rajotte, B Singh) *Elsevier*, Amsterdam, 1986, pp 279–86.
26 Ginsberg-Fellner F, Witt ME, Yagihaski S. Congenital rubella-syndrome as a model for type 1 (insulin-dependent) diabetes mellitus: increased prevalence of islet cell surface antibodies. *Diabetologia* 1984; **27**: 87–9.
27 Ginsberg-Fellner F, Witt ME, Fedun B. Diabetes mellitus and autoimmunity in patients with congenital rubella syndrome. *Rev Infect Dis* 1985; **7** (Suppl 1); S170–5.
28 White DO, Fenner F. *Medical Virology*, 3rd edn. Academic Press, New York, 1986, pp 419–26.
29 Ward KP, Galloway WH, Auchterlonie IA. Congenital cytomegalovirus infection and diabetes. *Lancet* 1979; **i**: 497.
30 Jenson AB, Rosenberg HS, Notkins AL. Pancreatic islet cell damage in children with fatal viral infections. *Lancet* 1980; **ii**: 354–8.
31 Fox GJ, Murphy JC. Cytomegalic virus-associated insulitis in diabetic *Octodon degus*. *Vet Pathol* 1979; **16**: 625–8.
32 Pak CY, Eun HM, McArthur RG, Yoon JW. Association of cytomegalovirus infection with autoimmune type 1 diabetes. *Lancet* 1988; **ii**: 1–4.
33 Pak CY, Cha CY, Rajotte RV, McArthur RG, Yoon JW. Human pancreatic islet cell-specific 38kD autoantigen identified by cytomegalovirus-induced mono-clonal islet cell autoantibody. *Diabetologia* 1990; **33**: 569–72.
34 Kilham L, Oliver, A. A latent virus of rats isolated in tissue culture. *Virology* 1959; **7**: 428–37.
35 Guberski DL, Thomas VA, Shek WR, et al. Induction of type 1 diabetes by Kilham's rat virus in diabetes-resistant BB/Wor rats. *Science* 1991; **254**: 1010–13.
36 Marliss EB (ed). The Juvenile Diabetes Foundation workshop on the sponta-neously diabetic BB rat: its potential for insight into human juvenile diabetes. *Metab Clin Exp* 1983; **32** (Suppl 1): 1–166.
37 Rossini AA, Mordes JP, Like AA. Immunology of insulin-dependent diabetes mellitus. *Annu Rev Immunol* 1985; **3**: 289–320.
38 Nakhooda AF, Like AA, Chappel CI, Wei CN, Marliss EB. The spontaneously diabetic Wistar rat (The 'BB' rat): studies prior to and during the development of the overt syndrome. *Diabetologia* 1978; **14**: 199–207.
39 Helmke K, Otten A, Willems W. Islet cell antibodies in children with mumps infection. *Lancet* 1980; **iii**: 211–12.
40 Gamble DR. Relation of antecedent illness to development of diabetes in children. *Br Med J* 1980; **2**: 99–101.
41 Ratzman KP, Strese J, Witt S, et al. Mumps infection and insulin-dependent diabetes mellitus (IDDM). *Diabetes Care* 1984; **7**: 170–3.
42 Onodera T, Jenson AB, Yoon JW, Notkins AL. Virus-induced diabetes mellitus: reovirus infection of pancreatic beta cells in mice. *Science* 1978; **301**: 529–31.
43 Onodera T, Toniolo A, Ray UR, et al. Virus-induced diabetes mellitus. *J Exp Med* 1981; **153**: 1457–65.
44 Onodera T, Toniolo A, Ray UR, et al. Virus-induced diabetes mellitus: autoim-

munity and polyendocrine disease prevented by immunosuppression. *Nature* 1982; **297**: 66–9.

45 Craighead JE, McLane MF. Diabetes mellitus: induction in mice by encephalomyocarditis virus. *Science* 1968; **162**: 913–15.

46 Yoon JW, McClintock PR, Onodera T, Notkins AL. Virus-induced diabetes mellitus: inhibition by a non-diabetogenic variant of encephalomyocarditis virus. *J Exp Med* 1980; **152**: 878–92.

47 Notkins AL, Yoon JW. Virus-induced diabetes. In: *Concepts in Viral Pathogenesis* (eds AL Notkins, MBA Oldstone) Springer-Verlag, New York, 1984, pp 241–7.

48 Ross ME, Onodera T, Brown KS, Notkins AL. Virus-induced diabetes mellitus. IV. Genetic and environmental factors influencing the development of diabetes after infection with the M variant of encephalomyocarditis virus. *Diabetes* 1976; **25**: 190–7.

49 Yoon JW, Onodera T, Notkins AL. Virus-induced diabetes mellitus. IX. Studies on virus passage and dose in susceptible and resistant strains of mice. *J Gen Virol* 1977; **37**: 225–32.

50 Bae YS, Eun HM, Yoon JW. Molecular identification of viral gene. *Diabetes* 1989; **38**: 316–20.

51 Bae YS, Eun HM, Pon RT, Yoon JW. Two amino acids, Phe-16 and Ala 776, on the polyprotein are most likely responsible for diabetogenicity of EMC virus. *J Gen Virol* 1990; **71**: 639–45.

52 Bae YS, Eun HM, Yoon JW. Genomic differences between the diabetogenic and nondiabetogenic variants of encephalomyocarditis virus. *Virology* 1989; **170**: 282–7.

53 Bae YS, Yoon JW. A single gene of the host and a single amino acid of a virus control the development of type 1 diabetes in mice. *Diabetes* 1991; **40** (Suppl 1): 296A.

54 Chariez R, Yoon JW, Notkins AL. Virus-induced diabetes mellitus. X. Attachment of encephalomyocarditis virus and permissiveness of cultured pancreatic beta cells to infection. *Virology* 1978; **85**: 606–11.

55 Onodera T, Yoon JW, Brown K, Notkins AL. Virus-induced diabetes mellitus: evidence for control by a single locus. *Nature* 1978; **274**: 693–6.

56 Yoon JW, Lesniak MA, Fussganger R, Notkins AL. Genetic differences in susceptibility of pancreatic β cells to virus-induced diabetes mellitus. *Nature* 1976; **264**: 178–80.

57 Buschard K, Hastrup N, Rygaard J. Virus-induced diabetes mellitus in mice and the thymus-dependent immune system. *Diabetologia* 1983; **24**: 42–6.

58 Yoon JW, McClintock PR, Bachurski CJ, Longstreth JD, Notkins AL. Virus-induced diabetes mellitus: no evidence for immune mechanisms in the destruction of beta cells by encephalomyocarditis virus. *Diabetes* 1985; **34**: 922–5.

59 Vialettes B, Baume D, Charpin C, DeMaeyer-Guignard J, Vague P. Assessment of viral and immune factors in EMC virus-induced diabetes: effects of cyclosporin A and interferon. *J Clin Lab Immunol* 1983; **10**: 35–40.

60 Baek HS, Yoon JW. Role of macrophages in the pathogenesis of encephalomyocarditis virus-induced diabetes in mice. *J Virol* 1990; **64**: 5708–715.

61 Baek HS, Yoon JW. Direct involvement of macrophages in destruction of β cells leading to the development of diabetes in virus-infected mice. *Diabetes* 1991; **40**: 269–74.

62 Morishima T, McClintock PR, Aulakh GS, Billups LC, Notkins AL. Genomic and receptor attachment differences between mengovirus and encephalomyocarditis virus. *Virology* 1982; **122**: 461–5.

63 Yoon JW, Morishima T, McClintock PR, Austin M, Notkins AL. Virus-induced

diabetes mellitus: mengovirus infects pancreatic beta cells in strains of mice resistant to the diabetogenic effect of encephalomyocarditis mice. *J Virol* 1984; **50**: 684–90.

64 Ross ME, Hayashi K, Notkins AL. Virus-induced pancreatic disease: alterations in concentration of glucose and amylase in blood. *J Infect Dis* 1974; **129**: 669–76.

65 Yoon JW, Onodera T, Notkins AL. Virus-induced diabetes mellitus: beta cell damage and insulin-dependent hyperglycemia in mice infected with Coxsackie virus B4. *J Exp Med* 1978; **148**: 1068–80.

66 Toniolo A, Onodera T, Jordan G, Yoon JW, Notkins AL. Virus-induced diabetes mellitus: glucose abnormalities produced in mice by the six members of the Coxsackie B virus group. *Diabetes* 1982; **32**: 496–9.

67 Yoon JW, Austin M, Onodera T, Notkins AL. Virus-induced diabetes mellitus: isolation of a virus from the pancreas of a child with diabetic ketoacidosis. *N Engl J Med* 1979; **300**: 1173–9.

68 Yoon JW, London WT, Curfman BL, Brown RL, Notkins AL. Coxsackie virus B₄ produces transient diabetes in nonhuman primates. *Diabetes* 1986; **35**: 712–16.

69 Yoon JW, Onodera T, Notkins AL. Virus-induced diabetes mellitus. IX. Replication of Coxsackie virus B3 in human pancreatic beta cell cultures. *Diabetes* 1978; **27**: 778–81.

70 Prince G, Jenson AB, Billups L, Notkins AL. Infection of human pancreatic beta cell cultures with mumps virus. *Nature* 1978; **27**: 158–61.

71 Yoon JW, Selvaggio S, Onodera T, Wheeler J, Jenson AB. Infection of cultured human pancreatic β cell with reovirus type 3. *Diabetologia* 1981; **20**: 462–7.

72 Champsaur H, Bottazzo G, Bertrams J, Assan R, Bach C. Virologic, immunologic and genetic factors in insulin-dependent diabetes mellitus. *J Pediatr* 1982; **100**: 15–20.

73 Gladisch R, Hoffmann W, Waldherr R. Myocarditis and insulitis in Coxsackie virus infection. *Z Kardiol* 1976; **65**: 873–81.

74 King ML, Shaikh A, Bidwell D, Voller A, Banatvala JE. Coxsackie B-virus specific IgM responses in children with insulin-dependent diabetes mellitus. *Lancet* 1983; **i**: 1397–9.

75 Banatvala JE, Schernthaner G, Schober E, et al. Coxsackie B, mumps, rubella and cytomegalovirus specific IgM responses in patients with juvenile-onset insulin-dependent diabetes mellitus in Britain, Austria and Australia. *Lancet* 1985; **i**: 1409–12.

76 Friman G, Fohlman J, Frisk G, et al. An incidence peak of juvenile diabetes: relation to Coxsackie B virus immune response. *Acta Paediatr Scand* 1985; **320** (Suppl): 14–19.

77 Foulis AK, Farquharsaon MA, Meager A. Immunoreactive α-interferon in insulin-secreting β cells in type 1 diabetes mellitus. *Lancet* 1987; **ii**: 1423–7.

78 Baekkeskov S, Aanstoot H-J, Christgau S, et al. Identification of the 64K autoantigen in insulin-dependent diabetes as the GABA-synthesizing enzyme glutamic acid decarboxylas. *Nature (Lond)* 1990; **347**: 151–6.

79 Roberts SS. New clues to IDDM origins: IDDM may arise from a case of mistaken identity in which the immune system mistakes a normal beta cell antigen for a virus. *Diabetes Care* 1992; **15**: 137–9.

80 Prabhakar BS, Haspel MV, McClintock PR, Notkins AL. High frequency of antigenic variants among naturally occurring human Coxsackie B4 virus isolates identified by monoclonal antibodies. *Nature* 1982; **300**: 374–6.

81 Prabhakar BS, Menegus MA, Notkins AL. Detection of conserved and nonconserved epitopes on Coxsackie virus B4: frequency of antigenic change. *Virology* 1985; **146**: 302–6.

82 Yoon JW. Role of viruses in the pathogenesis of IDDM. *Ann Med* 1991; **23**: 437–45.

83 Yoon JW, Bachurski CJ, McArthur RG. Concept of virus as an etiological agent in the development of IDDM. *Diabetes Res Clin Pract* 1986; **2**: 365–6.

84 Notkins AL, Yoon JW. Virus-induced diabetes in mice prevented by a live attenuated vaccine. *N Engl J Med* 1983; **306**: 486.

85 Pak CY, Yoon JW. Possible prevention of IDDM by vaccination with viral specific proteins. In: *Pediatric and Adolescent Endocrinology: Prediabetes* (ed Z. Laron) In press, 1993.

86 Oldstone MBA. Viruses as therapeutic agents. I. Treatment of nonobese insulin-dependent diabetes mice with vims prevents insulin-dependent diabetes mellitus while maintaining general immune competence. *J Exp Med* 1990; **101**: 2077–89.

87 Guberski DL, Butler L, Like AA. Environmental viral agents influence spontaneous and RT6 depletion induced diabetes (DB) in the BB/Wor rat. *Diabetes* 1990; **39**: 97A.

Chapter Six

The Role of Toxins

Roger Assan and Etienne Larger

Diabetes Department, Bichat Hospital, Paris, France

INTRODUCTION

Compelling epidemiological and experimental evidence indicates that environmental factors, such as chemical toxins, play an important role in the aetiology of at least some forms of insulin-dependent diabetes mellitus (IDDM). Concordance rates in monozygotic twins may be as low as 25–35%[1]. A significant minority of Caucasoid IDDM patients do not possess the human leucocyte antigen (HLA) DR or DQ risk alleles[2], particularly those patients with adult onset of the disease[3], and the presence of islet cell antibodies is less frequent in this subgroup of patients than in typical childhood diabetes and IDDM. Massive synchronous β cell necrosis can be, although rarely, the abrupt hallmark of recent IDDM in the absence of typical insulitis. Whether IDDM in such cases is synonymous of type 1 (autoimmune) diabetes is not merely a semantic debate. The low-dose streptozotocin model of diabetes in mice[4] demonstrates that toxin-induced islet damage can indeed trigger an autoimmune, T cell-mediated, genetically restricted IDDM.

Chemical toxins can precipitate IDDM through a variety of mechanisms. They can either poison β cells directly or trigger autoimmune mechanisms

Causes of Diabetes. Edited by R. D. G. Leslie
© 1993 John Wiley & Sons Ltd.

directed to the islets, or augment the diabetogenic properties of another agent such as a virus to hasten islet damage. Eventually a variety of chemical and pharmaceutical drugs can induce transient glucose intolerance through functional impairment of insulin secretion[5-8].

In this chapter, data from the well-established animal experimental models will be briefly discussed, in view of their contribution to the understanding of disease induction. IDDM following intoxication by pesticides and industrial toxins causing IDDM-like syndromes as well as drug-induced glucose intolerance in humans will then be considered.

EXPERIMENTAL MODELS OF TOXIN-INDUCED IDDM

STREPTOZOTOCIN

Steptozotocin (STZ) is a wide-spectrum antibiotic derived from *Streptomyces achromogenes*. It consists of a methylnitrosourea linked to D-glucose (2-deoxy-2-[methylnitrosoureido]-D-pyranose). Like its analogue chlorozotocin, STZ destroys selectively the β cells in rats, mice, dogs, monkeys and a variety of mammalian species[9]. Several models of STZ-induced diabetic syndromes exist, all informative in many ways for the understanding of human diabetic syndromes.

High-dose STZ Diabetes

A single dose of 50–200 mg STZ by intravenous (i.v.) or intramuscular (i.m.) injection in adult rats destroys the β cells. The cells are degranulated after a few hours, and then become necrotic, while non-β cells persist unchanged; insulitis does not appear. The blood glucose course is triphasic, with early transient hyperglycaemia (a few minutes) followed by hypoglycaemia (after 30 minutes) and eventually hyperglycaemia, insulinopenia and ketosis. The metabolic changes are typical of insulin lack (decreased glucose uptake and increased glucose production, excessive proteolysis and lipolysis, and the corresponding changes in enzyme activities, glucose transporter gene expression, etc.). These metabolic changes and the long-term alterations in collagen and micro-vessels have been intensively studied[9].

More informative for the present purpose are the studies concerning mechanisms of STZ toxicity, protective agents and islet regenerative ability[10,11].

Islets incubated *in vitro* and exposed to STZ show β cell necrosis preceded by degranulation and an acute drop in insulin content to less than 10% of normal. STZ exerts a direct effect on glucose-induced insulin secretion, a defect in oxygen consumption by the islets and depletion in nicotinamide adenine dinucleotide (NAD) and adenosine triphosphate (ATP) content, suggestive of an early mitochondrial dysfunction. Depletion of NAD appears central to the understanding of β cell destruction by STZ. Nicotinamide administration before and for 2 hours *after* STZ administration prevents the appearance of diabetes. Streptozotocin causes DNA strand breaks. This is followed by overstimulation of nuclear poly-(ADP-ribose)-synthetase and depletion of intracellular NAD. In addition, the levels of both reduced glutathione and superoxide dismutase in erythrocytes are decreased after STZ injection. Exogenous superoxide dismutase, administered before STZ, prevents the development of diabetes in this high-dose STZ model. The β cells have a low capacity for free radical scavenging, and the fragmentation of β cell DNA may result both from DNA alkylation and the accumulation of superoxide and OH· radicals.

Another phenomenon associated with STZ diabetes is the high tumour frequency in pancreatic islets, when STZ acute toxicity is prevented by concomitant administration of nicotinamide or poly-(ADP-ribose)-synthetase inhibitors. This treatment may cause abnormal DNA recombination resulting in the formation of a tumour-inducing gene. Such an oncogene was indeed discovered in β cell tumours, coding for a 145-amino acid protein and named *rig* (rat insulinoma gene). The same gene was found in DNA from a virus-induced hamster insulinoma and from spontaneous human insulinoma. Another gene coding for a 165-amino acid protein (*reg*—'regenerating gene') is expressed in islets of pancreatectomized, nicotinamide-treated rats, and appears specifically to regulate β cell proliferation[11].

Multiple Low-dose STZ Diabetes and Insulitis

Multiple injections of STZ (35–40 mg/kg per day for 5 days) produce, in appropriate strains of mice and rats, pancreatic insulitis progressing to nearly complete β cell destruction and gradual diabetes mellitus[4]. Insulitis is recognized 4–5 days after the last injection along with hyperglycaemia. A large reduction in both islet volume and number, as well as a decrease in insulin secretory responses to glucose, precede the peak of lymphocytic infiltration and are detected 24 hours after the first STZ injection. Destruction of β cells and hyperglycaemia become pronounced 10–25 days after the last injection, long after STZ is cleared from the bloodstream. Islets are infiltrated by T lymphocytes and macrophages. The A and D endocrine cells are normal. Type C viral particles are present within β cells, but not in either A or D cells, nor in inflammatory cells. Cellular autoimmunity is the pivotal cause of diabetes in this diabetic model. Alteration of macrophages and T cells (by irradiation, steroids, silica, and a variety of antibodies directed to crucial T cell surface molecules) prevents the development of insulitis and hyperglycaemia.

Anti-mouse lymphocyte serum and thymectomy prevent susceptibility to multiple low-dose (MLD) STZ and this is restored by syngeneic T cell replacement. Transfer of activated lymphocytes from MLD STZ animals produces diabetes in the recipients and this transfer is strain-restricted. Splenocytes from MLD STZ mice are toxic *in vitro* against a rat β cell line.

Islet transplantation experiments in syngeneic mice, where the islets and recipients were exposed to STZ in various combinations, show that both the transplants and recipients must be exposed to STZ to obtain insulitis in recipients, suggesting that STZ produces an islet neoantigen and that repeated stimulation by this neoantigen is needed to trigger the autoimmune process.

Perinatal STZ Diabetic Models

Both Portha and Weir and their collaborators have shown that STZ, when injected very early in life, produces acute transient diabetes, followed by incomplete remission, with the persistence of glucose intolerance and a selective loss of β cell secretory response to glucose[12–14].

STZ (35 mg/kg intraperitoneally (i.p.)) administered to female pregnant rats at the end of gestation induces in the male progeny a pronounced and persistent loss in pancreatic insulin, moderate fasting hyperglycaemia and a loss in β cell secretory response to glucose. Neonatal rats, injected with STZ 100 mg/kg i.v., exhibit an acute diabetes for the first 3 days of life, followed by incomplete remission, β cell regeneration and reaccumulation of pancreatic insulin stores. The β cell response to glucose is completely obtunded on day 1 after STZ, then reappears and increases as a function of age. This remission is incomplete and leads to glucose intolerance. Early insulin treatment during the early acute diabetic phase improves spontaneous remission by augmenting the recovery of pancreatic insulin stores and the β cell secretory response to glucose. STZ (90 mg/kg i.p.) administered to 2-day-old rats similarly induces acute transient hyperglycaemia followed by remission and then by non-ketotic diabetes. The β cell secretory responses to glucose are meagre, but enhanced by the concomitant administration of theophylline. The β cell responses to arginine and isoproterenol are preserved. But the concomitant administration of glucose and arginine fails to show the physiological potentiation of response to arginine by glucose. The α cell suppressibility by high glucose is altered and the δ cell responses to stimuli are excessive.

These variants of the perinatal STZ model provide the following important information: (1) islet β cells can regenerate, when lesioned early in life, from either ductular (Portha) or remnant insular cells (Weir); (2) there is a relative fragility of the β cell response to glucose compared with the integrity of β cell responses to arginine and other stimuli—a pattern which recalls that seen in NIDDM; (3) the progressive development of resistance to insulin, with the persistence of mild hyperglycaemia and hypoinsulinaemia, can be improved by insulin treatment; (4) no insulitis was detected after a single STZ injection in the perinatal period.

Clinical Relevance of the STZ Diabetic Models

High-dose STZ Model

While this is an important animal model for studying the short-term and long-term consequences of deep insulinopenia, it appears of limited clinical relevance. STZ, at doses of 0.5–2 g per patient i.v., is an efficient treatment for islet tumours, particularly gastrinomas and vipomas. Interestingly, STZ courses for the cure of islet tumours are associated with a low incidence of iatrogenic diabetes. A mild impairment of glucose tolerance was noted in six of 55 patients[15], in nine of 15 patients[16] (none of them requiring insulin therapy) and in no cases in two other studies[17,18]. We know (R. Garnier, unpublished) of two cases involving self-administration (suicide attempts) of 2 g and 4 g STZ respectively: no serious consequence on blood glucose levels occurred. The only discordant note here is the report of an insulinoma patient who developed circulating islet cell antibodies (ICA), antibody-dependent cytotoxicity to RIN cells *in vitro* and then IDDM 12 months after STZ treatment, given as five courses of STZ 850 mg per day i.v. for 5 days, over 5 months. The patient had no personal or familial history of IDDM; the HLA profile was not analysed and the presence of insulitis not verified[19]. This observation suggests a careful follow-up of ICA and glycaemia in STZ-treated patients, particularly in those with a high-risk genetic profile.

The MLD STZ and perinatal STZ models display exciting similarities to the potential role of environmental nitrosamines in the triggering of IDDM. In Iceland the traditional, festive, high intake of smoked/cured mutton during Christmas and New Year is correlated in time with an excessive incidence rate of IDDM, under the age of 15, in boys born in October and presenting high-risk HLA profiles. *N*-Nitroso compounds are abundant in this smoked/cured meat: 2 mg/kg of *N*-nitrosothiazolidine-4-carboxylic acid[20]. It was postulated that nitrosamines can damage the pancreatic β cells. This hypothesis was tested in CD1 mice fed with Icelandic, nitrosamine-rich, smoked/cured mutton before mating, during pregnancy, and in offspring from day 19, until 5 weeks later. Over 16% of the male progeny and 4.2% of the female progeny developed diabetes. The islet β cells were morphologically damaged, while lymphocytic infiltration of islets was infrequent[21]. *N*-Nitrosamines are present in a variety of foodstuffs and food additives[22]. They can be formed *in vivo* in man after ingestion of conventional foodstuffs such as fried bacon and spinach, and in nitrate/nitrite-rich drinking water. *In vivo* nitrosation is increased when gastric juice pH is increased. Contamination can occur in rubber industry workers. STZ itself is a nitrosamine. *N*-Nitrosomethyl urea and *N*-nitrosoethyl urea have proved to be diabetogenic. The rodenticide Vacor, as mentioned below, is chemically related to *N*-nitrosoureas and is diabetogenic. The pathogenic influence of industrial, alimentary and endogenous nitrosamines may therefore be wider than expected, their potential role in triggering IDDM being more easily unmasked in Iceland owing to concentration in space and time through the over-consumption of nitrosamine-rich foodstuffs. The same theory may be valid for betel nut chewing in the Middle East, which has been linked to diabetes[7].

ALLOXAN

Alloxan was the first diabetogenic toxin to be discovered; it was reported in wartime (1943), as beautifully related in McLetchie's inspired historical notes[23]. It was synthesized as early as 1818 by Brugnatelli and structurally analysed by Liebig. Thousands of papers have been devoted to this model of acute and/or chronic insulinopenic hyperglycaemia, which gave important insights into β cell physiology. Alloxan toxicity to the β cell is almost universal among vertebrates, from turtles to primates, with wide interspecies variability, with the notable exception of the guinea-pig. It is active by parenteral administration and may be toxic also when given orally or enterally. Toxicity is dose-dependent. The drug passes the placenta readily but no diabetes was detected in offspring following administration of diabetogenic doses to pregnant females, suggesting that alloxan did not reach diabetogenic concentrations in the fetus, perhaps due to a very short half-life in plasma, and to the prevailing temperature and pH. Furthermore, very young animals have a high resistance to the drug. No model equivalent to that of Portha and Weir has been described. Experiments using radiolabelled alloxan have suggested either a selective accumulation in the islets, or the opposite. Extrainsular toxicity of high alloxan doses can involve the kidney (acute tubular necrosis, sponge kidney) and the liver.

Toxicity is dose-dependent, although numbers remain unclear, owing to the use of either anhydrous or mono- or tetrahydrate alloxan—not always stated by authors. Schematically, in mice, doses of 150 mg/kg (i.p.) induce a complete selective necrosis of the β cells, while after injection of 125 mg/kg some β cells remain morphologically intact. The earliest change noted is a general swelling of β cells. An initial increase in granulation is followed by degranulation, mitochondrial swelling, vacuolization and nuclear pycnosis[24]. Lower doses (35–75 mg/kg in mice and rats) induce transient diabetes, partial β cell necrosis followed by β cell regeneration, δ cell hyperplasia and no change in absolute number of α cells[25]. The repeated administration of subdiabetogenic alloxan doses was not followed by the appearance of insulitis or other detectable autoimmune phenomena[4].

The blood glucose course after injection is triphasic: early transient hyperglycaemia (for 1–4 hours) is followed by hypoglycaemia (for up to 48 hours), which is sometimes severe or even lethal, and then permanent hyperglycaemia. The hypoglycaemic phase seems to result from a massive release of presynthesized insulin at the time of β cell necrosis. But *in vitro* perfused rat islets secrete insulin for the 2–3 minutes following exposure to the drug, this release being dependent on extracellular calcium concentration and associated with an increase in ^{45}Ca uptake by the islets, which suggests active hormone secretion induced by alloxan itself for the first few minutes of exposure. Later, the β cells are unable to respond to glucose by releasing insulin (or to repetitive alloxan pulses)[26].

Various hypotheses have been proposed for the mechanisms of alloxan toxicity, such as zinc chelation, α-amino acid deamination and decarboxylation, depletion of sulphydryl (SH) groups and interference with certain enzymes in the β cell. Our understanding of two main families of protective agents support two (not mutually exclusive) mechanistic theories.

On the one hand, glucose, mannose and several hexoses oppose the β cell toxicity of alloxan in direct proportion to their affinity with early transport and metabolism. The glucose α-anomer confers greater protection than the β-anomer, and the non-metabolized analogue 3-0-methylglucose provides even better protection than glucose, proportionate to their affinity for early transport and metabolism in the β cells. Mannoheptulose sensitizes the β cell to alloxan toxicity and abolishes the protection by hexoses[27]. Alloxan inhibits glucose utilization and oxidation and oxygen consumption by the islets. Methylglucose protects against this deleterious effect, which cannot be accounted for by a reduced glucose transport into islet cells. Glucokinase of β cells may be the primary target for alloxan with islet β cells, responsible for inhibition of the glucose-induced insulin secretion and probably also for the toxic effects. Alloxan inhibits the enzymatic activity of the islet (and liver) glucokinase below 10 μmol/l levels. The theory that alloxan interacts with thiol (SH) groups in the sugar binding site of the glucokinase molecule is supported by experimental data detailed by Lenzen and Panten[28].

On the other hand, reduced glutathione (GSH), dithiols and other SH radical containing compounds are potent inhibitors of alloxan toxicity, converting alloxan to dialuric acid. Alloxan depletes the glutathione stores in liver and islets, which leads to an increased generation of free radicals. Copper superoxide dismutase protects β cells against alloxan-induced toxicity[29], in agreement with this concept of increased free radical production due to alloxan. Free radicals eventually induce breaks in the DNA strands, which activate the poly-(ADP-ribose)-synthetase. The noxious interaction of glucokinase/alloxan increases the NADP/NADPH ratio and aggravates the shortage of reduced glutathione. While alloxan is widely taken up by the liver and islets, the selective sensitivity of islet β cells presumably reflects the poor GSH peroxidase activity, compared with the high potency of hepatocytes to synthesize GSH[30]. The inhibition of glucose oxidation, detailed above, contributes in turn to the regeneration of GSH.

Finally, other SH-containing enzymes (phosphofructokinase; calmodulin-dependent protein kinase) may also be altered by alloxan.

The clinical relevance of alloxan toxicity to the β cells is unclear, to date. Uric acid can be oxidized to alloxan and attempts have been made to establish a uric acid-induced diabetes in rabbits: the doses needed were high (1g/kg) and the prevalence of transient hyperglycaemia was low (one animal out of 12)—a fact which renders the hypothesis of uric acid-induced diabetes in man (relevant to syndrome X?) very weak. We are aware of three case records of children (16 months, 24 months and 5 years of age) who swallowed alloxan (120 mg, 120 mg and 5 g respectively) in the absence of medical consequences for the two younger ones and with no documented follow-up for the oldest, who ingested the highest dose (R. Garnier, personal communication).

DITHIZONE AND ORGANIC METAL COMPOUNDS: THE ZINC PARADOX

Zinc has a pivotal role in insulin storage within the β granule and is important, in a more general way, for islet β cell function[31]. Several zinc chelating agents can induce diabetes in experimental animals. Dithizone (diphenylthiosemicarbozone) and oxine (8-hydroxyquinoline) are diabetogenic in rabbits by parenteral and (in the case of dithizone) enteral routes[32,33]. Dithizone 25–50 mg/kg injected into rabbits induces diabetes in 95% of the animals; the diabetes is either ketotic or non-insulin-dependent. Morphological alterations in the islets are apparent, including cell degranulation and zinc depletion; islets become necrotic but no insulitis was noted. Diabetes can be prevented by the concomitant administration of reduced glutathione. Oxine, also a zinc chelator, induces transient diabetes in 10% of the animals injected. It has been suggested[34] that zinc chelators act as ionophores for zinc ions, dissociating insulin-zinc complexes in the granules, thus increasing intra-granular osmolarity, leading to disruption of the granules and eventually of the β cells.

In contrast, some organic compounds structurally related to dithizone induce preferential lesions of the α cells and severe, sometimes lethal, hypoglycaemia. Diethyldithiocarbamate 0.5–1.0 g/kg i.v. induces, in rabbits, transient hyperglycaemia followed by severe, irreversible hypoglycaemia with α cell necrosis, but no β cell alternation. Potassium ethyldithiocarbamate (xanthogenate) 200–350 mg/kg induces in rabbits a similar glucose course and similar α cell lesions, associated with β cell damage. We have investigated

15 compounds structurally related to thiosemicarbazone for their effects in rat islets cultured *in vitro*: a deficient insulin secretion, and for some of them a deficient glucagon secretion, was observed according to the compound used, these effects being proportionate to the dose and exposure time (R. Assan et al., unpublished).

Whether zinc deficiency, rather than osmotically induced β cell disruption, causes the deficit in insulin release is a matter of debate. Glucose intolerance and a reduced concentration of insulin have been reported in zinc-deficient animals but no difference in glucose tolerance was noted by others. Pancreatic slices from zinc-deficient rats release less insulin following glucose stimulation than slices from pair-fed controls.

On the other hand, an excess of exogenous zinc inhibits the basal and glucose induced insulin release from rat islets and perfused pancreas[31], a fact which may be due to some competition between the calcium and zinc ions. The divalent cations nickel, cobalt, manganese and magnesium exert an inhibitory effect on insulin release, and this inhibition decreases when calcium concentrations are increased.

These observations may have some limited clinical relevance. The low insulin levels in the pancreas and the excessive zincuria in recent-onset diabetic subjects are presumably consequences rather than causes of islet disease. Ergothioneine (thiol-histidine-betaine), a potent zinc chelator, has been found in higher concentrations in plasma from diabetic subjects than in controls[31]. Zinc-depleted patients subjected to long-term parenteral nutrition can develop glucose intolerance[35].

Retrospective surveys in industry workers have shown an increased incidence of diabetes in subjects exposed to metallic nickel powder, xanthogenate and methyl mercuric chloride (Minamata disease).

Some drugs structurally related to dithizone (e.g. Pyrilene, Dithiocarb) currently being assessed for the treatment of AIDS patients, should be tested for their potential deleterious effects on the glucose regulatory system.

PESTICIDES INDUSTRIAL TOXINS AND DRUGS

VACOR AND OTHER PESTICIDES

The Rodenticide Vacor

A clinical syndrome characterized by acute diabetic ketoacidosis associated with a toxic neuropathy developed in subjects who ingested (intentionally or accidentally) the poison N_3 pyridylmethyl-N'p-Nitrophenylurea (syn. PNU; RH 787; Vacor). Nearly 300 cases of diabetes have been recorded: over 250 cases in Korea, and more than 30 with severe insulinopenic diabetes in the

USA. This rodenticide had been developed for the control of warfarin-resistant rat populations. The LD_{50} is 4.7 mg/kg for rats, 700 mg/kg for chickens and 2000–4000 mg/kg for monkeys, suggesting relative safety in primates. In fact, severe and sometimes lethal human intoxication has occurred, due to ingestion of contaminated food or intentional (suicidal) ingestion[36–38].

Early symptoms of poisoning include digestive symptoms, mental confusion, cardiac arrythmias and pneumonitis. Severe orthostatic hypotension, peripheral and vesical neuropathy can occur later. Diabetic ketoacidosis is present in most cases, and occurring 2–7 days after intoxication. Patients, when they recover, need insulin therapy for several months or more. Extreme insulinopenia and hyperglucagonaemia are noted, and the C-peptide secretory response to stimuli is deficient. Exposure of islets of Langerhans to PNU results in a reduced glucose-induced insulin release, which is dose-dependent. In some patients who died shortly after intoxication, extensive necrosis of the islet β cells was noted, while α and δ cells were spared; no lymphocytic infiltration was observed, and the exocrine pancreas was normal. In some patients, ICA were transiently detected in serum, a mean of 1 year after the intoxication.[38]

Nicotinamide attenuates the suppression of the glucose-induced insulin release due to PNU. It has been suggested as an antidote to poisoning with this drug. The exact mechanisms by which Vacor causes β cell destruction remains elusive, but the protection by nicotinamide, and some structural similarities between the Vacor molecule and STZ and alloxan suggests some common features in their respective modes of action. Vacor has not been commercially available in France or in most European countries.

Pesticides Other than Vacor

Several pesticides, frequently used in agriculture and industry are diabetogenic when tested in animals, and also in humans (exposed due to health hazards or deliberate intoxication). They include DDT, diethylaminobenzene, hexachlorophene, malathion, dieldrin, Amitraz dissolved in xylene and fluoacetamide. For some of these pesticides (e.g. DDT), hyperglycaemia was associated with insulinopenia; for others (hexachlorophene, malathion) hyperlactataemia was present.

INDUSTRIAL SOLVENTS AND PRODUCTS

Interesting, sometimes unexpected, data can be derived from cases of acute intoxication, experiments in laboratory animals and long-term health surveys in industrial workers.

Drinking and Inhalation of Acetone in Factories

Inhalation of toluene (solvent abuse) induced hyperglycaemia associated with ketoacidosis. Exposure to methylene chloride (contained in a paint-stripper, Nitromors) in a confined atmosphere was followed by protracted hypergly-caemia for several months, requiring treatment. Individual cases of acute diabetes following intoxication with methylene chloride and ethylfluoroacetate have been published.

Experimental Exposure of Rats

Exposure to vapours of acrylonitrile and other acrylate analogues induces hyperglycaemia and glutathione depletion[39]. Exposure to methylisocyanate induces acute severe hyperglycaemic and lactic acidosis. Trisodium nitriloacetate added to drinking water induces chronic hyperglycaemia. Administration of cyclizine to rats induces hyperglycaemia and morphological alterations of the islet β cells[40].

Exposure of experimental rats to β-naphthylamine, benzidine, dioxin, benzylmethylpyrilene, sodium arsenite, cyclizine, chlorcyclizine and nitriloacetate proved toxic to the pancreas and induced either hyperglycaemia for days to weeks, islet cell tumours or exocrine pancreatic cancers.

Intoxication of laboratory animals by carbon monoxide induces hypergly-caemia, but literature on hyperglycaemia and/or pancreatitis following human carbon monoxide poisoning is surprisingly limited[41] in view of the well-documented effects of hypoxia on insulin secretion by the islets[42].

Health Surveys in Industrial Workers

In the USA, workers in the rubber industry[43], pulp and paper mill plants[44], oil refineries[45], dry cleaning and laundries[46] have a higher prevalence of diabetes and/or pancreatic cancer than the general US population.

Surveys of chemical workers exposed to various organic bromides, chloro-bromides and DDT found a significant excess mortality due to diabetes.

The incidence of diabetes mellitus in patients with the 'Spanish oil syndrome' (rapeseed oil) was 13%, versus 3.8% in the general population[47].

Few references are devoted to pancreatic damage following X-irradiation. We were notified by Dr José Timsit of two patients with nephroblastoma, treated and cured by heavy X-irradiation, who developed IDDM, some years later in the absence of a family history of diabetes, and without ICA or high-risk HLA genes.

IATROGENIC DIABETES

PENTAMIDINE

Pentamidine treatments are currently the most frequent causes of derangements of glucose homeostasis in emergency poison units (G. Garnier, personal commmunication), intensive care units and departments of infectious pathology. Hypoglycaemia, diabetes mellitus, or both syndromes occurring sequentially represent over 300 published case records[48].

Pentamidine (4,4'-diamidinophenoxypentane) is an efficient treatment of *Pneumocystis carinii* pneumonitis (PCP), when cotrimoxazole is poorly tolerated. Its use has exponentially expanded over a few years, as a cure or prophylaxis against PCP, a major opportunistic infection complicating the acquired immunodeficiency syndrome (AIDS).

Pentamidine isethionate is preferentially used at present, owing to its reduced toxicity and better solubility in water, but the mesylate salt is still widely used in spite of its high toxicity. The recommended dosage for parenteral use is 3 mg/kg per day as a slow i.v. infusion in 500 ml isotonic glucose solution, and the duration of the course should not exceed 1 week. Aerosolized pentamidine (300 mg per session) is used for prophylaxis of PCP in AIDS patients. Following administration, the drug disappears rapidly from the bloodstream; it is avidly taken up by tissues (including, in particular, the pancreas) and then excreted unmetabolized into the urine. Some degree of metabolism by the liver microsomes into inactive metabolites has been demonstrated *in vitro*. Severe alterations of blood glucose levels have been noted in 30–50% of several large cohorts of patients: hypoglycaemia precedes, in most instances, the onset of diabetes. Diabetes mellitus requires insulin treatment in about one half of cases. Some patients develop ketoacidosis or lactic acidosis. Factors predisposing to diabetes include high drug dosage, renal functional insufficiency, and severe shock and anoxia. PCP relapses result in high-risk iterative pentamidine courses. Pentamidine is nephrotoxic by itself and can precipitate latent renal insufficiency. The prevalence of dysglycaemic accidents due to pentamidine has decreased recently owing to a better awareness of the risk, a reduction in dosage from 4 mg to 3 mg/kg per day, and the switch from the mesylate to the isethionate salt. But it must be stressed that the use of pentamidine isethionate and of aerosolized pentamidine is not risk-free and can cause derangements in blood glucose homeostasis.

Pentamidine toxicity to β cells of the islets is central to the pathophysiology of glucose change. Inappropriate insulin levels in plasma have been documented which are either excessively high and unresponsive in the presence of hypoglycaemia, or reduced, with poor β cell response to stimuli, when diabetes is present. Selective lesions of the islet β cells were noted at autopsy of pentamidine-treated dysglycaemic AIDS patients. Derangements of blood glucose levels and/or insulin release, and selective lesions of the islet β cells, have been reproduced *in vivo* in rats subjected to experimental renal insufficiency, and selective lesions of islet β cells were observed *in vitro*, which were proportionate to the drug concentration and the time of exposure[49,50].

OTHERS

L-Asparaginase

The antileukaemic enzyme isolated from *Escherichia coli* and *Erwinia carotovora* is still widely used for the treatment of acute lymphoblastic leukaemia in children, usually in combination protocols with prednisone. This treatment can cause hyperglycaemia and insulinopenia, sometimes associated with ketoacidosis or hyperglycaemic hyperosmolar non-ketotic coma, and may be lethal. In a retrospective survey of 421 children with leukaemia, nearly 10% developed hyperglycaemia[51]. Those who were older than 10 years, exceeded ideal body weight by 20%, or had Down's syndrome were at higher risk. Similar hyperglycaemia occurred in children treated with L-asparaginase plus methotrexate, and in adults with acute myelogenous leukaemia treated with the enzyme. The *E.coli* enzyme appears more toxic to the pancreas than the *Erwinia* enzyme. The effect is most often reversed when the L-asparaginase is stopped. In rabbits, the enzyme also causes hyperglycaemia, which is more pronounced when associated with prednisone. The mechanisms (insulin resistance and/or insulin deficency; insulin deficiency due either to asparagine deprivation or to pancreatitis) are a matter of debate.

Mitotic Spindle Inhibitors

Colchicine, vincristine and vinblastine interfere with emiocytosis in the β and α islet cells, thus modifying the dynamics and magnitude of insulin and glucagon secretions *in vitro*. Moderate doses of vinblastine, administered to patients with Hodgkin's disease, induced minor effects on the plasma levels of insulin and glucose (A. L. Luycks and J. P. Carpentier, unpublished). In fasting rats, colchicine 0.2–0.5 mg/kg induced significant suppression of the insulin secretory response to glucose and impaired glucose tolerance.

Of 93 cases of acute suicidal intoxication by colchicine, 17 presented with severe dysglycaemia—diabetes in 12, and serious to severe hypoglycaemia in five—requiring treatment in all cases, but without ketoacidosis or a decisive influence on prognosis (Pr. Chantal Bismuth, personal communication).

The homo-harringtonine alkaloid from *Cephalotaxus hainanensis*, which is of possible therapeutic interest as an antileukaemic compound, has been reported to cause hyperglycaemia[52].

Drugs which Impair β Cell Function

Treatment with diazoxide, hydantoins, promethazine, trifluperazine, calcium channel blockers or diuretics can induce transient impairment of insulin release and hyperglycaemia. Hyperosmolar non-ketotic coma can be induced by diazoxide and by hydantoin administration. These therapeutic hazards have been known for years and will not be discussed further (Table 1).

More recently, theophylline overdose, over-treatments with β-mimetic agents, and suicidal intoxication with amphetamines, or dexfenfluramine have become an important cause of severe hyperglycaemia in patients admitted to emergency poison units (Pr. Chantal Bismuth and R. Garnier, unpublished). Treatment of severe shock with i.v. infusion of adrenaline and noradrenaline can be followed by sustained, protracted hyperglycaemia, requiring insulin therapy for days or even weeks. The antiarrythmic drug encainide caused episodes of hyperglycaemia in four patients out of 23. The expectorant Benylin, which contains the antihistamine diphenylamine, has been associated with hyperosmolar non-ketotic coma. Finally, overdosage of nalixidic acid has been associated with hyperglycaemia.

CORTICOSTEROIDS AND IMMUNOSUPPRESSIVE PROTOCOLS: INTERFERON-α

Hyperglycaemia and hyperglycaemic non-ketotic coma are classic complications of corticosteroid treatment[53]. It has been suggested that treatment with cyclosporin A (CyA) and FK-506 can both impair insulin secretion *in vitro* and precipitate hyperglycaemia *in vivo*. We have analysed a consecutive series of 586 liver transplant recipients where the immunosuppressive protocol consisted of corticosteroids and azathioprine combined with either CyA or FK-506. Diabetes was present in 52 (8.8%), preceding the transplantation in 21 and diagnosed after transplantation in the remaining 31. The diabetes required insulin treatment in all but one of the 52. Post-transplant hyperglycaemia was associated with a family history of diabetes in one half of the post-transplant diabetic group (R Assan et al., unpublished). Similar observations have been made in renal transplant recipients[54].

Treatment with recombinant interferon-α2b, currently being tested for the treatment of chronic hepatitis C infection, was followed in one case by the development of IDDM 4 months after starting treatment. Hyperglycaemia was associated with seroconversion to ICA positive and the patient had a

119

Table 1 Drugs which have been reported to cause hyperglycaemia. Modified after the list published in *Diabetes* 1979; **28**: 1045

Diuretics and antihypertensive agents
Chlorthalidone
Clonidine
Diazoxide
Furosemide
Metalazone
Thiazides
Bumetamide
Clopamide
Clorexolone
Ethacrynic acid
Calcium channel blockers

Psychoactive agents
Chlorprothixene
Haloperidol
Lithium carbonate
Phenothiazines
   Chlorpromazine
   Perphenazine
   Clopenthixol
Tricyclic antidepressants
   Amitriptyline
   Desipramine
   Doxepin
   Imipramine
   Nortriptyline
Marijuana
Carbomazepine

Immunosuppressive agents
Corticosteroids
FK-506 } in combination
Cyclosporin A } with corticosteroids

Hormonally active agents
Adrenocorticotrophin
Tetracosactrin
Glucagon
Glucocorticoids (natural and synthetic)
Oral contraceptives
Somatotrophin and biosynthetic analogues
Thyroid hormones
Calcitonin
Medroxyprogesterone
Prolactin
Somatostatin and analogues

Miscellaneous
Isoniazid
Nicotininc acid
Encainide
Cimetidine
Edetic acid
Ethanol
Heparin
Mannoheptulose
Nalidixic acid
Niridazole
Pentamidine
Phenolphthalein
Thiabendazole
Reverse transcriptase inhibitors
Diphenylamine (Benylin)
Cyproheptadine
Carbon monoxide

Antineoplastic agents
Alloxan
L-Asparaginase
Streptozotocin
Chlorozotocin
Cyclophosphamide
Megestrol acetate
Colchicine
Taxus alkaloids
Vincristine, vinblastine

Catecholamines and other neurologically active agents
Diphenylhydantoin
Adrenaline
Isoproterenol
L-Dopa
Noradrenaline
Buphenine
Fenoterol
Propranolol (Inderal)
Analgesic, antipyretic and anti-inflammatory agents
Indomethacin
Acetaminophen (overdose amounts)
Aspirin (overdose amounts)
Morphine

Industrial toxic agents
Carbon disulphide
Nickel chloride, chromium, heavy metals
Vacor and other pesticides
Dithizone and zinc chelators
Acrylonitrile and analogues
Acetone, exposure to solvent vapours
Methylene chloride

family history of diabetes with at least two HLA DR and DQ high-risk alleles[55].

DRUG-INDUCED PANCREATIC DIABETES

Pancreatic diabetes due to chronic alcoholic pancreatitis or tropical malnutrition pancreatitis has been widely described elsewhere and will not be discussed here, except to say that the role of cassava and cyanide (CNH) remains debatable. The experiments where transient hyperglycaemia followed the acute administration of CNH in rats do not, in our opinion, clearly demonstrate a role for CNH in causing pancreatic damage.

More relevant to this review are observations that reverse transcriptase inhibitors, given to AIDS patients, can induce hyperamylasaemia and/or clinical pancreatitis associated with diabetes (F Pichon and PN Gowen, unpublished observations). DDI (Didanosine, Bristol) treatment was followed by pancreatitis in 7% of cases, by transient hyperglycaemia in 0.18% and by diabetes in 0.04% of cases. Administration of DDC (Zalcitabine, Roche) to several thousand patients was followed in 10 cases by amylasaemia, and in three by clinical pancreatitis.

CONCLUSIONS

Can one (or a few) leading concepts emerge from this hotch-potch of experimental models, toxicological anecdotes, occupational and therapeutic hazards, sufficient to support hypotheses regarding the triggering of IDDM (and also of NIDDM)? Can these conditions provide schemes for the elaboration of efficient protective agents? Until recently the low-dose STZ rat model and observations on nitrosamine-rich foodstuffs monopolized our attention. Induction of pancreatic neoantigens by nitrosourea and nitrosamine derivatives remains an attractive hypothesis, albeit superseded by the cow's-milk hypothesis. We will probably encounter in the years ahead other unexpected mechanisms, such as the postulated arginine NADP-dependent pathway of nitrogen oxide synthesis in islets, which may be important in some diabetic models[56].

With regard to protective agents, nicotinamide is presently of great interest, owing to encouraging experiments in which it may have prevented IDDM in animal models and possibly in prediabetic (pre-IDDM) children. On the other hand, the low free radical scavenging capacity of islets is well known. Some subjects (such as AIDS patients and other patients with wasting syndromes) are greatly depleted of glutathione: in these patients, the effects of superoxide dismutase and supplementation with glutathione precursors deserve, we think, further reassessment.

ACKNOWLEDGEMENTS

We wish to express our gratitude, for strong bibliographic support and for communication of personal cases, to the following people: Dominique Assan, Mrs M. Pancaldi, Dr R. Garnier, Prs Brière, Ch. Bismuth and H. Bismuth, Drs P. Le Bozec, J. Timsit, Pr. B. Messing, Drs F. Pichon, P. N'Gowen, Beatrice Deruti-Windsor and finally Françoise Rieuse, who prepared the manuscript.

REFERENCES

1 Barnett AH, Eff C, Leslie RDG, Pyke DA. Diabetes in identical twins: a study of 200 pairs. *Diabetologia* 1981; **20**: 87–93.
2 Caillat-Zucman S, Garchon HJ, Timsit J, et al. Age-dependent HLA heterogeneity of type 1 insulin-dependent diabetes mellitus. *J Clin Invest* 1992; **90**: 2242–2326.
3 Wilson RM, Van'Der Minne P, Deverill I, et al. Insulin-dependence: problems with the classification of 100 consecutive patients. *Diabetic Med* 1985; **2**: 167–72.
4 Like AA, Rossini AA. Streptozotocin-induced pancreatic insulitis: new model of diabetes mellitus. *Science* 1976; **193**: 415–17.
5 Toniolo A, Onodera T, Yoon JW, Notkins AL. Induction of diabetes by cumulative environmental insults from viruses and chemicals. *Nature* 1980; **288**: 383–5.
6 Wilson GL, Ledoux SP. The role of chemicals in the etiology of diabetes mellitus. *Toxicol Pathol* 1989; **17**: 317–63.
7 Alberti KGMM, Boucher BG, Hitman GA, Taylor R. Diabetes mellitus: mechanism of B cell destruction in IDDM; the role of toxins. In: *The Metabolic and Molecular Basis of Acquired Diseases* (eds RD Cohen, B Lewis, KGMM Alberti, AM Denman) Baillière-Tyndall, London, 1990, pp 789–91.
8 Ferner RE. Drug-induced diabetes. In *Baillière's Clin Endocrinol Metab* 1992; **6**: 849–66
9 Dulin WE, Soret MG. Chemically and hormonally induced diabetes. In: *The Diabetic Pancreas* (eds BW Volk, KE Welman) Plenum Press, New York, 1978, pp 425–37.
10 Dulin WE, Wyse BM. Studies on the ability of compounds to block the diabetogenic activity of streptozotocin. *Diabetes*, **18**: 459–66.
11 Okamoto H, Yamamoto H, Takasawa S, et al. In: *Lessons from Animal Diabetes* (eds E Shafrir, AE Renold) Libbey, London, 1988, pp 149–57.
12 Portha B, Levacher C, Picon L, Rosselin G. Diabetogenic effect of streptozotocin in the rat during the perinatal period. *Diabetes* 1974; **23**: 889–95.
13 Giroix MH, Portha B, Kergoat M, Bailbe D, Picon L. Glucose insensitivity and amino-acid hypersensitivity of insulin release in rats with non-insulin dependent diabetes. *Diabetes* 1983; **32**: 445–51.
14 Weir GC, Clore ET, Zmachinski C, Bonner-Weir S. Islet secretion in a new experimental model of non-insulin dependent diabetes. *Diabetes* 1981; **30**: 590–5.
15 Broder LE, Carter SK. Chemotherapy of malignant insulinomas with streptozotocin. *Ann Intern Med* 1973; **79**: 108–18.
16 Sadoff L. Patterns of IV glucose tolerance before and after treatment with streptozotocin in patients with cancer. *Chemother Rep* 1972; **56**: 61–69.
17 Ruszniewski P, Hochlaf S, Rougier P, Mignon M. Chimiothérapie intraveineuse

par streptozotocine et 5-FU des métastases hépatiques du syndrome de Zollinger-Ellison. *Gastroenterol Clin Biol* 1991; **15**; 393–6.

18 Moertel CG, Lefkopoulo M, Lipsitz S, Hahn RG, Klaasen D. Streptozotocin–doxorubicin, streptozotocin–5FU or chlorozotocin in the treatment of advanced islet-cell carcinoma. *N Engl J Med* 1992; **326**: 512–23.

19 Shulz B, Hemke B, Zander E, Ziegler B. Auto-immune reactions in a patient with malignant insulinoma treated by multiple low dose streptozotocin. *Exp Clin Endocrinol* 1991; **95**: 77–82.

20 Helgason T, Jonasson MR. Evidence for a food-additive as a cause of ketosis-prone diabetes. *Lancet* 1981; **ii**: 716–20.

21 Helgason T, Ewen SWB, Ross IS, Stowers JM. Diabetes produced in mice by smoked-cured mutton. *Lancet* 1982; **ii**: 1017–22.

22 Bittel R. Composés *N*-nitrosés: origine, effets cancérogènes, incidence de l'alimentation et du mode de vie. *Med Nutr* 1988; **24**: 295–9.

23 McLetchie NGB. Alloxan diabetes: the sorcerer and his apprentice. *Diabetologia* 1982; **23**: 72–5.

24 Wellmann KF, Volk BW, Lazarus SL, Brancato P. Pancreatic B cell morphology and insulin content of normal and alloxan-diabetic rabbits and their offspring. *Diabetes* 1969; **18**: 138–45.

25 McEvoy RC, Hegre OD. Morphometric quantitation of the pancreatic insulin, glucagon and somatostatin-positive cell populations in normal and alloxan-diabetic rats. *Diabetes* 1977; **26**; 1140–6.

26 Weaver DL, McDaniel ML, Naber SP, Barry D, Lacy PE. Alloxan stimulation and inhibition of insulin release from isolated rat islets of Langerhans. *Diabetes* 1978; **25**: 1205–14.

27 Rossini AA, Arcangeli MA, Cahill GF. Studies of alloxan toxicity to the beta cell. *Diabetes* 1975; **24**: 516–22.

28 Lenzen S, Panten U. Alloxan: history and mechanism of action. *Diabetologia* 1988; **31**: 337–42.

29 Thaete LG, Crouch RK, Buse MG, Spicer SS. The protective role of copper–zinc superoxide dismutase against alloxan-induced diabetes: morphological aspects. *Diabetologia* 1985; **28**: 677–82.

30 Malaisse WJ, Malaisse-Lagae F, Sener A, Pipeleers DG. Determinants of the selective toxicity of alloxan to the pancreatic B cells. *Proc Natl Acad Sci USA* 1981; **79**: 927–30.

31 Figlewicz DP, Formby B, Hodgson AT, Schmid G, Grodsky GM. Kinetics of ^{65}zinc uptake and distribution in fractions from altered rat islets of Langerhans. *Diabetes* 1980; **29**: 767–773.

32 Okamoto K. Drugs producing diabetes through damage of the insulin secreting cells. *Pharmacol Rev* 1970; **22**: 485–518.

33 Kadota I, Kawachi I. Diabetogenic action of analogues of 8-hydroxy quinolines. *Proc Soc Exp Biol Med*, **101**: 365–70.

34 Epand RM, Stafford AR, Tyers M, Nieboer E. Mechanism of action of diabetogenic zinc-chelating agents: model system studies. *Mol Pharmacol* 1984; **27**: 366–74.

35 Wolman SL, Anderson GH, Marliss EB, Jeejeeboy KN. Zinc in total parenteral nutrition: requirements and metabolic effects. *Gastroenterology* 1979; **76**: 458–63.

36 Hayes WJ. Synthetic organic rodenticides. In: *Pesticides Studied in Man*. Williams & Wilkins, Baltimore, 1982, pp 494–519.

37 Miller LV, Stokes JD, Silpipat C. Diabetes mellitus and autonomic dysfunction after Vacor rodenticide ingestion. *Diabetes Care* 1978; **1**: 73–6.

38 Karam JH, Lewitt PA, Young CW, et al. Insulinopenic diabetes after rodenticide

(Vacor) ingestions: a unique model of acquired diabetes in man. *Diabetes* 1980; **29**: 971–8.

39 Vodicka P, Gut I, Frantik E. Effects of inhaled acrylic derivatives in rats. *Toxicology* 1990; **65**: 209–21.

40 Hruban Z, Rubenstein AH, Slesers S. Alterations in pancreatic beta cells induced by cyclizine. *Lab Invest*, 1972; **26**: 270–7.

41 Penney DG. Acute carbon monoxide poisoning: animal models. A review. *Toxicology*, 1990; **62**: 123–60.

42 Dionne KE, Colton CK, Yarmush MC. Effects of hypoxia on insulin secretion by isolated rat and canine islets of Langerhans. *Diabetes*, 1993; **42**: 12–21.

43 Andjekolovic D, Taulbee J, Symons M. Mortality experience of a cohort of rubber workers, 1964–1973. *J. Occupational Med.*, 1976; **18**: 7–14.

44 Schwartz E. A proportionate mortality ratio analysis of pulp and paper/mill workers in New Hampshire. *Br J Ind Med*, 1988; **45**: 234–8.

45 Marsh GM, Enterline PE, McGraw D. Mortality pattern among petroleum refinery and chemical plant workers. *Am J Ind Med*, 1991; **19**: 29–42.

46 Katz RM, Jowet D. Female laundry and dry cleaning workers in Wisconsin: a mortality analysis. *Am J Publ Health*, 1981; **71**: 305–7.

47 Saenz A, Rojas-Hidalgo E, Cordon E, Irquierdo MG, del Valle M. Hyperglycemia and toxic oil syndrome in Spain. *Diabetes Care*, 1991; **14**: 424.

48 Perronne C, Bricaire F, Leport C, et al. Hypoglycemia and diabetes mellitus following parenteral pentamidine mesylate treatment in AIDS patients. *Diabetic Med*, 1990; **7**: 585–9.

49 Boillot D, Int'Veld P, Sai P, et al. Functional and morphological modifications induced in rat islets by pentamidine and other diamidines in vitro. *Diabetologia*, 1985; **28**: 359–64.

50 Assan R, Assan D, Delaby J, Debussche X, Toublanc M. Pentamidine-induced dysglycemia: experimental models in rats in vivo. *Diabete Metab* 1993 (in press).

51 Land VJ, Sutow WW, Fernbach DJ, Lane DM, Williams T. Toxicity of L-asparaginase in children with advanced leukemia. *Cancer (Brussels)*, 1972; **30**: 339–47.

52 Sylvester RK, Lobell H, Ogden W, Stewart JA. Homo-harringtonine-induced hyperglycemia. *J Clin Oncol*, 1989; **7**: 392–5.

53 Arieff AI, Carroll J. Non-ketotic hyperosmolar coma with hyperglycemia. *Medicine*, 1972; **51**: 73–94.

54 Von Kiparski A, Frei D, Uhlschmid G, Largiader F, Binswanger U. ·Post-transplant diabetes mellitus in renal allograft recipients. *Nephrol Dial Transplant*, 1990; **5**: 220–5.

55 Fabris P, Betterle C, Floreani A, et al. Type 1 diabetes developed during interferon alpha treatment for chronic hepatitis C. *Lancet*, 1992; **ii**: 340–46.

56 Schmidt HHHW, Warner TD, Ishii K, Sheng H, Mural F. Insulin secretion from pancreatic B cells caused by L-arginine-derived nitrogen oxides. *Science*, 1992; **255**: 721–3.

Chapter Seven

Nutritional Factors

G. Dahlquist

Department of Paediatrics, Umeå University, Umeå, Sweden

INTRODUCTION

In the search for triggers of the autoimmune β cell destructive process that may lead to insulin-dependent diabetes mellitus (IDDM) one focus of interest has been different nutrients, including possible toxic food additives, and energy intake. That different eating habits could hide risk factors for IDDM is indicated by descriptive epidemiological studies; incidence rates of IDDM show large geographical and temporal variations even in genetically stable populations (for references see Chapter 2). Further indirect evidence of a relationship between food or nutrient intake and incidence of IDDM includes: the incidence rate of the disease during periods of relative starvation, such as during times of war, is reduced[1,2]; incidence rates of IDDM among migrants from the islands of Western Samoa to Auckland, where eating habits differ mainly as to protein intake are increased[3]; incidence in Icelandic males born in October, i.e. 9 months after a period of traditionally high intake of nitrosamine-rich foods, including smoked mutton, is increased[4]; there is a correlation between the mean incidence of childhood IDDM and the mean consumption of unfermented cow's milk[5]. Such ecological studies provide weak support for causal relationships but during the last

Causes of Diabetes. Edited by R. D. G. Leslie

decade a number of animal experiments, together with individually based analytical epidemiological studies, have strengthened the argument that different nutrients have a causal relationship to IDDM.

BREAST-FEEDING AND FORMULA-FEEDING HABITS AND RISK FOR IDDM

In 1984 a Danish study[6] compared IDDM incidence data from Norway and Sweden with reports on the breast-feeding habits of these respective populations and found an inverse relationship between the incidence of IDDM and the percentage of children breast-fed less than 3 months. In the same report, a case–control study, using healthy siblings as controls, indicated that a short duration of breast-feeding was a risk factor for IDDM developing before 18 years of age. Following that report a number of epidemiological case–control studies (see Table 1) have verified that breast-fed children had a decreased risk of IDDM compared with those not breast-fed, and that a long duration of breast-feeding can protect from IDDM. A clear trend in decrease of the adjusted odds ratio for IDDM by duration of breast-feeding was found in a careful study from the Colorado IDDM registry[10].

Initially, it was proposed that breast milk offered protection to the newborn infant against possible disease triggers, such as infectious agents, through its

Table 1 Breast-feeding habits and risk for IDDM as recorded in epidemiological case–control studies. The odds ratios indicate either a relative increase in risk for IDDM if >1.0 or a decrease in risk if <1.0. NS denotes a statistically non-significant effect

Measured variable		Odds ratio[a]	No. of cases	Population	Reference
Breast-feeding < 3 months		1.8	266	Danish	6
Breast-feeding < 3 months		1.7	339	Swedish	7
Breast-feeding > 3 months		0.3	107	Finnish	8
Breast-feeding	no	1.4	194	Australian (whites)	9
Breast-feeding	no	1.3 (NS)	161	Canadian	10
Breast-feeding	yes	0.7	268	US	11
Breast-feeding	yes	0.5	158	US (whites)	12
Breast-feeding	yes	0.5 (NS)	79	US (blacks)	12

[a]An odds ratio is used in case–control studies as a measure of effect of exposure on the risk of developing a disease. In the case of a low prevalent disease such as IDDM it is equal to the probability of disease occurrence in an exposed group relative to that of an unexposed group of individuals (relative risk).

content of specific secretory immunoglobulin A (IgA) antibodies and cytotoxic T and B lymphocytes[6]. An alternative interpretation could be that an early cessation of breast-feeding will lead to an early introduction of foreign antigens—mainly cow's milk proteins—and significant relationships have also been reported in case–control studies between risk for IDDM and an early introduction of cow's milk formula[8,13]. In addition, patients with IDDM have increased levels of IgA class antibodies towards cow's milk proteins, e.g. β-lactoglobulin[13,14] and bovine serum albumin (BSA)[15]. Experimental studies in BioBreeding (BB) rats also support the hypothesis that cow's milk proteins may act as triggers of IDDM. Elliot and Martin in 1984 found that feeding diabetes-prone BB rats a mixture of amino acids instead of intact proteins significantly decreased the incidence of diabetes, whereas the addition of 1% skimmed milk powder to the amino acid mixture diet increased the incidence of diabetes[16]. Furthermore, it was shown that the skimmed milk powder diet increased the risk for diabetes in the offspring of the BB rat, particularly when it was fed to the mother and pups during the weaning period[17]. Experimental studies in another animal model for the autoimmune form of diabetes, the non-obese diabetic (NOD) mouse, also showed protection from diabetes by a diet in which the sole amino acid source was hydrolysed casein[18]. Both NOD mice and BB rats have been shown to have high levels of antibodies to BSA[19,20]. It was recently shown that BSA shared an amino acid sequence (ABBOS) with certain DR and DQ class II major histocompatibility complex (MHC) proteins and that antibodies against this BSA region could cross-react with a β cell membrane protein[15]. These findings led to the theory that the ABBOS peptide is immunogenic but only in individuals carrying the diabetes-associated HLA class II haplotypes. If the ABBOS peptide is introduced into a leaky immature gut it could induce an immune reaction; this reaction could be further boosted, even after gut maturation, by the β cell surface protein sharing an epitope with ABBOS. Thus the ABBOS-specific immune response might induce β cell destruction. In support of this theory it was found that IDDM children had much higher serum concentrations of IgG anti-BSA antibodies, which were also ABBOS-specific, when compared with healthy control children[21].

Thus both experimental and epidemiological studies indicate a relationship between the risk of IDDM and an early introduction of cow's milk proteins that may act as one possible trigger of autoimmunity. However, further animal and human studies are needed before this hypothesis is accepted and only a large prospective intervention study may prove a causal relationship between the early introduction to cow's milk proteins and the risk of developing IDDM. It is, however, important to point out that the introduction of cow's milk protein is unlikely to be the only trigger of autoimmunity against the β cell.

POSSIBLE NUTRITIONAL RISK FACTORS AFTER
THE WEANING PERIOD

It remains unclear from animal experiments whether exposure to intact proteins must occur early in life or during weaning, in order to act as a trigger for diabetes. Experiments with the BB rat have demonstrated an effect of casein-based diets given after the weaning period[22]. There are very few studies of humans because of the obvious difficulties of estimating or manipulating children's eating habits. In an epidemiological case–control study mothers of children with diabetes of recent onset were questioned regarding the frequencies of intake of different foods and compared to age- and sex-matched control children[23]. Thirty-six food items were classified as to their content of proteins, fat, carbohydrates, mono- and disaccharides, nitrosamine and nitrates, vitamin C and fibres. (The frequency of intake of different nutrients were categorized in three levels.) There was a dose–response relationship between the frequency of intake of foods rich in proteins, especially proteins from meat, and IDDM risk (Figure 1). A relationship between solid food proteins and risk for IDDM in childhood, if true, might not be due solely to protein fragments acting as triggers of the

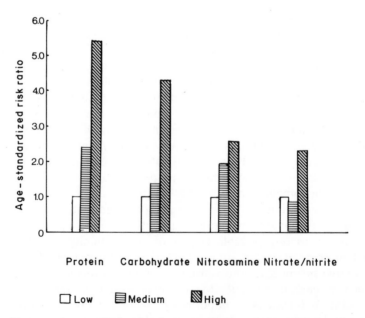

Figure 1 Dose–response relationship between the age-standardized risk ratio for IDDM and three levels of frequency of intake of foods rich in protein, carbohydrate, nitrosamine and nitrate/nitrite

β cell autoimmune destructive process but could also result from a high intake of proteins which could promote an ongoing β cell destructive process, since protein-rich foods will stimulate the β cell.

NITROSAMINES

There is a dose–response relationship between the odds ratio for IDDM and frequency of intake of foods rich in nitrosamine (Figure 1)[23]. As proteins and nitrosamine are found in the same foods the two nutrients were standardized for each other and possible confounders such as age, sex, maternal education and family history of IDDM; the significant associations between nitrosamine intake and IDDM remained. Animal studies have shown that nitrosamine compounds are toxic to the β cell both in mice[24] and Chinese hamsters[25]. Furthermore streptozotocin, which in repeated low doses induces an auto-immune type of diabetes in experimental animals, is chemically related to the nitrosamines and smoked mutton which has been held responsible for the October rise in IDDM risk in Iceland alluded to earlier, is rich in nitrosa-mines. For further details on the toxic effect of nitrosamines see Chapter 6.

CARBOHYDRATE

Carbohydrate intake, especially mono- and disaccharides, might induce IDDM[26]. Studies in BB rats, however, did not find any relationship between the source and amount of carbohydrate and the incidence of IDDM[27]. In a Swedish case–control study[23] there was an increased risk for IDDM in patients with a high intake of complex carbohydrates but not in those with a high intake of mono- and disaccharides (Figure 1). The frequent intake of foods such as complex carbohydrates stress the β cell and accords with the experimental findings that β cells when stimulated by glucose are more susceptible to the cytotoxic action of interleukin 1[28]. Alternatively, foods rich in carbohydrate may also be rich in wheat gliadin, which is potentially harmful to the β cell in BB rats[16].

VITAMINS

Vitamins are important nutritional factors, and both nicotinamide (a vitamin B) and vitamin E would modify the β cell destructive process in experimental animals perhaps by acting as free oxygen radical scavengers. Such effects are, however, related to pharmacological doses of the respective vitamins. There is no evidence at present that a deficiency of either of these vitamins is a risk factor for IDDM, so this issue will not be discussed further.

Neither the results obtained in experimental animals nor those obtained in case–control studies in humans are without shortcomings, and causal relationships between nutrients and risk of IDDM in man remain unproven. Long-term prospective follow-up studies are needed in humans to determine the relationship between eating habits and risk for IDDM.

NUTRITIONAL STATUS AND IDDM RISK

A reduced incidence of IDDM was observed during the war years 1940–1945 in Germany[1] and in northern Sweden[2]. The descriptive epidemiological studies from Finland[29] and Estonia[30] show huge differences in incidence rates between these genetically similar populations and point to a connection between high socio-economic wealth and IDDM risk. Wealth is closely related to nutritional status and therefore to risk for IDDM. The increase in incidence rate among migrant populations may indicate a similar connection with nutritional status[3]. One possible mechanism for such an association could be that caloric excess during the early years of life will lead to accelerated growth. An increased growth rate is clearly a risk factor for IDDM as indicated by the well-known incidence peak repeatedly shown in descriptive epidemiological studies during the pubertal growth spurt in both boys and girls. Similarly in a recent case–control study analysing prospectively recorded growth charts of children who later became diabetic and comparing them with age-matched controls[31], there was an increased linear growth 1–5 years before the onset of diabetes. Growth could precipitate the onset of IDDM because of the increased peripheral insulin resistance associated with puberty.

These associations between early nutritional status and risk for IDDM must still be regarded as speculative rather than causally proven. Environmental factors, such as dietary factors, are likely to interact with genetic factors[32].

CONCLUDING REMARKS

An association between nutritional factors and the aetiology of IDDM is best documented with regard to a short duration of breast-feeding; the mechanism behind this association may be an early introduction of cow's milk proteins. Other associations with the aetiology of IDDM include a high frequency of intake of protein-rich and nitrosamine-rich foods and an early excess calorie intake. It is possible that in the genetically susceptible individual several non-genetic exposures can act as *initiators* for an autoimmune process that may be *accelerated* by other exposures and *precipitated* by still different non-genetic risk factors. If the cause of IDDM is multifactorial then we do not need to look for a common mechanism for these risk factors, since, for example, nitroso compounds may act at the β cell level by a different mechanism from cow's milk antigens or viruses. A high growth rate or an increased total energy load could accelerate an already ongoing autoimmune destructive process or, alternatively, by decreasing insulin sensitivity precipitate the clinical onset of the disease. It is also possible that different nutritional risk factors may be of different importance in different age groups, as indicated by a multivariate analysis of different identified risk factors, including dietary factors[33].

Finally, it must be emphasized that more studies are needed, including long-term prospective intervention studies in high-risk groups, before advice to the general population regarding a change in eating habits could be used for primary prevention.

REFERENCES

1 Dörner G, Thoeke H, Mohnike A, Schneider H. High food supply in perinatal life appears to favour the development of insulin-treated diabetes mellitus (IDDM) in later life. *Exp Clin Endocrinol* 1985; **85**: 1–6.

2 Hägglöf B, Holmgren G, Wall S. Incidence of insulin-dependent diabetes mellitus among children in a north-Swedish population 1938–1977. *Hum. Hered* 1982; **32**: 408–17.

3 Elliot RB, Pilcher C, Edgar BW. Geographic IDDM in Polynesia and Macronesia: the epidemiology of insulin-dependent diabetes in Polynesian children born and reared in Polynesia, compared with Polynesian children resident in Auckland, New Zealand. *Diabetes in the Young Bulletin* 1989; **20**: 16.

4 Helgason T, Jonasson MR. Evidence for a food additive as cause of ketosis-prone diabetes. *Lancet* 1981; **ii**: 716–20.

5 Scott FW. Cow milk and insulin-dependent diabetes mellitus: is there a relationship? *Am. J. Clin Nutr* 1990; **51**: 489–91.

6 Borch-Johnsen K, Mandrup-Poulsen T, Lachan-Christiansen B, et al. Relation between breast-feeding and incidence rates of insulin-dependent diabetes mellitus. *Lancet* 1984; **ii**: 1083–6.

7 Blom L, Dahlquist G, Nyström L, Sandström A, Wall S. The Swedish childhood diabetes study: social and perinatal determinants for diabetes in childhood. *Diabetologia* 1989; **32**: 7–13.

8 Virtanen SM, Räsänen L, Aro A, et al. Infant feeding in Finnish children <7 yr of age with newly diagnosed IDDM. *Diabetes Care* 1991; **14**: 415–17.

9 Glatthaar Ch, Whittall DE, Welborn TA, et al. Diabetes in Western Australian children: descriptive epidemiology. *Med J Aust* 1988; **148**; 117–23.

10 Siemiatycki J, Colle E, Campbell S, Dewar RAD, Belmonte MM. Case–control study of IDDM. *Diabetes Care* 1989; **12**: 209–16.

11 Mayer EJ, Hamman RF, Gay EC, et al. Reduced risk of IDDM among breast-fed children. *Diabetes* 1988; **37**: 1625–32.

12 Kostraba JN, Dorman J, La Porte R, et al. Early infant diet and risk of IDDM in blacks and whites. *Diabetes Care* 1992; **15**: 626–31.

13 Dahlquist G, Savilahti E, Landin-Olsson M. An increased level of antibodies to beta-lactoglobulin is a risk determinant for early-onset type I (insulin-dependent) diabetes mellitus independent of islet cell antibodies and early introduction of cow's milk. *Diabetologia* 1992; **35**: 980–4.

14 Savilahti E, Åkerblom HK, Tainio V-M, Koskimies S. Children with newly diagnosed insulin-dependent diabetes mellitus have increased levels of cow's milk antibodies. *Diabetes Res* 1988; **7**: 137–40.
15 Martin JM, Trink B, Daneman D, Dorsch H-M, Robinson BH. Milk proteins in the etiology of insulin-dependent diabetes mellitus (IDDM). *Ann Med* 1991; **23**: 447–52.
16 Elliot RB, Martin JM. Dietary protein: a trigger of insulin-dependent diabetes in the BB rat? *Diabetologia* 1984; **26**: 297–9.
17 Daneman D, Fishman L, Clarson C, Martin JM. Dietary triggers of insulin-dependent diabetes in the BB rat. *Diabetes Res* 1987; **5**: 93–7.
18 Ellio RB, Reddy SN, Bibby NJ, Kida K. Dietary prevention of diabetes in the non-obese diabetic mouse. *Diabetologia* 1988; **31**: 62–4.
19 Beppu H, Winter WE, Atkinson MA, et al. Bovine albumin antibodies in NOD mice. *Diabetes Res* 1987; **6**: 67–9.
20 Scott FW, Clontier HE, Solligny J, et al. Diet and antibody production in the diabetes-prone BB rat. In: *Diabetes 1988: Proceedings of the 13th International Diabetes Federation Congress* (eds R Larkins, P Zimmet, D Chisholm) Elsevier, Amsterdam, 1988.
21 Karjalainen J, Martin JM, Knip M et al. A bovine albumin peptide as a possible trigger of insulin-dependent diabetes mellitus. *N Engl J Med* 1992; **327**; 302–7.
22 Scott FW. Diet as a prerequisite in development of insulin-dependent diabetes. *Nutr Today* 1987; **22**: 43.
23 Dahlquist G, Blom L, Persson L-Å, Sandström A, Wall S. Dietary factors and the risk of developing insulin dependent diabetes in childhood. *Br Med J* 1990; **300**: 1302–6.
24 Helgason T, Ewen SW, Ross JS, Stowers JM. Diabetes produced in mice by smoked/cured mutton. *Lancet* 1982; **ii**: 1017–22.
25 Wilander G, Gunnarsson R. Diabetogenic effects of *N*-nitrosomethylurea in the Chinese hamster. *Acta Pathol Microbiol Immunol Scand* 1975; **83**: 206–12.
26 Yudkin J. Infant feeding and diabetes (Letter). *Lancet* 1972; **ii**: 1424.
27 Scott FW, Elliott RB, Kolb H. Diet and autoimmunity: prospects of prevention of type I diabetes. *Diabetes Nutr Metab* 1989; **2**: 61–73.
28 Nerup J, Mandrup-Poulsen T, Molvig J, et al. Mechanisms of pancreatic B-cell destruction in type I diabetes. *Diabetes Care* 1988; **11**: 16–23.
29 Reunanen A, Åkerblom HK, Tuomilehto J. High incidence of insulin-dependent diabetes mellitus in children in Finland. *Arctic Med Res* 1988; **47** (Suppl 1): 535–9.
30 Kalits J, Podar T. Incidence and prevalence of type I (insulin-dependent) diabetes in Estonia in 1988. *Diabetologia* 1988; **33**: 346–9.
31 Blom L, Persson L-Å, Dahlquist G. A high linear growth and risk for diabetes. *Diabetologia* 1992; **35**; 528–33.
32 Kostraba JN, Cruickshanks KJ, Lawler Heavner J, et al. Early exposure to cow's milk and solid foods in infancy, genetic predisposition, and risk of IDDM. *Diabetes* 1993; **42**: 288–95.
33 Dahlquist G, Blom L, Lönnberg G. The Swedish childhood diabetes study: a multivariate analysis of risk determinants for diabetes in different age groups. *Diabetologia* 1991; **34**: 757–62.

Chapter Eight

Environmental Factors in Pregnancy and Infancy Influencing Insulin-dependent Diabetes Mellitus

R. B. Elliott
*Paediatrics Department, School of Medicine, University of Auckland,
Auckland, New Zealand*

INTRODUCTION

The discovery that antibodies signalling islet destruction appear years ahead of the onset of insulin-dependent diabetes has shifted the emphasis on aetiopathogenesis away from the weeks or months prior to disease onset, to a much earlier age. The youngest age at which some evidence of immune-mediated destruction of islet β cells can be detected has not yet been defined, but a number of observations on the effects of some intrauterine and infantile events on subsequent diabetes suggest that the disease may have its origins in very early life.

Causes of Diabetes. Edited by R. D. G. Leslie
© 1993 John Wiley & Sons Ltd.

DISPROPORTIONATE INFLUENCE OF MATERNAL AND PATERNAL DIABETES

The contribution of mothers and fathers to the risk of offspring developing diabetes should be equal, given the autosomal inheritance of known associated genetic human leucocyte antigen (HLA) risk markers. Despite this, the risk to the child (2.6%)[1] is two to three times less if the mother is diabetic than if the father has the disease[2], implying a strong parental non-genetic imprinting.

If this disproportion of maternal/paternal influence was due to the underlying immunological status associated with diabetes, one would expect more non-diabetic fathers of diabetic children to express islet cell antibodies than non-diabetic mothers of such children. Such is not the case (Table 1).

Table 1 Islet cell antibody status of non-diabetic parents of 163 insulin-dependent diabetic children

	Proband		
	Female	Male	Total
Both parents ICA-negative	143	145	288
Father alone ICA ≥ 10 units	10	4	14
Mother alone ICA ≥ 10 units	9	12	21
Both parents ICA ≥ 10 units	1	0	1

Thus 13.4% mothers and 9.2% fathers ICA 'positive'.

Diabetic mothers' non-genetic imprinting could be due to selective fetal toxicity of disordered carbohydrate metabolism on those fetuses most genetically prone to develop diabetes. However, one could equally well propose a benign protective influence of the diabetic state which suppresses the expression of diabetes in such fetuses in their later extrauterine existence. Offspring born to mothers who subsequently develop diabetes are more likely to become diabetic than the offspring of mothers already diabetic[3].

In this context, it is of interest that DR3/4 diabetic patients more often share DR3 with their mother (and DR4 with their father) than can be explained by chance—a phenomenon suggesting interaction *in utero* between mother and fetus[4]. Similarly, certain alleles (VNTR) near the insulin gene are preferentially inherited from the father in HLA DR4-positive diabetics, again suggesting fetal–maternal interaction or genomic imprinting[5].

ONTOGENY OF 'DIABETIC' SERUM MARKERS

The ontogeny of the immunological markers of diabetes provides strong evidence that the aetiopathogenesis of the disease occurs in very early life. Permanent diabetes occurring in infancy is a rare event, and islet cell antibodies, which mark immunological events in the islets of Langerhans which may lead to diabetes, are not found at birth except when these are of maternal origin. The time course of appearance of such circulating antibodies in a group of first-degree relatives of insulin-dependent diabetes mellitus (IDDM) siblings or parents, studied longitudinally, is shown in Figure 1.

This suggests that the immunological processes associated with diabetes first occur in very early childhood, and rarely commence thereafter. Epidemics of common childhood viral diseases, such as mumps, measles and Cocksackie B4, have been reported in association with increased incidence of diabetes at later ages, but from the above these infections can only be regarded as accelerating the clinical onset of the disease in children already predisposed. The winter peak of diabetes incidence found in cold climate countries may also be produced by such a process.

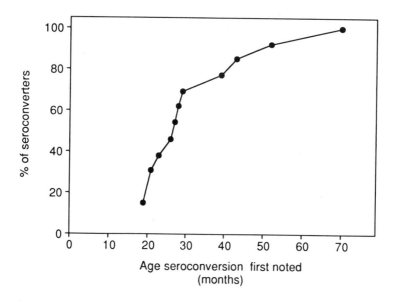

(No child in cohort studied so far has seroconverted after 70 months)

Figure 1   Age at which ICA conversion (i.e. <5 units to >10 units) occurred in a cohort of infant first-degree relatives studied longitudinally

VIRAL INFECTIONS

Rubella is the only known maternal infection which can produce diabetes in the offspring[6], although other maternally or neonatally transmitted viruses such as cytomegalovirus have been suggested as possible diabetogenic agents[7].

About a third of the long-term survivors of congenital rubella develop diabetes, half of whom show insulin dependence and develop the disease predominantly in childhood. Those with milder forms of congenital rubella tend to develop the non-insulin-dependent disease.

Congenital rubella may be associated with insulitis[8], and islet cell antibodies have been reported in some of those with IDDM[9] but there is no excess of family history of diabetes. The heterozygous DR3/DR4 genotype predominates but DR3 is the commonest genetic association with the rubella/ diabetes syndrome[10]. Individuals with DR3 show low response to viral antigens[11], which may plausibly explain both the predisposition to chronic rubella viral invasion in the fetus and the predisposition to diabetes.

Children dying from neonatal viral infections not infrequently show β cytolysis, and inflammatory infiltrates around the islets, but association with similar non-fatal infections with later diabetes is unproven. The case of fatal Cocksackie B_4 infection associated with the onset of diabetes in an older child[12] makes viral aetiology a possibility in some individuals. Experimental infection with encephalomyocarditis virus (among others) in some species of animals may result in acute diabetes, so similar aetiological agents cannot be discounted in humans in very early life.

DIET

There is circumstantial evidence that early infant diet may affect IDDM onset in later life. Prolonged exclusive breast-feeding is partially protective against the risk of subsequent diabetes imposed by being a first-degree relative of an IDDM patient[13]. The reasons for this may be a delay in the introduction of a putative diabetogen into the weaning diet, or some protective moiety in human milk itself. As cow's milk is the predominant weaning food in high diabetes incidence countries, it's involvement as a diabetogen has been studied in animal models of Type 1 diabetes, and to a lesser extent in humans. In the NOD mouse, and the BB rat models of Type 1 diabetes, an elemental diet containing the amino acids found in cow's milk given from weaning prevents diabetes[14,15]. A diet containing cow's milk protein or peptides does not[16]. The elemental diet must be introduced early in the animal's life to be protective. There is evidence that introduction of the elemental diet to the dam from the time of conception until the time of weaning is partially protective to the offspring even when they are fed a diabetogenic diet from weaning (Figure 2).

Whether or not a human counterpart of these phenomena exists is unknown. Young children with recently diagnosed diabetes have higher levels of milk protein antibodies than their non-diabetic sibs or non-diabetic norman children of the same age[17]. Recently antibodies to a specific epitope found in bovine albumin (ABBOS) have been found almost exclusively in recently diagnosed diabetic children. This epitope is shared with a surface antigen which islet β cells can be made to express[18].

Studies of migrant Polynesian children suggests that infant or maternal diet could be reasonably associated with the change in diabetic incidence[19] found

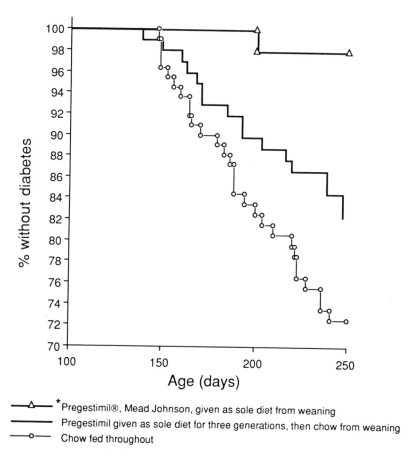

—△— *Pregestimil®, Mead Johnson, given as sole diet from weaning
——— Pregestimil given as sole diet for three generations, then chow from weaning
—○— Chow fed throughout

Figure 2 The effect of an elemental diet on subsequent development of diabetes in NOD mice (females only)

after migration, though whether this is related to the change in maternal or infant cow's milk intake in an aetiological fashion is unclear.

Maternal diets containing nitrate pickled mutton[20] or coffee have been espoused as increased risk factors, but the evidence is based on statistical association only.

MOTHER–CHILD BLOOD GROUP INCOMPATIBILITY

From Sweden[21] has come the intriguing observation that rhesus or ABO incompatibility is associated with increased subsequent risk of diabetes in the child odds risk (OR) (OR = 1.61, as compared with OR = 3.9 of maternal diabetes). This association is stronger the younger the child at diabetes onset (OR = 3.86 for onset less than 5 years), or the more severe the clinical effects of the maternal antibodies.

For a long time it has been known that children dying from erythroblastosis fetalis exhibit hyperplasia of the islets of Langerhans, and it may be speculated that this in some way predisposes to later diabetes.

The same Swedish authors identified lesser associations between maternal non-smoking (OR = 1.54), maternal age above 35 (OR = 1.36) and Caesarean section (OR = 1.32) and diabetes in the offspring.

REFERENCES

1 Tuomilehto J, Lounainaa R, Tuomilehto W, et al. Epidemiology of childhood diabetes mellitus in Finland: background of a nationwide study of type 1 (insulin dependent) diabetes mellitus. *Diabetologia* 1992; **35**: 70–6.
2 Dahlquist C, Blum L, Tuveno T, et al. The Swedish Childhood Diabetes Study. *Diabetologia* 1989; **32**: 2–6.
3 Warran JH, Martin BC, Kroleuski AS. Risk of IDDM in children of diabetic mother decreases with increasing maternal age at pregnancy. *Diabetes* 1991; **40**: 1679–84.
4 Deschamps J, Hors J, Clerget Darpoux F, et al. Excess of maternal HLA DR3 antigens in HLA DR3, 4 positive type 1 (insulin dependent) diabetic patients. *Diabetologia* 1990; **33**: 425–30.
5 Julier C, Hyer RN, Davies J, et al. Insulin IGF2 region on chromosome 11p encodes a gene implicated in HLADR4 dependent diabetes susceptibility. *Nature* 1991; **354**: 155–9.
6 Menser MA, Forrest JM, Bransby RD. Rubella infection and diabetes mellitus. *Lancet* 1978; **i**: 57–60.
7 Pak CY, McArthur RG, Eun HU, Yoon JW. Association of cytomegalovirus infection with autoimmune type 1 diabetes. *Lancet* 1988; **ii**: 2–4.
8 Gepts W. Pathologic anatomy of the pancreas in juvenile diabetes mellitus. *Diabetes* 1965; **14**: 619–33.

9 Schopfer K, Matter L, Flueler U, Werder E. Diabetes mellitus, endocrine auto-antibodies and prenatal rubella infection (Letter). *Lancet* 1982; **ii**: 159.
10 Rubinstein P, Walker ME, Fedun B, et al. The HLA system in congenital rubella patients with and without diabetes. *Diabetes* 1982; **31**: 1088–91.
11 Southern P, Oldstone MB. Medical consequences of persistent viral infection. *N Engl J Med* 1983; **314**: 359–67.
12 Notkins AL, Yoon J, Onodera T, Jenson AB. Virus-induced diabetes mellitus: infection of mice with variants of encephalomyocarditis virus coxsackievirus B4 and reovirus type 3. *Adv Exp Med Biol* 1979; **119**: 137–46.
13 Virtanen SM, Räsänen L, Aro A, et al. Infant feeding in Finnish children less than 7 yr of age with newly diagnosed IDDM: Childhood Diabetes in Finland Study Group, *Diabetes Care* 1991; **14**: 415–17.
14 Elliott RB, Martin JM. Dietary protein: a trigger of insulin-dependent diabetes in the BB rat? *Diabetologia* 1984; **26**: 297–9.
15 Elliott RB. Dietary prospects of prevention of type I diabetes. *Diabetes Nutr Metab* 1989; **2**: 67–71.
16 Elliott RB, Bibby NJ. Dietary triggers of diabetes in the NOD mouse. In: *Frontiers in Diabetes Research. Lessons from Animal Diabetes III* (ed E Shafrir) Smith-Gordon & Co Ltd, London, 1991, pp 195–7.
17 Savilahti E, Akerblom HK, Tainio V-M, Koskimies S. Children with newly diagnosed insulin dependent diabetes mellitus have increased levels of cow's milk antibodies. *Diabetes Res* 1988; **7**: 137–40.
18 Dosch HM, Karjalainen J, Morkowski J, Martin JM, Robinson BH. Nutritional triggers of IDDM. In: *Pediatric and Adolescent Endocrinology* (ed Z Laron). Karger, Basel, Switzerland, 1992, pp 202–17.
19 Elliott RB Epidemiology of diabetes in Polynesia and New Zealand. *Pediatr Adolesc Endocrinol* 1992; **21**: 66–71.
20 Helagson T, Jonasson MR. Evidence for a food additive as a cause of ketosis-prone diabetes. *Lancet* 1981; **ii**: 716–20.
21 Dahlquist G, Källen B. Maternal–child blood group incompatibility and other perinatal events increase the risk for early-onset type 1 (insulin-dependent) diabetes mellitus. *Diabetologia* 1992; **35**: 671–5.

Chapter Nine

Towards Prevention of Insulin-dependent Diabetes Mellitus

Ellen Connor and Noel Maclaren
Department of Pathology and Laboratory Medicine, University of Florida College of Medicine, Gainesville, Florida, USA

INTRODUCTION

Realization of the ability to prevent insulin-dependent diabetes mellitus (IDDM) would herald the end of a common chronic disease with distressing morbidity and mortality, which persists despite all currently available treatment modalities. IDDM places enormous financial and personnel demands upon dialysis and transplantation services in Western countries and is responsible for much human suffering worldwide. Although an effective means for IDDM prevention has long been sought, its development has been hampered by the imprecision of IDDM prediction and the potential side effects of available treatment. Successful prediction and prevention of IDDM requires an understanding of the natural history of the disease[1].

Progression to IDDM is a variable phenomenon with exacerbations and remissions of insulitis determining the possible time courses (Figure 1). Stage 1

Causes of Diabetes. Edited by R. D. G. Leslie
© 1993 John Wiley & Sons Ltd.

of the pathogenic process is a genetic predisposition to IDDM, apparently with a normal structural and functional islet cell mass. IDDM is clearly a polygenic disease with variable penetrance. However, apart from the class II human leukocyte antigen (HLA) DQ/DR alleles recognized to be linked with IDDM, other diabetes genes have yet to be unequivocally identified[2]. The IDDM associated DR3 or DR4 alleles are carried by 50% of Caucasian patients in the USA, while DR1, DR16 and DR8 are also known to predispose persons to IDDM[3]. Conversely, DR15, DR11 or DR14 alleles confer protection from the development of the disease[4].

Class II major histocompatibility complex (MHC) molecules are heterodimers of α and β chains which present medium-length peptide (8–10 amino acids) antigens to T cells for immune recognition and specific antigen binding. The presented antigens are bound by a unique T cell receptor which is formed from products encoded by rearrangements of variable, diversity, constant and joining genes. For certain antigens, specific families of T cell receptor variable genes are selected preferentially on the basis of their reactivity. Understanding the mechanisms of antigen presentation and receptor interaction in the context of a patient's class II HLA alleles should elucidate the mechanism by which HLA phenotypes predispose to IDDM and potentially improve IDDM prediction.

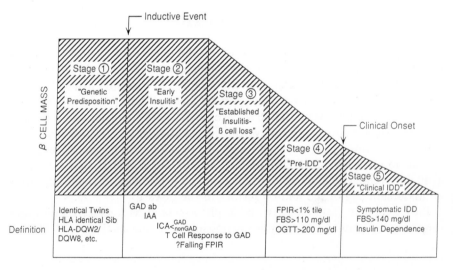

Figure 1   A pathogenic model for insulitis and IDD. (Copyright © Harwood Academic Publishers GmbH)

The highest IDDM risk is seen for the non-diabetic sibling with an identical twin affected by IDDM (approximately one in three chance of IDDM). The next highest risk is for an HLA identical sibling of an IDDM proband (approximately one in seven chance), or one sharing only one HLA haplotype (one in 15). In the general population, individuals with certain HLA DQ phenotypes, such as HLA DQ2/DQ8, have a risk of a developing IDDM of about one in 20. These DQ antigens have no positively charged aspartic acid residues at β chain position 57 but do have an arginine at residue 52 of the DQ α chain[5,6]. These variant amino acid substitutions affect the antigen-binding cleft conformations. It remains to be determined why these HLA encode susceptibility to IDDM; however, they must have importance in maintaining tolerance to self or have a role in the inductive events that initiate the pathogenic sequence leading to IDDM[7]. Although these DQ alleles are strongly represented in IDDM, the majority of persons with them will never actually develop IDDM. Accordingly, the possibilities are that an environmental factor is needed to initiate insulitis and that multiple genes affect IDDM susceptibility. Our eventual ability to intervene in genetically susceptible individuals will be directly correlated with advances in gene mapping for IDDM.

Silent, early insulitis heralds the onset of Stage 2 in the pathogenic sequence of events leading to β cell destruction in genetically susceptible individuals, as autoreactive lymphocytes begin to converge on the pancreatic islets. The stage begins with the putative inductive immunization event, whether it is one involving an islet cell autoantigen or a molecular environmental mimic of a self antigen. Autoantibodies to insulin (IAA), to a variety of islet cell constituent antigens including the lower molecular weight isoform of glutamic acid decarboxylase (GAD_{65}) and to other antibodies are demonstrable[8], but might be expected to fluctuate during the early course of insulitis. Established insulitis, or Stage 3 in the pathway to the development of IDDM, initiates the loss of β cell mass. Abnormal T cell responses to GAD, as well as diminishing first-phase insulin release (FPIR) to an intravenous glucose tolerance test (IVGTT) challenge, can be demonstrated as the loss of insulin secretory cells evolves. Insulitis can be followed by recovery and improvement in β cell function, by an arrested but permanent loss of β cell function without continuing deterioration, or by further loss of the remaining β cell function leading to a state of preclinical diabetes (stage 4; Figure 2). As we define the pathogenic process, symptomatic IDDM or Stage 5 is the end result of a pancreatic assault, with classical symptoms and a fasting blood glucose greater than 140 mg/dl heralding the loss of most of the normal β cell mass.

At each of these stages there are many opportunities for therapies aimed at the prevention of clinical IDDM. All approaches depend upon our imperfect ability to predict impending IDDM. Whereas this topic has been covered elsewhere, we would like to review briefly our own experience with prediction, since what follows is based upon these insights. In our study of more

THE NATURAL HISTORY OF EVENTS
LEADING TO INSULIN-DEPENDENT DIABETES

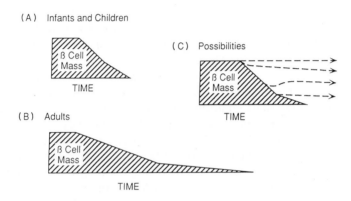

Figure 2 Possible outcomes of insulitis

than 4800 family members of probands with IDDM, we have demonstrated an increased risk of IDDM development in those relatives who were less than 20 years of age when ICA was first detected, who had high titres of ICA (with increasing risk for ICA between 20 and 80 JDF units) and who were members of multiplex families[9]. These findings permit us to assign risks for IDDM development among non-diabetic relatives of IDDM probands over a 5-year period.

A 72% risk for IDDM development within 5 years is indicated by the presence of ICA >80 JDF units and an FPIR to IVGTT of less than the first percentile of normal age-adjusted controls. A moderate risk of 60% is conferred by the simultaneous presence of ICA and insulin autoantibodies (IAA). ICA positivity of 40–80 JDF units without concurrent IAA carries a risk of 30% in this population of relatives. Family members with an ICA between 20 and 40 JDF units or IAA positivity have a disease risk of 15% over 5 years, while the isolated finding of an ICA <20 JDF units carries a risk of only 3%—the expected frequency of the disease in our normal population. The data on IDDM prediction in the general population is less well developed; however, in our own studies of more than 10 000 school children in Florida, we are impressed that our ability to predict diabetes is not very different from that for the population of relatives of IDDM probands, especially when we perform additional tests on those initially found to be antibody-negative[10].

Using the model of multistaged development of IDDM, we can outline a counterattack against the β cell autoimmune process which results in insulinopenia. In the following sections of this chapter, we will consider each stage of IDDM development and examine appropriate strategies for present and future collaborative multicentre trials.

STAGE ONE: GENETIC PREDISPOSITION

Prevention of IDDM in genetically susceptible individuals includes avoidance of suspected environmental triggers. Avoidance of the inductive agent could be pursued by a specific dietary manipulation, or through active immunizations if viruses can be proven to be causal. Dietary strategies include maintenance of ideal body weight, since obesity is recognized to be a stressor of islet cell function. Dietary restriction of protein has also been proposed, given the reported benefits of vegetarian or restricted protein chow diets in the BB rat model of diabetes[11]. Dietary protein manipulation has also been reported to prevent diabetes in the NOD mouse, and recent epidemiological evidence in humans has also suggested a link between milk protein ingestion and diabetes. Interestingly, BB rats which did not have cow's milk intake during the first 8–12 weeks of life did not develop diabetes[12]. Anti-bovine serum albumin antibodies were isolated from BB rats, and the antibodies demonstrated binding to a 69 kDa β cell protein. A similar reactivity has been reported in humans using sera from newly diag-nosed patients with IDDM[13], although this has yet to be confirmed by other groups. Further studies will be necessary before families with genetic predisposition or immune markers for IDDM can be reasonably advised to restrict cow's milk protein exposure[14]. Meanwhile, one prospective study will address the hypothesis that ingestion of cow's milk in early life can lead to the absorption of intact bovine serum albumin (BSA) and immunization to this molecule, whereupon an activated immune system will encounter a molecular mimic of BSA on β cells and initiate damage. The study will be carried out in Finland, where breastfeeding will be followed by introduction of a non bovine-based infant formula in all children less than 9 months of age. This concept of IDDM being the result of BSA exposure is, however, in conflict with the concept of defective oral tolerance induced by repeated feeding of BSA in rodents or humans predisposed to IDDM.

Vaccination against viruses suspected of initiating insulitis could be a feasible strategy in IDDM prevention. Sequence homology between the P-2 protein of Coxsackie viruses and GAD suggests that molecular mimicry between the two could be the culprit in early insulitis, as the immune responses to the virus claim casualties in the islets. Indeed, some reports of increased Coxsackie B titres in patients with new-onset IDDM have been reported[15], although other studies did not find differences in titres of IDDM patients and their family members[16]. Additional evidence of a possible viral insult initiating insulitis is provided by sequence homology of insulin with retroviral antigen p73 in the NOD mouse[17] and the recognition of an autoantibody in pre-IDDM reacting with a 37 kDa molecule with homology to a retroviral antigen.

Gene therapy, with transfection of protective DQ genes of the affected α or β chains to genetically susceptible individuals, may eventually have a role in early IDDM prevention. In NOD mice, transgenic insertions of the IE α chain gene as well as substitutions of the serine at position 57 of the IA β chain with aspartic acid or of a histidine for a proline at residue 56 completely prevented diabetes[18]. For the moment it is not possible to reduplicate such genetic manipulations by gene transfections in either man or mouse. It is, however, possible to effect much the same result through the creation of stable bone marrow chimeras using bone marrow stem cell reconstitutions of NOD mice with normal FI cells. Such would presumably be possible for humans; however, the risks for allogeneic bone marrow transplantation would be unacceptable at present.

Finally, there may be a place for genetic counselling after molecular HLA DR/DQ typing for patients with IDDM, individuals at risk for IDDM, and their prospective spouses who are contemplating parenthood.

STAGE TWO: EARLY INSULITIS

Potential early insulitis management includes the aforementioned dietary adjustments and the use of appropriate vaccines. Specific immune manipulation may become possible once the effects of immune dysregulation appear. Antigen-driven β cell damage could be minimized by islet cell antigen-specific therapies, such as induction of oral tolerance or the use of blocking immunizations.

Oral administration of insulin as well as GAD_{65} has been demonstrated to delay the onset of diabetes in NOD mice, with a disproportionate effect in females[19]. The effect is transferable with spleen cells and the mechanism is believed to rely on active immunoregulation and to affect bystander immune responses ongoing in the islets as well. In this respect the effect is organ- but not antigen-specific. We believe that this approach should also be feasible and nontoxic in humans, and are making plans to initiate such a multicentre trial at the time of writing.

Blocking immunizations of insulin, GAD_{65} or heat shock protein 65 kDa are also being actively investigated by our group in NOD mice to assess their potential in humans. The role of immune enhancement mechanisms in diabetes prevention should also be considered as potential therapy in the presence of early insulitis. Administration of adjuvants containing tuberculin antigens or cytokines such as tumour necrosis factor α (TNFα), tumour growth factor β (TGFβ), interleukin (IL-7 or IL-10) might be candidates. NOD mice are powerfully protected from diabetes by administration of TNFα, by complete Freund's adjuvant, or by recombinant IL-1 or IL-2[20]. The specific interactions of self or molecular mimic antigens in the context of the MHC and the specific T cell receptor offer another potential site for future interventions. These interactions could be interrupted by the administration of blocking antigens which occupy the MHC receptor but do not stimulate T helper cells. The subject is complex but is an area of active research in other autoimmune diseases.

Alternatively, administration of antibodies to the class II MHC, to CD4 accessory molecules, or to the T cell receptor may also be effective. In the BB rat and the NOD mouse, administration of anti-class II MHC antibodies convincingly prevents diabetes, but the risk of potential side effects precludes use of the approach in humans. Lytic antibodies to CD4 prevent diabetes in NOD mice, but again this approach appears to be too risky in humans. More recently, IDDM prevention has been demonstrated in NOD mice by Cooke and colleagues using anti-CD4 antibodies that are not lytic to CD4$^+$ (helper) T cells[21]. Here the antibody may be given transiently in early life with the induction of β cell tolerance thereafter. Presumably immunological tolerance to other antigens, such as those from infectious agents, might be a concern in humans.

STAGE THREE: PROGRESSIVE INSULITIS

Signs of progressive insulitis herald the need for more intense counterassault and protection of the β cell mass under autoimmune siege. 'β cell rest' could be employed to reduce the antigen load being seen by the immune system and give the β cells a period for recovery. A number of investigators have shown that not only diabetes but the insulitis lesion itself can be interrupted by administering prophylactic daily insulin injections[22]. We have performed such studies in NOD mice, while investigators at the Joslin Clinic have further applied the approach to prevent diabetes in humans. The preliminary results from that study are encouraging and indicate that the approach is safe. We have begun a similar pilot study in human subjects. Our index patient was a 4-year-old twin sibling of an IDDM proband, in whom we hoped to inhibit the ongoing insulitis process. She had been found to be ICA, IAA and GAD antibody-positive and had impaired FPIR to intravenous glucose.

Progressive insulitis would also be an indication for other intense interventional strategies. Antioxidant therapy could be employed to reduce the oxidant damage by free radicals within the islets. Although the free radical damage may not be an initiating event in IDDM, it is likely that the release of free radicals from activated macrophages within the insulitis lesions would accelerate the process of β cell destruction. Nicotinamide, an inhibitor of poly-(ADP-ribose)-synthetase and a free radical scavenger, has been used with encouraging results in NOD mice as well as in pilot studies in human relatives of patients with IDDM and ICA-positive children from normal populations. In a collaborative trial between centres in Denver and New Zealand, 14 children with ICA positivity >80 JDF units, impaired FPIR and a first-degree relative with IDDM were given oral nicotinamide twice daily. Only one of these 14 developed diabetes in a 2-year period, while all of six control patients developed IDDM[23]. However, more of these at-risk children have apparently developed IDDM since the initial report.

Specific vitamin therapy similarly might be helpful to reduce β cell damage by free radicals from insulitis. Vitamin E, or α-tocopherol, has been recognized for its antioxidant properties[24]. The mechanism of action of vitamin E is the interruption of lipid peroxidation following free radical damage. The effects of vitamin E can be potentiated by ascorbic acid or vitamin C[25]. In addition, ascorbic acid acts directly on singlet oxygen, the superoxide radical and lipid peroxides. β-Carotene and vitamin A administration should also be considered to minimize the effects of singlet oxygen[26]. Finally, progressive insulitis should be the target of the same antigen-specific therapies and immune enhancement mechanisms discussed above for early insulitis.

STAGE FOUR: PRE-IDDM

The pre-IDDM state offers the last opportunity for diabetes prevention. Accordingly, the therapies selected should be focused on salvaging β cell function and halting the rampant immune attack. Non-specific immunotherapies, already employed with some promising results, could be utilized in insulitis management.

Specifically, cyclosporin A has been demonstrated to inhibit IL-2 production and release from CD4$^+$ and CD8$^+$ T cells, while azathioprine, a known purine antagonist capable of halting the development of natural killer and cytotoxic T cells[27], is another agent to consider. Cyclosporin has had some efficacy in slowing progression to IDDM or inducing remission in newly found IDDM, although the remissions are not permanent[28]. However, the risk of toxic nephropathy, characterized by tubular fibrosis and an uncertain chance of recovery, delegates the use of cyclosporin to only those instances in which a very great likelihood of IDDM is thought to exist.

An increased risk of nephropathy among 192 patients with autoimmune diseases who received cyclosporin A has been recently described[29]. Of the patients studied, 152 had received cyclosporin for IDDM intervention at diagnosis. Forty-one patients had proven nephropathy; of these 25 were patients with IDDM. Use of dosages greater than 5 mg/kg per day was significantly associated with nephropathy. Thus the use of cyclosporin for IDDM prevention may carry significant risks[29]. Azathioprine has been shown to affect β cell stabilization in the pre-IDDM state or early IDDM, without evidence of increased lymphoma or infection occurrences in study patients to date at our institution, although these side effects remain potential concerns. In particular, those patients with early IDDM given doses of up to 3 mg/kg per day or a total of 150 mg per day have prolonged C-peptide secretion and thus decreased exogenous insulin requirements 1 year or longer following study entry[30]. Prolonged remission in newly diagnosed patients correlated particularly with initial and persistent relative lymphopenia (absolute count <1800) during azathioprine therapy[31].

The opportunity to arrest free radical damage in pre-IDDM would again be an indication for the use of nicotinamide, vitamins E, C and A and β-carotene. In addition, the successful use of probucol, an antioxidant free radical scavenger, in the prevention of IDDM in the BB Wistar rat makes its use in pre-IDDM a possibility. When fed probucol from the time of weaning to 160 days of age, BB Wistar rats had greater than a 20% reduction in the incidence of IDDM and developed IDDM at a later age[32].

Nitric oxide has recently been found to be suppressible by an analogue of L-arginine, aminoguanidine, which inhibits the inducible form of nitric oxide synthetase. We believe that nitric oxide may prove to be a significant mediator of β cell destruction in IDDM; thus this finding may be of great clinical potential, particularly since it should be relatively safe[33]. The drug also inhibits the Amadori reaction and thus will prevent non-enzymatic glycations once hyperglycaemia appears. β Cell rest induced by early or prophylactic insulin therapy may also prove to be effective even at this late stage of the disease[34]. Prophylactic subcutaneous insulin will soon be administered to patients with pre-IDDM in a multicentre US trial with this principle in mind, with hypoglycaemia as the principal side effect of potential concern. A worrisome possibility raised by one group is that immunization by insulin might precipitate diabetes itself. However, a lack of increased incidence of IDDM was reported in psychiatric patients who received insulin 'shock therapy' between the years 1934 and 1962[35]. A lingering question remains as to appropriate duration of daily insulin prophylactic therapy. That is to say, in any given patient not developing IDDM, would the protective effect be permanent after therapy is stopped or would the therapy be merely masking diabetes? Obviously, this would need to be tested by interrupting therapy for a few days and monitoring subsequent blood glucose levels.

STAGE FIVE: CLINICAL IDDM

Early detection of new patients with IDDM, although too late for preventive therapy, can enable the physician to intervene and preserve residual β cell function. We now know that early and aggressive insulin therapy minimizes the effects of glucose toxicity on the β cells. Perhaps β cell rest with attendant reduction in expression of surviving islet cell antigens might be a factor in this response. Aminoguanidine therapy could be indicated in minimizing glucose toxicity. Reduction of continuing insulitis should also be a goal of therapy, utilizing non-specific immunotherapies such as cyclosporin, azathioprine, FK-506, methotrexate or anti-CD5-ricin. A recent evaluation of the use of up to 10 mg/m^2 of methotrexate showed reduction in symptoms in young patients with juvenile rheumatoid arthritis (JRA) with 6 months of therapy. In contrast to azathioprine, this agent has effects on both T and B cells. The most frequently seen side effects were mild gastrointestinal upset, haematuria, pyuria, alterations in leucocyte differentials, and transient liver enzyme elevations[36]. However, lasting remissions of JRA have not been reported in paediatric or adult populations, and the report of hepatic fibrosis in a child with JRA receiving methotrexate makes its use warrant caution[37].

FK-506 is another powerful weapon in the immunosuppressive arsenal and has been used with variable results in transplant patients. However, like cyclosporin, this drug is also known to cause significant nephrotoxicity, rendering it less favourable for IDDM prevention than the longer-studied cyclosporin A[38]. Anti-CD5-ricin is a subject of interest in IDDM prevention, but remains to be studied in long-term IDDM preventive trials. The CD5 antigen is present on T cells, as well as on those B cell subsets purported to be involved in insulitis provocation, and ricin is a plant toxin to which the antibody has been conjugated. Early reports are promising[39] but the potential for side effects remains.

The gravity of unopposed insulitis leading to IDDM is clear. Certainly, the need for precise, early detection of a worldwide population at risk for IDDM is unquestioned. As our methods of risk detection continue to improve, investigators worldwide could add IDDM to the list of preventable childhood diseases through cooperative interventional trials.

TRIALS TO PREVENT IDDM

Interventional trials for diabetes prevention should meet certain criteria (Table 1). A trial should be timely and feasible, yielding results at surrogate endpoints that are conclusive. Multicentre participation and comprehensive central patient and trial registries are desirable; multicentre collaboration will be essential to compile statistically meaningful patient populations. Standardization of selection criteria and outcome assessment must be accomplished. Interventional methods should be stage-dependent, based on a comprehensive evaluation of staging. The inherent risks of side effects from therapy can

Table 1 Recommendations for diabetes intervention trials

1. Timely enrollment of participants
2. Feasible study designs
3. Relative yields are high to minor risk groups
4. Intervention methods are stage-dependent
5. Surrogate outcomes are measured
6. Multicentre participation is necessary
7. Standardized criteria for patient selection
8. Standardized outcome measures
9. Comprehensive patient and trial registries

thus be weighed against accurate risks of IDDM development (Table 1). A patient at low but increased risk by virtue of genetic predisposition might be prudently advised to make low-risk dietary and immunization adjustments, while a patient with low first-phase insulin release and high titres of ICA and IAA could reasonably be advised of the potential benefits of more intensive strategies known to have some appreciable side effects.

CONCLUSIONS

Improvements in the prediction of IDDM, coupled with advances in molecular biology and immunology that have elucidated the immunological destructive processes culminating in IDDM, now allow us to gather our efforts in collaborative interventional trials. These trials will require large patient populations to be conclusive; prevention of IDDM in the twenty-first century will be the achievement of a global collaboration.

REFERENCES

1 Maclaren NK. How, when, and why to predict insulin dependent diabetes. *Diabetes* 1988; **37**: 1591–4.
2 Winter WE, Obata M. Heritable origins of type I (insulin-dependent) diabetes mellitus: immunogenetic update. *Growth Genet Horm* 1991; **7**(2): 1–6.
3 Maclaren NK, Henson V. The genetics of insulin-dependent diabetes. *Growth Gene Horm* 1986; **2**(1): 1–4.
4 Maclaren, NK, Riley WJ, Skordis N, et al. Inherited susceptibility to insulin-dependent diabetes is associated with HLA-DR1, while DR5 is protective. *Autoimmunity* 1988; **1**: 197–205.
5 Dorman JS, LaPorte RE, Stone RA, et al. Worldwide differences in the incidence of type I diabetes are associated with amino acid variation at position 57 of the HLA-DQb chain. *Proc Natl Acad Sci USA*, 1990; **87**: 7370–4.
6 Todd JA. Genetic control of autoimmunity in type 1 diabetes. *Immunol Today* 1990; **11**: 122–8.

7 Lundin KE, Qvigstad E, Ronningen KS, et al. Antigen-specific T cells restricted by HLA-DQw8: importance of residue 57 of the DQ beta chain. *Hum Immunol* 1990; **24**: 397–405.

8 Atkinson MA, Maclaren NK, Scharp DW, et al. 64,000 Mr autoantibodies as predictors of insulin-dependent diabetes. *Lancet* 1990; **335**: 1357–60.

9 Riley WJ, Maclaren NK, Krisher J, et al. A prospective study of the development of diabetes in relatives of patients with insulin-dependent diabetes. *N Engl J Med* 1990; **323**: 1167–72.

10 Maclaren NK, Horne G, Riley WJ, et al. The predictability of insulin dependent diabetes in United States school children. (Unpublished data.)

11 Elliott RB, Martin JM. Dietary protein: a figure of insulin-dependent diabetes in the BB rat? *Diabetologia* 1984; **26**: 297.

12 Daneman D, Fishman L, et al. Dietary triggers of IDD in the BB rat. *Diabetes Res* 1987; **5**: 93–7.

13 Karjalainen J, Martin JM, et al. A bovine serum albumin peptide as a possible trigger of insulin-dependent diabetes mellitus. *N Engl J Med* 1992; **327**: 302–7.

14 Maclaren NK, Atkinson M. Is insulin-dependent diabetes mellitus environmentally induced? *N Engl J Med* 1992; **327**: 348–9.

15 Vague P, Vialettes B, Prince MA, De Micco P. Coxsackie B viruses and autoimmune diabetes. *N Engl J Med* 1981; **305**: 1157.

16 Riley WJ, Maclaren NK, Rand K, Bejar R. Inherited autoimmunity versus Coxsackie B4 in insulin-dependent diabetes. *Diabetes* 1980; **29**: 211a.

17 Serreze DV, Leiter EH, Kuff EL, Jardieu P, Ishizaka K. Molecular mimicry between insulin and retroviral antigen p73: development of cross-reactive autoantibodies in sera of NOD and C57BL/KsJ db/db mice. *Diabetes* 1988; **37**: 351.

18 Lund T, O'Reilly L, Hutchings P, et al. Prevention of insulin-dependent diabetes in non-obese diabetic mice by transgenes encoding modified I-A beta chain or normal I-E alpha chain. *Nature* 1990; **345**: 727–9.

19 Dong J, Muir A, Schatz D, et al. Oral administration of insulin prevents diabetes in NOD mice. *Diabetes Res Clin Pract* 1991; **14**: S55.

20 Jacob CO, Aiso S, Michie SA, et al. Prevention of diabetes in nonobese diabetic mice by tumour necrosis factor (TNF): similarities between TNF-alpha and interleukin 1. *Proc Natl Acad Sci USA* 1990; **87**: 968–72.

21 Proceedings of the 12th International Immunology and Diabetes Workshop, 1993. Prevention of diabetes but not insulitis in NOD mice injected with non-depleting anti-CD4. AR Hayward, M Shriber, A Cooke and H Waldmann, p 61.

22 Shah SC, Malone JI, Simpson RN. A randomized trial of intensive insulin therapy in newly diagnosed insulin-dependent diabetes mellitus. *N Engl J Med* 1989; **320**: 550–4.

23 Elliott RB, Chase HP. Prevention or delay of type 1 (insulin-dependent) diabetes mellitus in children using nicotinamide. *Diabetologia* 1991; **34**: 362–5.

24 Halliwell B. Oxygen radicals and metal ions: potential antioxidant intervention strategies. *Ann Int Med* 1987; **107**: 526–45.

25 Frei B, England L, Ames BN. Ascorbate is an outstanding antioxidant in human blood plasma. *Proc Natl Acad Sci USA* 1989; **86**: 6377–81.

26 Burton GW, Ingold KU. Beta-carotene: an unusual type of lipid antioxidant. *Science* 1984; **224**: 569–73.

27 Adorini L, Barnaba V, Bona C, et al. New prospectives on immunointervention in autoimmune diseases. *Immunol Today* 1990; **11**: 383–6.

28 Bougneres P-F, Landers P, Boisson C, et al. Limited duration of remission of insulin dependency in children with recent overt type I diabetes treated with low-dose cyclosporin. *Diabetes* 1990; **39**: 1264–72.

29 Feutren, G, Mihatsch MJ. Risk factors for cyclosporine-induced nephropathy in patients with autoimmune diseases. *N Engl J Med* 1992; **326**: 1654–60.

30 Silverstein J, Maclaren NK, Riley WJ, et al. Immunosuppression with azathioprine and prednisone in recent onset insulin dependent diabetes mellitus. *N Engl J Med* 1988; **319**: 599–604.

31 Silverstein J, Maclaren N, Riley W, et al. Lymphopenia dictates metabolic response to azathioprine in new onset IDD. *Diabetes Res. Clin. Pract.* 1991; **14**: S53.

32 Drash AL, Rudert WA, Borquaye S, et al. Effect of probucol on development of diabetes mellitus in BB rats. *Am J Cardiol* 1988; **62**: 27B–30B.

33 Corbitt JA, McDaniel ML. Does nitric oxide mediate autoimmune destruction of beta cells? *Diabetes* 1992; **41**: 897–903.

34 Atkinson MA, Maclaren NK, Luchetta R. Insulitis and diabetes in NOD mice are reduced by prophylactic insulin therapy. *Diabetes* 1990; **39**: 933–7.

35 Bock T, Pederson CR, Josefsen K, et al. No risk of diabetes after insulin-shock treatment. *Lancet* 1992; **339**: 1504–6.

36 Giannini EH, Brewer EJ, Kuzmina N, et al. Methotrexate in resistant juvenile rheumatoid arthritis. *N Engl J Med* 1992; **326**: 1043–9.

37 Keim D, Ragsdale C, Heidelberger K, et al. Hepatic fibrosis with the use of methotrexate for juvenile rheumatoid arthritis. *J Rheumatol* 1990; **17**: 846–8.

38 Schreiber SL, Crabtree GR. The mechanism of action of cyclosporin A and FK506. *Immunol Today* 1992; **13**: 136–42.

39 Skyler JS, Byers V, Einhorn et al. Effects of CD-5 immunoconjugate (H65-RTA) on pancreatic islet beta cell function in type I diabetes mellitus (IDDM). *Diabetes Res Clin Pract* 1991; **14**: S54.

Part II

Non-insulin-dependent Diabetes Mellitus

Chapter Ten

The Genetic Aspects of Non-insulin-dependent Diabetes Mellitus

M. McCarthy and G. A. Hitman

Medical Unit, Royal London Hospital, London, UK

INTRODUCTION

It is the conventional wisdom that non-insulin-dependent diabetes mellitus (NIDDM) has a strong genetic basis: in other words that a large part of the variability in blood glucose levels seen within and between populations is determined by genotype rather than environment. If this is the case, and the number of genes involved is relatively small, it should prove possible, in theory at least, to predict individual risk of future NIDDM from a knowledge of that individual's genotype. However, at this stage knowledge of the specific genetic determinants of glucose intolerance remains poor and our understanding of the complex interactions of genes and environment which lead to glucose intolerance is rudimentary.

Causes of Diabetes. Edited by R. D. G Leslie
© 1993 John Wiley & Sons Ltd.

IS NIDDM A GENETIC DISEASE?

The evidence for a strong genetic element in the development of NIDDM comes from a range of studies of different designs.

TWIN STUDIES

Since monozygotic (MZ) twins share all of their genes and dizygotic (DZ) twins only 50%, the marked differences in concordance rates for NIDDM between MZ and DZ twin pairs provide strong evidence for a genetic element[1-3]. This assumes that the environments of MZ and DZ twin pairs are equally similar, which may not be entirely true[4], so that heritability calculated from such studies represents an upper estimate. Early twin studies failed to recognize the distinction between IDDM and NIDDM but found that concordance was in general greater for MZ than DZ twins and for elderly-onset diabetes over early-onset diabetes[5]. The classic studies from King's College Hospital suggested MZ concordance rates close to 100% but were undoubtedly subject to ascertainment bias which inflated this result[1]. Newman's study of twin pairs ascertained without bias from US Army recruiting records suggested a 'snapshot' rate of concordance amongst MZ twins of 58%: with follow-up, however, most of those pairs initially discordant became concordant[6].

POPULATION STUDIES

The high prevalence of NIDDM in certain isolated populations, such as the Nauruan islanders[7] and the apparent transmission within families, is supportive of a genetic basis of disease. Neel[8] has proposed the 'thrifty genotype' hypothesis to explain the persistence at high frequencies of genotypes that so clearly result in an adverse phenotype in modern societies, on the grounds that those same genes have, by promoting efficient energy storage, previously proven beneficial in times of food shortage.

Further evidence is provided by migration studies: individuals from the Indian subcontinent have relatively high prevalence rates of NIDDM whether in India[9,10] or as migrants[11-14]. Migrant Indian groups typically have higher prevalence rates than indigenous or other immigrant populations resident in those same locations. However, migrant populations do not immediately acquire all of the environmental attributes of their new homes, so these effects may partly reflect dietary and cultural as well as genetic factors.

Amongst the strongest backing for genetic input derives from studies of genetic admixture. Serjeantson reported that the prevalence of NIDDM in Nauruan islanders over 60 years was 83% in full-blooded Nauruans but only 17% in those islanders demonstrated on human leucocyte antigen (HLA) typing to have foreign genetic admixture[15]: since there were no apparent differences in environment between the two groups, this is indicative of a protective effect of foreign genotypes on the development of diabetes. Similar findings have been reported in Pima Indians[16] and also in other Amerindian groups, where the degree of native American admixture parallels the prevalence of NIDDM[17,18].

FAMILY STUDIES

The familial aggregation of NIDDM is striking but may reflect shared environmental as well as genetic effects: at the turn of the century, tuberculosis and leprosy were considered genetic diseases because of their apparent familial aggregation. Köbberling has reported that 38% of siblings of patients with NIDDM and 21% of their parents themselves suffer from NIDDM (compared with 6.3% and 9.2% of controls)[19]. Estimates of the prevalence of NIDDM in the offspring of conjugal diabetic parents have ranged widely according to the ethnic group under study and the assumptions made as to age-related penetrance[20–23]. In southern Indians, Viswanathan and colleagues have reported that if one parent is diabetic then 36% of the offspring will be diabetic, while if both are diabetic the figure is 50% (and can be predicted to reach 63% by the age of 60)[23].

HOW MANY GENES ARE INVOLVED?

Twin, family and population studies indicate a genetic basis for NIDDM but do not imply a model for that genetic predisposition. Given the phenotypic heterogeneity evident amongst NIDDM patients in the clinic (with regard to obesity, requirement for insulin and age of onset, for example), and the demonstration from physiological studies that defects both of insulin action and insulin secretion are necessary before diabetes is manifest, it is not unduly pessimistic to suspect that NIDDM may be a heterogeneous disease (or group of diseases) at the genetic level as well. Such considerations bear directly on the practicalities and likely success of the various strategies which might be employed in the search for diabetes susceptibility genes.

Some of the possible models for the genetic contribution to NIDDM are shown in Figure 1. The single-gene model (A) may, as described below, be applicable to subtypes of NIDDM such as maturity-onset diabetes of the young (MODY)[24]. The second model (B) implies that a number of different genes contribute to the development of NIDDM both within an individual (polygenic) and/or within a population (multigenic). The last model (C)

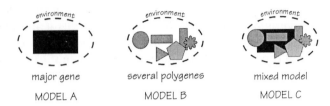

Figure 1 Possible models for the genetic basis of NIDDM. The major gene is represented by the dark rectangle, and minor genes or polygenes by the grey polygons. For further details see text

suggests that a significant part of the genetic basis is provided by a major gene, the expression of which is influenced by a number of modifier genes.

A number of different approaches have been employed in an attempt to define the relevance of each model in NIDDM. The observed bimodality of glucose levels in many populations at high risk of diabetes[25-27] has been taken as evidence that segregation at a single locus determines glucose levels. Although consistent with such an explanation, it is equally likely that bimodality represents distortion of a continuous distribution by the deleterious effects of hyperglycaemia on β cell function[28], leading to rapid transition from the 'tolerant' to the 'intolerant' mode.

Several studies have attempted to discern likely major gene effects by inspection of the patterns of affection within families—what might be termed 'informal' segregation analysis. The observation that 38% of the siblings of diabetic probands were themselves diabetic[19] is consistent with an autosomal dominant gene, and the rather low (around 50%) prevalence of diabetes in the offspring of conjugal diabetic parents[20-22] has been considered as evidence against recessivity. However, such analyses fail to take full account of the effects of age on penetrance of disease and fail to extract the maximum information from the data.

Since genetic load in a pedigree or individual might be expected to be reflected in terms of an early age of onset, the analysis of those families characterized by an unusually early onset of NIDDM might emphasize the effects of genes over those of environment. Tattersall and Fajans were the first to describe the concept of MODY, identifying a subset of NIDDM pedigrees displaying early onset of NIDDM and an apparent autosomal dominant inheritance[22,29]. However, physiological[30] and genetic[30-32] studies suggest that even under these restrictive criteria MODY is a heterogeneous, multigenic entity. O'Rahilly has described pedigrees in which early-onset diabetes was associated with a high probability that both parents were affected[33,34]: this 'gene dosage' effect would be consistent with a co-dominant single gene, but also with multigenic or polygenic models of inheritance.

Formal segregation analysis[35] is the preferred technique in simple Mendelian disease for determining the mode of inheritance: in the case of NIDDM, there are considerable methodological difficulties which arise from the late onset of disease, the absence of a biochemical marker for future diabetes and the premature mortality caused by NIDDM.

In Nauruans, reports of segregation analysis have suggested a dominant or co-dominant autosomal model, although this was not compared to a purely polygenic model[36,37]. Elston in his study of Oklahoma Indians deduced evidence for a major gene largely from the bimodality but failed to discriminate between dominance or recessivity[38].

Our studies in southern Indians, using the programs POINTER and COMDS, suggest that the inheritance of 'everyday' NIDDM is not best explained by simple models of inheritance. Amongst single-gene models, a co-dominant model provided a significantly better fit to the data than did a dominant or recessive model: however, more satisfactory descriptions of the data were provided by a polygenic model (in the case of POINTER) or a two-gene model (in the case of COMDS) (reference 39 and M. McCarthy, unpublished).

In keeping with these findings, Rich has pointed out that the risks for diabetes amongst the relatives of NIDDM subjects decline in a non-linear fashion as the degree of genetic relationship becomes more remote. Single-locus models fail to explain these results adequately, whereas multifactorial models (involving a combination of major and polygenes) produce a relative risk function in keeping with the observed non-linearity[40].

Thus simple models of inheritance in which one or two genes determine glucose levels may be a feature of certain subtypes of NIDDM (MODY, Pimas, Nauruans) while the situation in everyday NIDDM may be considerably more complex.

WHICH KINDS OF GENES MIGHT BE INVOLVED?

The search for the genetic determinants of NIDDM is complicated enormously by the fact that the basic biochemical defect(s) underlying glucose intolerance have not been established. Indeed, if, as seems probable, NIDDM is a polygenic/multigenic disease with significant genetic/environmental interactions there may be a number of distinct pathophysiological routes to glucose intolerance. A clue that this may be so comes from the diversity of inherited diseases which include diabetes within their phenotype[41]: these range from conditions in which diabetes arises from a primary pancreatic defect (e.g. cystic fibrosis) to those with a manifest defect of insulin action (e.g. leprechaunism).

A great deal of effort has been expended in physiological studies which have attempted to define the 'primary' lesion in NIDDM[42-47] and in particular to determine whether a defect of insulin action or insulin secretion is pre-eminent. Subjects with established NIDDM demonstrate defects in both these parameters: indeed glucose intolerance *ipso facto* implies inadequate insulin secretion for the prevailing degree of glycaemia. Furthermore, hyperglycaemia itself can lead to deterioration in insulin secretion and action[28] such that it is impossible to distinguish primary and secondary effects in those already glucose-intolerant. The results of studies which have looked at differing prediabetic populations, in an effort to separate primary and secondary effects, have yielded mixed results with advocates for the primacy both of insulin action and insulin secretion[48].

What clues do these studies provide in the search for potential diabetes susceptibility genes? Genes coding for proteins felt to constitute the glucose 'sensor' of the β cell (e.g. GLUT2, glucokinase[49], ATP-sensitive potassium channel) are excellent candidates, particularly since insulin release to non-glucose secretagogues may be relatively preserved in NIDDM[50]. Genes involved in β cell development and regeneration (e.g. 'reg'[51]) may be important given evidence that β cell function can be irreversibly compromised by prenatal influences[52,53]. Genes contributing to obesity (as yet unidentified) could be important modifier genes for NIDDM. The fairly consistent finding that defects in non-oxidative glucose disposal (which effectively equates with glycogen synthesis) are seen in first-degree relatives of NIDDM subjects[42,44,54] indicates that glycogen synthase or other enzymes in the glycogen synthetic pathway would be worthy of study.

HOW TO FIND THE GENES

A variety of different methodological approaches have been employed in the search for genetic determinants of diabetes: each has merits and disadvantages which need to be appreciated if the often inconsistent results of these studies are to be understood.

Most studies to date have relied on the candidate gene approach and looked for (a) differences between diabetic and controls in the allele frequencies at markers (e.g. restriction fragment length polymorphisms (RFLP)) linked to the candidate gene under consideration (population association studies), and/or (b) linkage between such polymorphic markers and glucose intolerance within pedigrees segregating for diabetes (linkage family studies).

POPULATION ASSOCIATION STUDIES

In the case of population association studies the interpretation of a positive finding is that the marker is linked to a disease susceptibility gene (by implication the candidate gene). However, it is important to realize that the maintenance of a positive association between a marker and disease requires both that (i) the marker be linked to the disease susceptibility gene and (ii) there be linkage disequilibrium between alleles at the marker and the disease locus: the absence of an association does therefore not automatically exclude a candidate gene from involvement in the development of disease. False negative results can also occur where a number of disease-predisposing mutations in the candidate gene are each in linkage disequilibrium with a different marker allele, or simply when the study has insufficient power to detect a difference (particularly likely if the disease-predisposing mutation is in linkage disequilibrium with the more common marker allele[55]).

A more serious pitfall is that population association studies are prone to generate false positive results, arising from unsuspected stratification in the diabetic and control populations (e.g. poor ethnic matching of the two groups) or to survivor effects (where it might be genes for longevity rather than diabetes which are being detected). Despite these caveats, under the right circumstances[55] population studies have the capacity to detect subtle genetic effects (e.g. a minor modifying gene effect) which linkage studies would fail to expose (see below). Subphenotyping of diabetic populations (for example, choosing those of early onset, those with a strong family history, or those with the greatest insulin insensitivity) may increase the chances of demonstrating a true positive effect.

In summary, population association studies are best regarded as a guide to possible genetic effects that require verification by other techniques.

LINKAGE STUDIES

The problems of linkage analysis in complex diseases have been elegantly discussed elsewhere[56]. Principally these are that, for everyday NIDDM, at least, the late age of onset and premature mortality complicates the collection of multigenerational families appropriate for linkage analyses; the late age of onset renders the correct designation of those with normal glucose tolerance uncertain; and that the mode of inheritance (which needs to be specified for linkage analysis) is unknown. To a considerable extent, these difficulties are overcome in the study of MODY, which explains why these families have been extensively used in the study of NIDDM: however, the relevance of MODY to NIDDM remains to be established.

The identification of classes of highly polymorphic markers throughout the genome (variable number of tandem repeats (VNTR) and di/tri/ tetranucleotide repeats e.g. CA repeats[57]) has permitted the construction of dense maps of polymorphic markers which can be used to screen the entire genome for regions linked to the disease of interest, thereby avoiding the need to identify candidate genes. This approach has been termed blind linkage or positional cloning and has proved enormously successful in a number of conditions[58]. Application to a single well-characterized pedigree with MODY has recently identified a region on chromosome 20q linked to glucose intolerance[59,60]. Blind linkage studies in animal models of diabetes may also identify regions linked to disturbed glucose metabolism so that syneteic regions can be studied in man. Such methodology has the capacity to identify new, hitherto unsuspected genes influencing glucose tolerance, the relevance of which can be tested in subjects with everyday NIDDM.

Although often regarded as the critical test for a candidate gene, linkage analysis is highly susceptible to genetic heterogeneity[61] such as may apply in NIDDM: it may be difficult to gather sufficient families to derive evidence for positive linkage when much of the diabetes is not linked to the gene under study (either caused by other genes or environmental effects). Even fairly significant contributions to NIDDM (of the order of 30%) might easily be missed by linkage studies. Only if a particular candidate gene is a major disease susceptibility gene for NIDDM in a particular set of families should linkage analysis have the capacity to detect this linkage (provided sufficient numbers of families are gathered and provided appropriate models for the mode of inheritance and age-related penetrance are employed).

With reference to Figure 1, therefore, linkage analysis is the most appropriate tool for detecting major gene effects as seen in models A and C. However, linkage analysis in NIDDM is most unlikely to provide evidence for the polygenes of model B or the modifying genes of model C: clues to these genes may come from well-designed population association or molecular screening studies.

MOLECULAR SCREENING TECHNIQUES

Given the methodological difficulties of population association and linkage studies, techniques permitting more direct detection of mutations in genes have been developed. Direct sequencing of candidate genes in cohorts of diabetic patients and controls is one option but entails considerable effort. Newer techniques such as polymerase chain reaction—single-strand conformational polymorphisms: (PCR–SSCP)[62] and denaturing gradient gel electrophoresis (DGGE)[63] allow rapid screening of large numbers of diabetic patients and controls in the search for mutations. With SSCP, single base-pair differences in DNA sequence can be detected with 80–100% efficiency, these changes being manifest as differential mobility of the single-stranded PCR product as it migrates through a non-denaturing polyacrylamide gel. Any SSC polymorphisms identified can be sequenced and their likely contribution to disease assessed. If an SSCP-identified variation plays a role in the development of NIDDM it should be possible to demonstrate:

1. That it leads to a change in the primary structure of the protein (or else significant change in the promoter region).

2. That it be seen more commonly in diabetic patients than controls.
3. Ideally, that there is evidence of co-segregation with disease within pedigrees (though this may be difficult to demonstrate for a minor/ modifying gene).
4. That expression of the altered sequence produces abnormalities of transcription or function of the mutated protein.

SHOULD NIDDM BE THE AFFECTED PHENOTYPE TO BE STUDIED?

Given the complex genetic basis of diabetes there may be merit in examining 'intermediate traits' (insulin secretion or insulin resistance) in the hope that these may be simpler to dissect. There is strong evidence, in certain populations at least, that insulin levels (and by implication insulin sensitivity) show familial aggregation[64] and that this may be controlled by a major gene[65,66]. Such an approach would be analogous to that taken by genetic epidemiologists working on coronary artery disease[67]. Recognizing the multiplicity of genetic and environmental determinants for atheroma, the task has been simplified by study of intermediate traits such as low-density lipoprotein (LDL) cholesterol, high-density lipoprotein (HDL) cholesterol and blood pressure. There are, however, important complicating factors when this approach is applied to glucose intolerance. Not least of these is the complex feedback effects of early glucose intolerance on the intermediate traits which underlie it: these are mediated by both physiological (e.g. glucotoxicity[28]) and behavioural (dietary modification, weight change, medication) mechanisms and clearly make the hierarchical relationship of intermediate traits and the major disorder difficult to resolve.

The evidence that NIDDM may be only one manifestation of a group of conditions (including hypertension, dyslipidaemias and vascular disease: syndrome X[68]), resulting from underlying insulin resistance[69], further distorts the relationship of the intermediate trait (insulin level) to the disease phenotype (NIDDM).

WHICH GENES ARE INVOLVED?

The diabetes literature is replete with well over 250 studies of candidate genes and their possible roles in NIDDM, but it is fair to summarize that at an optimistic estimate those candidate genes so far tested account for perhaps 5–10% of the inherited predisposition to NIDDM. For convenience the genes studied are subdivided into four categories, although it should be borne in mind that the classification is somewhat arbitrary.

PRIMARY EFFECT ON β CELL FUNCTION

Insulin Gene

❧ Defects in the insulin gene and in insulin processing have been shown to lead to glucose intolerance in certain rare pedigrees[70]. Population studies in a variety of ethnic groups (Danes[71], Caucasians[72], Japanese[73] and southern Indians[74]) have suggested an association with the class 3 allele of the hypervariable region 5' to the insulin gene, but a number of other studies (in Nauruans[15], Pimas[75], Japanese[76-78], US blacks[79], Mexican-Americans and Tunisians[80]) have failed to support these findings. Linkage analysis studies in MODY and NIDDM have been negative[30,72,81-83]. Sequence studies[84-86] have failed to detect any mutations within the coding region of the insulin gene in over 100 diabetic patients using SSCP and DGGE. However, a minority role for the insulin gene cannot be excluded, particularly given evidence that the polymorphism in the hypervariable region itself may effect insulin gene transcription[87] and the suggestion that alleles at the hypervariable region may determine insulin levels in non-diabetic subjects[88-90].

Amylin

The fact that the majority of patients with NIDDM demonstrate deposition of amyloid protein in their islets[91] led to the identification of amylin (or islet amyloid polypeptide, IAPP) as the monomeric component of islet amyloid. Amylin is co-processed and co-secreted with insulin by β cells[92]; it has been shown to produce insulin resistance albeit at pharmacological doses[93,94]. However, the sequence of the amylin extracted from human islet amyloid is identical with normal amylin[95], and nucleotide sequencing of the coding region of the amylin gene has demonstrated no differences between diabetic patients and controls[96]. Population studies in Caucasians[97] and southern Indians[98] and one linkage study[97] have been negative. A role for amylin as a primary susceptibility gene is effectively excluded.

HLA

Conventional dogma has it that the genetic determinants of NIDDM and IDDM are distinct[99] and that as such HLA has no role in the genetic susceptibility to NIDDM. A number of lines of study suggest that this may not be the case:

1. HLA haplotypes associated with IDDM in Finnish families predict the development of glucose intolerance (with the clinical features of NIDDM) amongst elderly Finnish men[100].

2. Studies in a variety of non-Caucasian populations reveal associations between NIDDM and alleles at HLA Class I and II loci[15,101-106].
3. Associations have been demonstrated between gestational diabetes mellitus and HLA alleles[107] despite the fact that gestational diabetes mellitus is principally a marker for future NIDDM rather than IDDM.
4. HLA DR4 determines the risk of NIDDM in families with IDDM[108].
5. There is an increased risk of IDDM in siblings of an IDDM proband if there is a parent with NIDDM[109,110].

As might be expected if HLA were only a modifying gene for NIDDM, linkage studies in MODY[30] and NIDDM[83,111] have been negative.

The significance of these findings to NIDDM remains uncertain at this stage. Undoubtedly, a proportion of patients initially identified as having NIDDM on clinical grounds can be demonstrated to have a pathology more akin to IDDM, albeit slowly evolving[112]. This does not appear to explain the data in the Finnish elderly men[100], who were mostly diet-controlled with C-peptide values typical of NIDDM and minimal progression of glucose intolerance on follow-up. One possibility which deserves study is that subclinical autoimmune β cell damage (determined in part by HLA haplotype) which fails to progress to IDDM may deplete β cell mass to the extent that glucose intolerance (to all clinical appearances, NIDDM) supervenes with the advent of age- and/or obesity-related insulin resistance.

PRIMARY EFFECT ON INSULIN ACTION

Insulin Receptor Gene

Defects in the insulin receptor gene can also lead to glucose intolerance, as seen in families demonstrating syndromes of extreme insulin resistance[113]. Again, results of population association studies have been inconsistent. McClain and colleagues[114] demonstrated associations between alleles at an Sst1 polymorphism and diabetes; associations have also been reported in Welsh[115] and Chinese–American subjects[116] when haplotypes derived from a number of RFLPs were constructed. There have been many negative population[117-125] and linkage studies[82,83,120-122,126-129] in a variety of ethnic groups. Kusari[130] has sequenced the insulin receptor gene in an individual homozygous for the Sst1 allele identified by McClain[114] and found it to be identical with the published sequence. Recent sequencing and molecular screening studies have demonstrated a number of mutations present at low frequency in diabetic subjects[121,126,131-133] but few of these have as yet met the criteria outlined earlier which would confirm a pathogenetic role in NIDDM. At this stage, it seems likely that abnormalities in the insulin receptor gene account for less than 1% of the inherited predisposition to NIDDM.

Glucose Transporter 1

Given that GLUT1 is the glucose transporter responsible for basal glucose uptake into brain and other tissues, it seems an implausible candidate for NIDDM: defects might be expected to have serious adverse consequences early in life. Reports from one group of an association between diabetes and an allele at an Xba1 RFLP in Caucasians and Japanese[134] have not been substantiated in other studies[116,135–137]. Sibpair analysis[138] and linkage analysis in NIDDM and MODY have proved negative[37,129,139,140] and a contribution of GLUT1 to NIDDM appears unlikely.

Glucose Transporter 4

GLUT4 is the insulin-responsive glucose transporter, responsible for insulin-stimulated glucose uptake into fat and muscle. Defects in GLUT4 activity or expression might underlie the defective glucose transport into peripheral tissues seen in NIDDM[141]. Population association studies have failed to demonstrate an association[142–144] and linkage was excluded in a panel of 91 Caucasian families[139]. SSCP studies have identified a Val to Ile mutation in exon 9 in three of 160 diabetic patients, in a further three of 42 particularly insulin-resistant diabetic patients and in four of 200 controls[131,145,146]. With further study this mutation may be shown to contribute to glucose intolerance in a small number of subjects, but the fact that the vast majority of diabetic patients have normal GLUT4 sequence as judged by SSCP means that it is not a major genetic factor.

Glycogen Synthase

The consistent finding in a number of studies that normoglycaemic first-degree relatives of subjects with NIDDM have a defect of non-oxidative glucose disposal has focused attention on the glycogen synthetic pathway[42,44]. Glycogen synthase activity is reduced in diabetic patients[147] but this may be secondary to reduced activation of glycogen synthase by glycogen synthase phosphatase[148–150]. RFLPs generated by Xba1 restriction have been shown to associate with diabetes in Finns[151–152] but recent sequence studies of glycogen synthase and glycogen synthase phosphatase have failed to reveal any significant mutations in the coding sequences of diabetic subjects[153]. Other proteins in the glycogen synthetic pathway have not been studied.

EFFECT ON β CELL FUNCTION AND INSULIN ACTION

Glucose Transporter 2

GLUT2 is expressed predominantly in β cell and liver and as such abnormalities in this gene could plausibly lead to both defective insulin secretion and apparent insulin insensitivity in the liver[154-156]. Mixed results of population association studies (positive in Caucasians[157]; negative in Caucasians and US blacks[142,158,159]) and negative linkage studies[139] suggest that GLUT2 is not a major gene for diabetes susceptibility but further studies remain to be done.

Glucokinase

Glucokinase has for some time been considered as a highly plausible candidate gene for NIDDM[49]. Expressed in liver and β cells it is responsible for the phosphorylation of glucose to glucose-6-phosphate. In contrast to other hexokinases it has a high K_m value and is not inhibited by glucose-6-phosphate; thus, given that glucose transport into the cell is generally not rate-limiting, rates of glucose phosphorylation vary in tandem with glucose levels within the physiological range. In the β cell, this has led to the suggestion that glucokinase is a critical element of the 'glucose sensor'[49], and that in the liver glucokinase is an important arbiter of hepatic glucose flux. Defects in glucokinase could therefore produce abnormalities of insulin secretion as well as apparent insulin insensitivity at the hepatic level.

Identification of two CA repeats straddling the glucokinase gene[160,161] has permitted these hypotheses to be tested. Groups in Oxford[32] and France[162] have provided unequivocal evidence of linkage between these markers and glucose intolerance in approximately 50% of families segregating for what is described variously as early-onset NIDDM or MODY. An increasing number of distinct mutations[163-165] have been identified in these pedigrees, and expression studies[166] demonstrate that the degree of suppression of activity and affinity of the expressed protein correlate with the severity of glucose intolerance. Members of families carrying these mutations[163,166,167] have a marked β cell secretory defect consistent with an alteration in the setpoint for insulin secretion in the islet; unlike the typical subject with NIDDM, insulin sensitivity and body mass index are normal. The features of glucose intolerance in those families demonstrating linkage to glucokinase are that it is mild (often not reaching WHO criteria for diagnosis of diabetes) and only slowly progressive: the French group have recently described this as 'familial hyper-glycaemia linked to glucokinase' to emphasize the distinction from NIDDM.

So far only a few studies have reported results in populations with classic NIDDM. Positive population association results have been reported in Mauritian Creoles[168] (although the possibilities of a spurious result must be high in such an ethnically mixed group), in US Blacks[169], and south Indians[170], and negative results in Mauritian Indians[168] and Caucasians[171]. Linkage analyses in families with NIDDM have thus far proved negative[170,172,173]), with little evidence for a contribution to glucose intolerance in more than a small minority of families.

It seems unlikely at this stage that glucokinase contributes to more than a small percentage of the inherited predisposition to diabetes mellitus (perhaps 1–5%). However, this represents significantly more than any other candidate gene so far identified and these findings increase considerably our knowledge of potential pathophysiological bases of glucose intolerance.

Mitochondrial

One explanation for the excess of maternal transmission of NIDDM observed in some populations[52,174–176] would be maternal inheritance of mitochondrial DNA mutations. These could lead to defects in oxidative metabolism and hence to defects of glucose sensing at the β cell and of insulin action in other tissues. Diabetes mellitus has been reported in patients with mitochondrial DNA mutations[177]. More recently there have been two reports that, in families segregating for a syndrome of diabetes and sensorineural hearing loss, linkage can be demonstrated between glucose intolerance and defects in mitochondrial DNA[178,179]. In one study the prevalence of these mutations was estimated to be less than 1% in NIDDM[178].

LOCI ARISING FROM POSITIONAL CLONING

Adenosine Deaminase

The RW pedigree is a massive well-characterized pedigree segregating for MODY and (in certain branches of the family) for late-onset NIDDM as well. As mentioned earlier, this family has been studied by two groups who using 'positional cloning' have produced strong evidence for linkage between early-onset glucose intolerance and a region of chromosome 20q close to the adenosine deaminase (ADA) gene[59,60]. The gene responsible has not been identified and seems to be a rare cause of glucose intolerance since studies in other pedigrees indicate linkage to ADA in only a small number of families with MODY and NIDDM[31,173]. It is to be hoped that, despite this, characterization of the responsible gene will provide new insights into the pathophysiology of glucose intolerance.

GENES AND ENVIRONMENT: AN INTERACTION

All the evidence cited above has sought to emphasize the role which genes are likely to play in the development of NIDDM. It is, however, impossible to consider genetic effects in isolation since the effects of disease susceptibility loci are clearly extensively modified by the prevailing environment.

The significant role of the environment is evident in migration studies (e.g.

Chinese migrants to Mauritius[180]), in the rapid, 'epidemic' increase in the prevalence of NIDDM in Pimas and Nauruans over the course of half a century[16] and by the fact that the concordance for NIDDM in MZ twins is substantially less than 100%[3,6]. Many studies have sought to define those environmental factors which are most critical: age, obesity and levels of exercise seem to be the dominant forces[7,181,182]. In particular, the relationship of obesity and diabetes is so strong that the genetic and environmental determinants of the two may be difficult to divorce. Obesity is itself strongly influenced by genetic factors[183,184] in the context of a permissive environment, and these genes (as yet unidentified) could be considered as modifying genes for diabetes.

In the absence of a clear understanding of the specific genetic determinants of glucose intolerance, even less is known about the ways in which genes and environment may interact to lead to glucose intolerance. It is safe to assume, however, by analogy with studies of hyperlipidaemias, that these interactions will be complex. For example, the E4 isoform of apolipoprotein E is only associated with high lipid levels in populations with a high dietary fat intake[67]. Furthermore, while in the general population the E2E2 genotype is associated with a low plasma cholesterol, a small proportion of such individuals have marked (type III) hyperlipidaemia, due to interaction of apoE genotype and other (genetic and/or environmental) factors, as yet unknown[67].

The difficulty of distinguishing genetic and environmental effects is emphasized by evidence that environmental influences operating in the intrauterine period can mimic genetic effects. Studies in a number of populations have indicated that transmission of NIDDM from parent to child is more likely through the maternal than the paternal line[174-176] and a number of explanations have been advanced for this.

Genetic mechanisms, including genetic imprinting and transmission through mitochondrial DNA (see above), may offer partial explanation. However, there is evidence for 'epigenetic' mechanisms such that a fetus raised in the uterus of a hyperglycaemic mother is predisposed to the later development of NIDDM. Pettitt found that the prevalence of NIDDM in the offspring of Pima mothers was significantly greater if the mother was diabetic at the time of pregnancy than if the mother developed diabetes only after the pregnancy (45% versus 8.6% in the 20–24-year age group[52]). A number of animal models of gestational diabetes have reproduced this effect. Female rats rendered hyperglycaemic by low-dose streptozotocin[185] and by glucose infusion[186] produce offspring that themselves display mild glucose intolerance. Since the intolerance of the offspring is often exacerbated by pregnancy, glucose intolerance can be 'transmitted' to subsequent generations. The precise mechanism of this effect is as yet unclear as studies of the offspring have suggested insulin resistance in some cases[187] and failure of insulin secretion in others[188].

Recent work by Hales and Barker has suggested that predisposition to later glucose intolerance can also follow intrauterine and perinatal malnutrition. In studies of elderly men born in Hertfordshire they have reported that a high prevalence of glucose intolerance in later life is associated with a history of low birth weight[189]. The 'thrifty phenotype' hypothesis[53] advocates that poor nutrition in pregnancy and early life is responsible for a prioritisation of nutrient supply which diverts limited resources to neurological development at the expense of the viscera (including the β cells). Given their limited capacity to regenerate after the first years of life, such an individual is left with a suboptimal complement of β cells. Provided this individual remains thin and relatively insulin-sensitive, normal glucose homeostasis can be maintained; however, insulin resistance consequent on advancing age, obesity or pregnancy may render this β cell insufficiency manifest as diabetes. This hypothesis is fully consistent with a major genetic contribution to NIDDM, especially as the majority of low birth-weight high-risk subjects in the studies of Hales and colleagues did not develop glucose intolerance in later life. The candidate genes would still be those described, although those involved in β cell replication and growth might assume more importance (see Chapter 15).

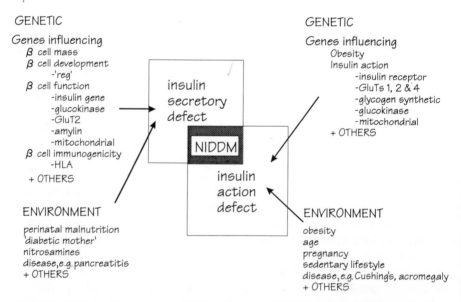

GENETIC

Genes influencing
  β cell mass
  β cell development
    -'reg'
  β cell function
    -insulin gene
    -glucokinase
    -GluT2
    -amylin
    -mitochondrial
  β cell immunogenicity
    -HLA
  + OTHERS

ENVIRONMENT

perinatal malnutrition
'diabetic mother'
nitrosamines
disease,e.g.pancreatitis
+ OTHERS

GENETIC

Genes influencing
  Obesity
  Insulin action
    -insulin receptor
    -GluTs 1, 2 & 4
    -glycogen synthetic
    -glucokinase
    -mitochondrial
  + OTHERS

ENVIRONMENT

obesity
age
pregnancy
sedentary lifestyle
disease,e.g.Cushing's, acromegaly
+ OTHERS

insulin secretory defect

NIDDM

insulin action defect

Figure 2   Genes and environment and their contribution to NIDDM. In rare instances single genes alone can lead to NIDDM, but in the majority of instances it seems likely that NIDDM arises from a combined defect of β cell function and insulin action, either of which can in principle have a genetic or environmental basis

CONCLUSION

Any attempt, given our present state of knowledge, to produce a 'grand unified' theory for the development of NIDDM can only be provisional (Figure 2) particularly given likely ethnic differences in the genetic and environmental determinants of glucose intolerance. Clearly, genetic influences play a major part in the development of NIDDM. It seems likely that genes influencing both insulin secretion and insulin action are involved. Everyday NIDDM is likely to be a heterogeneous condition in which the specific genetic determinants differ between individuals and between populations; only a minority of these determinants have been identified thus far. Genetic effects interact with environmental influences which can have dramatic effects on the expression of any inherited predisposition. Little is known about the ways in which these interactions occur, but there seems no doubt that they are interdependent. What is yet to be resolved is whether there is a major gene for NIDDM which can explain part of the genetic predisposition to the disease or whether NIDDM is a truly polygenic disease.

REFERENCES

1 Barnett AH, Eff C, Leslie RDG, Pyke DA. Diabetes in identical twins: a study of 200 pairs. *Diabetologia* 1981; **20**: 87–93.
2 Harvald B, Hauge M. Selection in diabetes in modern society. *Acta Med Scand* 1963; **173**: 459–65.
3 Matsuda A, Kusuya T. Concordance rate of type 2 (non-insulin-dependent) diabetes among monozygotic and dizygotic twins. *Diabetologia* 1992; **35** (Suppl 1): A139.
4 Hunt SC, Hasstedt SJ, Kuida H, et al. Genetic heritability and common environmental components of resting and stressed blood pressures, lipids and body mass index in Utah pedigrees and twins. *Am J Epidemiol* 1989; **129**: 625–38.
5 Then Berg H. The genetic aspect of diabetes mellitus. *J Am Med Assoc* 1939; **112**: 1091.
6 Newman B, Selby J, King M-C, et al. Concordance for type 2 (non-insulin-dependent) diabetes mellitus in male twins. *Diabetologia* 1987; **30**: 763–8.
7 Zimmet P. Type 2 (non-insulin-dependent) diabetes: an epidemiological overview. *Diabetologia* 1982; **22**: 399–411.
8 Neel JV. The thrifty genotype revisited. In: *The Genetics of Diabetes Mellitus* (eds J Köbberling, R Tattersall) Academic Press, London, 1982, pp 283–93.
9 Ramachandran A, Jali MV, Mohan V, Snehalatha C, Viswanathan M. High prevalence of diabetes in an urban population in south India. *Br Med J* 1988; **297**: 587–9.
10 Ramachandran A, Snehalatha C, Dharmaraj D, Viswanathan M. Prevalence of glucose intolerance in Asian Indians: urban–rural difference and significance of upper body adiposity. *Diabetes Care* 1992; **15**: 1348–55.

11 Zimmet P, Taylor R, Ram P, et al. Prevalence of diabetes and impaired glucose tolerance in the biracial (Melanesian and Indian) population of Fiji: a rural–urban comparison. *Am J Epidemiol* 1983; **118**: 673–88.
12 Mather HM, Keen H. The Southall Diabetes Survey: prevalence of diabetes in Asians and Europeans. *Br Med J* 1985; **291**: 1081–4.
13 Marine N, Edelstein O, Jackson WPU, Vinik AI. Diabetic hyperglycaemia and glycosuria among Indians, Malays and Africans (Bantu) in Cape Town, South Africa. *Diabetes* 1969; **18**: 840–57.
14 Poon-King T, Henry MV, Rampersad F. Prevalence and natural history of diabetes in Trinidad. *Lancet* 1968; **i**: 155–60.
15 Serjeantson S, Owerbach D, Zimmet P, Nerup J, Thoma K. Genetics of diabetes in Nauru: effects of foreign admixture, HLA antigens and the insulin-gene-linked polymorphism. *Diabetologia* 1983; **25**: 13–17.
16 Knowler WC, Pettitt DJ, Saad MF, Bennett PH. Diabetes mellitus in the Pima Indians: incidence, risk factors and pathogenesis. *Diabetes Metab Rev* 1990; **6**: 1–27.
17 Brosseau JD, Eelkema RC, Crawford AC, Abe TA. Diabetes among the three affiliated tribes: correlation with degree of Indian inheritance. *Am J Public Health* 1979; **69**: 1277–8.
18 Gardner LI, Stern MP, Haffner SM, et al. Prevalence of diabetes in Mexican Americans: relationship to percentage of gene pool derived from native American sources. *Diabetes* 1984; **33**: 86–92.
19 Köbberling J, Tillil H. Empirical risk figures for first degree relatives of non-insulin-dependent diabetics. In: *The Genetics of Diabetes Mellitus* (eds J Köbberling, R Tattersall) Academic Press, London, 1982, pp 201–9.
20 Cooke AM, Fitzgerald MG, Malins JM, Pyke Da. Diabetes in children of diabetic couples. *Br Med J* 1966; **2**: 674–6.
21 Kahn CB, Soeldner JS, Gleason RE, et al. Clinical and chemical diabetes in offspring of diabetic couples. *N Engl J Med* 1969; **281**: 343–7.
22 Tattersall RB, Fajans SS. Prevalence of diabetes and glucose intolerance in 199 offspring of thirty-seven conjugal diabetic parents. *Diabetes* 1975; **24**: 452–62.
23 Viswanathan M, Mohan V, Snehalatha C, Ramachandran A. High prevalence of type 2 (non-insulin-dependent) diabetes among the offspring of conjugal type 2 diabetic parents in India. *Diabetologia* 1985; **28**: 907–10.
24 Tattersall RB. Mild familial diabetes with dominant inheritance. *Q J Med* 1974; **170**: 339–57.
25 Zimmet, P, Whitehouse S. Bimodality of fasting and two-hour glucose tolerance distributions in a Micronesian population. *Diabetes* 1978; **27**: 793–800.
26 Raper LR, Taylor R, Zimmet P, Milne B, Balkau B. Bimodality in glucose tolerance distributions in the urban Polynesian population of Western Samoa. *Diabetes Res* 1984; **1**: 19–26.
27 Rushforth NB, Bennett PH, Steinberg AG, Burch TA, Miller M. Diabetes in the Pima Indians: evidence of bimodality in glucose tolerance distributions. *Diabetes* 1971; **20**: 756–65.
28 Rossetti, L, Giaccori A, De Fronzo RA. Glucose toxicity. *Diabetes Care* 1990; **13**: 610–30.
29 Tattersall R, Fajans S. A difference between the inheritance of classic juvenile-onset and maturity-onset type diabetes of young people. *Diabetes* 1975; **24**: 44–53.
30 Fajans S. Scope and heterogeneous nature of MODY. *Diabetes Care* 1990; **13**: 49–64.

31 Froguel Ph, Velho G, Fang S, et al. Heterogeneity of maturity-onset diabetes of the young (MODY) genetics: linkage analysis of the adenosine deaminase gene region in 23 French families. *Diabetes* 1992; **41** (Suppl 1): 91A.

32 Hattersley AT, Turner RC, Permutt MA, et al. Linkage of type 2 diabetes to the glucokinase gene. *Lancet* 1992; **339**; 1307–10.

33 O'Rahilly S, Spivey RS, Holman RR, et al. Type II diabetes of early onset: a distinct clinical and genetic syndrome? *Brit Med J* 1987; **294**: 923–5.

34 O'Rahilly S, Turner R. Early onset type 2 diabetes vs. maturity onset diabetes of youth: evidence for the existence of two distinct diabetic syndromes. *Diabetic Med* 1988; **5**: 224–9.

35 Lalouel JM, Morton NE. Complex segregation analysis with pointers. *Hum Hered* 1981; **31**: 312–321.

36 Serjeantson S, Zimmet P. Diabetes in the Pacific: evidence for a major gene. In: *Diabetes Mellitus: Recent Knowledge on Aetiology, Complications and Treatment* (eds S Baba, M Gould, P Zimmet) Academic Press, Sydney, 1984, pp 23–40.

37 Serjeantson SW, Zimmet P. Genetics of non-insulin dependent diabetes mellitus in 1990. *Baillière's Clin Endocrinol Metab* 1991; **5**: 477–93.

38 Elston RC, Namboodiri KK, Nino HV, Pollitzer WS. Studies on blood and urine glucose in Seminole Indians: indications for segregation of a major gene. *Am J. Hum Genet*, 1974; **26**: 13–34.

39 McCarthy MI, Hitman GA, Morton N, et al. Type 2 diabetes in South Indians is a polygenic disease: preliminary results of a family study. *Diabetic Med* 1992; **9** (Suppl 1): A23.

40 Rich SS. Mapping genes in diabetes: genetic epidemiological perspective. *Diabetes* 1990; **39**: 1315–19.

41 Rimoin D, Rotter J. Genetic syndromes associated with diabetes and glucose intolerance. In: *The Genetics of Diabetes Mellitus* (eds J. Köbberling, R Tattersall) Academic Press, London, 1982, pp 149–81.

42 Eriksson J, Franssila-Kallunki A, Ekstrand A, et al. Early metabolic defects in persons at increased risk for non-insulin-dependent diabetes mellitus. *N Engl J Med* 1989; **321**: 337–43.

43 O'Rahilly S, Turner R, Matthews D. Impaired pulsatile secretion of insulin in relatives of patients with non-insulin-dependent diabetes. *N Engl J Med* 1988; **318**: 1255–30.

44 Shulman G, Rothman D, Jue T, et al. Quantitation of muscle glycogen synthesis in normal subjects and subjects with non-insulin-dependent diabetes by ^{13}C nuclear magnetic resonance spectroscopy. *N Engl J Med* 1989; **322**: 223–228.

45 Ward K, Johnston CLW, Beard JC, Benedetti TJ, Porte D. Abnormality of islet B-cell function, insulin action and fat distribution in women with histories of gestational diabetes: relationship to obesity. *J Clin Endocrinol Metab*, 1985; **61**: 1039–45.

46 Efendic S, Hanson U, Persson B, Wajngot A, Luft R. Glucose tolerance, insulin release and insulin sensitivity in normal-weight women with previous gestational diabetes mellitus. *Diabetes* 1987; **36**: 413–19.

47 Dornhorst A, Chan SP, Gelding SV, et al. Ethnic differences in insulin secretion in women at risk of future diabetes. *Diabetic Med* 1992; **9**: 258–62.

48 Turner R, O'Rahilly S, Levy J, Rudenski A, Clark A. Does type II diabetes arise from a major gene defect producing insulin resistance or β-cell dysfunction? In: *Genes and Gene Products in the Development of Diabetes Mellitus* (eds J. Nerup, T Mandrup-Poulsen, B Hökfelt) Elsevier, Amsterdam, 1989, pp 171–80.

49 Matschinsky FM. Glucokinase as glucose sensor and metabolic signal generator in pancreatic beta-cells and hepatocytes. *Diabetes* 1990; **39**: 647–52.

50 Efendic S, Luft R, Wajngot A. Aspects of the pathogenesis of type 2 diabetes. *Endocr Rev* 1990; **5**: 395–409.

51 Okamoto H, Yamamoto H, Takasawa S, et al. Molecular mechanism of degeneration, oncogenesis and regeneration of pancreatic B-cells of islets of Langerhans. In: *Frontiers in Diabetes Research: Lessons from Animal Diabetes II* (eds E Shafrir, AE Renold) John Libbey and Co, London, 1988, pp 149–57.

52 Pettitt DJ, Aleck KA, Baird HR, et al. Congenital susceptibility to NIDDM: role of intrauterine environment. *Diabetes* 1988; **37**: 622–8.

53 Hales CN, Barker DJP. Type 2 (non-insulin-dependent) diabetes mellitus: the thrifty phenotype hypothesis. *Diabetologia* 1992; **35**: 595–601.

54 Vaag A, Henriksen JE, Beck-Nielsen H. Defect in insulin activation of glycogen synthase in skeletal muscles in first-degree relatives to patients with type 2 (non-insulin-dependent) diabetes mellitus. *Diabetologia* 1991; **34** (Suppl 1): A70.

55 Cox NJ, Bell GI. Disease associations: chance, artifact or susceptibility genes? *Diabetes* 1989; **38**: 947–50.

56 O'Rahilly S, Wainscoat JS, Turner RC. Type 2 (non-insulin-dependent) diabetes mellitus: new genetics for old nightmares. *Diabetologia* 1988; **31**: 407–14.

57 Hearne CM, Ghosh S, Todd JA. Microsatellites for linkage analysis of genetic traits. *Trends Genet* 1992; **8**: 288–94.

58 Collins FS. Positional cloning: let's not call it reverse anymore. *Nature Genet* 1992; **1**: 3–6.

59 Bell GI, Xiang K-S, Newman MV, et al. Gene for non-insulin-dependent diabetes mellitus (maturity onset diabetes of the young subtype) is linked to DNA polymorphism on human chromosome 20q. *Proc Natl Acad Sci USA* 1991; **88**: 1484–8.

60 Bowden DW, Gravius TC, Akots G, Fajans SS. Identification of genetic markers flanking the locus for maturity-onset diabetes of the young on human chromosome 20. *Diabetes* 1992; **41**: 88–92.

61 Lander ES, Botstein D. Mapping complex genetic traits in humans: new methods using a complete RFLP linkage map. *Cold Spring Harbor Symp Quant Biol* 1986; **LI**: 49–62.

62 Orita M, Suzuki Y, Sekiya T, Hayashi K. Rapid and sensitive detection of point mutations and DNA polymorphisms using the polymerase chain reaction. *Genomics* 1989; **5**: 874–9.

63 Gray MR. Detection of DNA sequence polymorphisms in human genomic DNA by using denaturing gradient gel blots. *Am J Hum Genet* 1992; **50**: 331–46.

64 Martin BC, Warram J, Rosner B, et al. Familial clustering of insulin sensitivity. *Diabetes* 1992; **41**: 850–4.

65 Bogardus C, Lillioja S, Nyomba BL, et al. Distribution of in vivo insulin action in Pima Indians as mixture of three normal distributions. *Diabetes* 1989; **38**: 1423–32.

66 Schumacher MC, Hasstedt SJ, Hunt SC, Williams RR, Elbein SC. Major gene effect for insulin levels in familial NIDDM pedigrees. *Diabetes* 1992; **41**: 416–23.

67 Humphries S, Dunning A, Tybjærg-Hansen A, Talmud P. The use of molecular biology techniques to analyse a multifactorial trait: atherosclerosis as an example. In: *Genes and Gene Products in the Development of Diabetes Mellitus* (eds J Nerup, T Mandrup-Poulsen, B Hökfelt) Elsevier, Amsterdam, 1989; pp 359–71.

68 Reaven G. Role of insulin resistance in human disease. *Diabetes* 1988; **37**: 1595–1607.

69 Ferranini E, Haffner SM, Mitchell BD, Stern MP. Hyperinsulinaemia: the key

feature of a cardiovascular and metabolic syndrome. *Diabetologia* 1991; **34**: 416–22.

70 Gabbay K. The insulinopathies. *N Engl J Med* 1980; **302**: 165–7.

71 Owerbach D, Nerup J. Restriction fragment length polymorphism of the insulin gene in diabetes mellitus. *Diabetes* 1982; **31**: 275–7.

72 Hitman G, Jowett N, Williams L, et al. Polymorphisms in the 5′ flanking region of the insulin gene and non-insulin-dependent diabetes. *Clin Sci* 1984; **66**: 383–8.

73 Nomura M, Iwama N, Mukai M, et al. High frequency of class 3 allele in the human insulin gene in Japanese type 2 (non-insulin-dependent) diabetic patients with a family history of diabetes. *Diabetologia* 1986; **29**: 402–4.

74 Kambo P, Hitman G, Mohan V, et al. The genetic predisposition to fibrocalculous pancreatic diabetes. *Diabetologia* 1989; **32**: 45–51.

75 Knowler W, Pettitt D, Vasquez B, et al. Polymorphisms in the 5′ flanking region of the human insulin gene: relationships with non-insulin-dependent diabetes mellitus, glucose and insulin concentrations and diabetes treatment in the Pima Indians. *J Clin Invest* 1984; **74**: 2129–35.

76 Awata T, Shibisaki Y, Hirai H, et al. Restriction fragment length polymorphism of the insulin gene region in Japanese diabetic and non-diabetic subjects. *Diabetologia* 1985; **28**: 911–13.

77 Haneda M, Kobayashi M, Maegawa H, Shigeta Y. Low frequency of the large insertion in the human insulin gene in Japanese. *Diabetes* 1986; **35**: 115–18.

78 Takeda J, Seino Y, Fukumoto H, et al. 1986; The polymorphism linked to the human insulin gene: its lack of association with either IDDM or NIDDM in Japanese. *Acta Endocrinol (Copenh)* 1986; **113**: 268–71.

79 Elbein S, Rotwein P, Permutt A, et al. Lack of association of the polymorphic locus in the 5′-flanking region of the human insulin gene and diabetes in American Blacks. *Diabetes* 1985; **34**: 433–9.

80 Frazier ML, Ferrell RE, Arem R, Chamakhi S, Field JB. Restriction fragment length polymorphism of the human insulin gene region among type II diabetic Mexican Americans and Tunisians. *Res Commun Chem Pathol Pharmacol* 1986; **52**: 371–86.

81 Elbein SC, Corsetti L, Goldgar D, Skolnick M, Permutt MA. Insulin gene in familial NIDDM: lack of linkage in Utah Mormon Pedigrees. *Diabetes* 1988; **37**: 569–76.

82 Elbein SC, Ward WK, Beard JC, Permutt MA. Familial NIDDM: molecular-genetic analysis and assessment of insulin action and pancreatic B-cell function. *Diabetes* 1988; **37**: 377–82.

83 Cox NJ, Epstein PA, Spielman RS. Linkage studies on NIDDM and the insulin and insulin-receptor genes. *Diabetes* 1989; **38**: 653–8.

84 Raben N, Barbetti F, Cama A, et al. Normal coding sequence of insulin gene in Pima Indians and Nauruans, two groups with highest prevalence of type II diabetes. *Diabetes* 1991; **40**: 118–22.

85 Raben N, Barbetti F, Gejman P, et al. Denaturing gradient gel electrophoresis exonerates the enhancer/promoter region of the insulin gene in hyperinsulinaemic Pimas, Nauruans and Mexican Americans. *Diabetes* 1991; **40** (Suppl 1): 93A.

86 Olansky L, Janssen R, Welling C, Permutt MA. Variability of the insulin gene in American Blacks with NIDDM: analysis by single strand conformational polymorphisms. *Diabetes* 1992; **41**: 742–9.

87 Tadkeda J, Ishii S, Seino Y, Imamoto F, Imura H. Negative regulation of human insulin gene expression by the 5′-flanking region in non-pancreatic cells. *FEBS Lett* 1989; **247**: 41–5.

88 Weaver JU, Kopelman PG, Hitman GA. Central obesity and hyperinsulinaemia

in women are associated with polymorphism in the 5' flanking region of the human insulin gene. *Eur J Clin Invest* 1992; **22**: 265–70.

89 Cocozza S, Riccardi G, Monticelli A, et al. Polymorphism of the 5' end flanking region of the insulin gene is associated with reduced insulin secretion in healthy individuals. *Eur J Clin Invest* 1988; **18**: 582–6.

90 Amos CI, Cohen JC, Srinivasan SR, et al. Polymorphisms in the 5' flanking region of the insulin gene and its potential relation to cardiovascular disease risk: observation in a biracial community. The Bogalusa Heart Study. *Atherosclerosis* 1989; **79**: 51–7.

91 Clark A. Islet amyloid and type 2 diabetes. *Diabetic Med* 1989; **6**: 561–7.

92 Kahn SE, D'Alessio DA, Schwartz MW, et al. Evidence of cosecretion of islet amyloid polypeptide and insulin by beta-cells. *Diabetes* 1990; **39**: 634–8.

93 Bretherton-Watt D, Gilbey SG, Ghatei MA, et al. Very high concentrations of islet amyloid polypeptide are necessary to alter the insulin response to intravenous glucose in man. *J Clin Endocrinol & Metab* 1992; **74**: 1032–5.

94 Steiner DF, Ohagi S, Nagamatsu S, Bell GI, Nishi M. Is islet amyloid polypeptide a significant factor in pathogenesis or pathophysiology of diabetes? *Diabetes* 1991; **40**: 305–9.

95 Cooper GJS, Willis AC, Clark A, et al. Purification and characterization of a peptide from amyloid-rich pancreases of type 2 diabetic patients. *Proc Natl Acad Sci USA* 1987; **84**: 8628–32.

96 Nishi M, Bell GI, Steiner DF. Islet amyloid polypeptide (amylin): no evidence of an abnormal precursor sequence in 25 type 2 (non-insulin-dependent) diabetic patients. *Diabetologia* 1990; **33**: 628–30.

97 Cook JTE, Patel PP, Clark A, et al. Non-linkage of the islet amyloid polypeptide gene with type 2 (non-insulin-dependent) diabetes mellitus. *Diabetologia* 1991; **34**: 103–8.

98 McCarthy MI, Hitman GA, Mohan V, et al. The islet amyloid polypeptide gene and non-insulin dependent diabetes mellitus in South Indians. *Diabetes Res Clin Pract* 1992; **18**: 31–4.

99 World Health Organization Study Group. Diabetes mellitus. *WHO Tech Rep Ser*, no 727.

100 Tuomilehto-Wolf E, Tuomilehto J, Hitman GA, et al. The genetic susceptibility to diabetes (non-insulin-dependent and insulin-dependent diabetes mellitus) and glucose intolerance is located in the HLA region on chromasome 6. *Br Med J* 1993; in press.

101 Briggs B, Jackson W, DuToit E, Botha M. The histocompatibility (HLA) antigen distribution in diabetes in Southern African Blacks (Xhosa). *Diabetes* 1980; **29**: 68–71.

102 Williams R, Knowler W, Butler W, et al. HLA-A2 and type 2 (non-insulin-dependent) diabetes mellitus in Pima Indians: an association of allele frequency with age. *Diabetologia* **21**: 460–3.

103 Omar M, Hammond M, Motala A, Seedat M. HLA class 1 and II antigens in South African Indians with NIDDM. *Diabetes* 1988; **37**: 796–9.

104 Bhatia K, Patel M, Gorogo M. Type 2 (non-insulin-dependent) diabetes mellitus and HLA antigens in Papua New Guinea. *Diabetologia* 1981; **27**: 370–2.

105 Kirk R, Ranford P, Serjeantson S, et al. HLA, complement C2, C4, properdin factor B and glyoxylase types in South Indian diabetetics. *Diabetes Res Clin Pract* 1984; **1**: 41–7.

106 Serjeantson S, Ryan D, Ram P, Zimmet P. HLA and non-insulin dependent diabetes in Fiji Indians. *Med J Aust* 1981; **1**: 462–3.

107 Freinkel N, Metzger BE, Phelps RL, et al. Gestational diabetes mellitus: heterogeneity of maternal age, weight, insulin secretion, HLA antigens and islet cell antibodies and the impact of maternal metabolism on pancreatic beta-cell and somatic development on the offspring. *Diabetes* 1985; **34** (Suppl 2): 1–7.

108 Rich SS. Shared genetic susceptibility of type 1 (insulin-dependent) and type 2 (non-insulin-dependent) diabetes mellitus: contributions of HLA and haptoglobin. *Diabetologia* 1991; **34**: 350–5.

109 Chern MM, Anderson VE, Barbosa J. Empirical risk for insulin-dependent diabetes (IDD) in sibs: further definition of genetic heterogeneity. *Diabetes* 1982; **31**: 1115–18.

110 Wagener DK, Sachs JM, LaPorte RE, Macgregor JM. The Pittsburgh study of insulin-dependent diabetes mellitus: risk for diabetes among relatives of IDDM. *Diabetes* 1982; **31**: 136–44.

111 McCarthy MI, Hitman GA, Mohan V, et al. HLA is not a major gene for type 2 diabetes in South India. *Diabetic Med* 1992; **9** (Suppl 2): p 4.

112 Groop L, Groop P-H, Koskimies S. Relationship between β cell function and HLA antigens in patients with type 2 (non-insulin-dependent) diabetes. *Diabetologia* 1986; **29**: 757–60.

113 Taylor SI, Cama A, Accili D, et al. Molecular genetics of insulin resistant diabetes mellitus. *J Clin Endocrinol Metab* 1991; **73**: 1158–63.

114 McClain D, Henry R, Ullrich A, Olefsky J. Restriction-fragment-length polymorphism in insulin-receptor gene and insulin resistance in NIDDM. *Diabetes* 1988; **37**: 1071–5.

115 Morgan R, Bishop A, Owens DR, et al. Allelic variants at insulin-receptor and insulin gene loci and susceptibility to NIDDM in Welsh population. *Diabetes* 1990; **39**: 1479–84.

116 Xiang K-S, Cox N, Sanz N, et al. Insulin-receptor and apolipoprotein genes contribute to development of NIDDM in Chinese Americans. *Diabetes* 1989; **37**: 17–23.

117 Sten-Linder M, Vilhelmsdotter S, Wedell A, et al. Screening for insulin receptor gene DNA polymorphisms associated with glucose intolerance in a Scandinavian population. *Diabetologia* 1991; **34**: 265–70.

118 Takeda J, Seino Y, Yoshimasa Y, et al. Restriction fragment length polymorphism (RFLP) of the human insulin receptor gene in Japanese: its possible usefulness as a genetic marker. *Diabetologia* 1986; **29**: 667–9.

119 Elbein S, Corsetti L, Ullrich A, Permutt A. Multiple restriction fragment length polymorphisms at the insulin receptor locus: a highly informative marker for linkage analysis. *Proc Natl Acad Sci USA* 1986; **83**: 5223–7.

120 Hitman G, Karir P, Mohan V, et al. A genetic analysis of type 2 (non-insulin-dependent) diabetes mellitus in Punjabi Sikhs and British Caucasoid patients. *Diabetic Med* 1987; **4**: 526–30.

121 Elbein S. Molecular and clinical characterization of an insertional polymorphism of the insulin-receptor gene. *Diabetes* 1989; **38**: 737–43.

122 O'Rahilly S, Trembath R, Patel P, et al. Linkage analysis of the human insulin receptor gene in type 2 (non-insulin-dependent) diabetic families and a family with maturity onset diabetes of the young. *Diabetologia* 1988; **31**: 792–7.

123 Oelbaum RS, Bouloux PMG, Li SR, et al. Insulin receptor gene polymorphisms type 2 (non-insulin-dependent) diabetes mellitus. *Diabetologia* 1991; **34**: 260–4.

124 Raboudi S, Mitchell B, Stern M, et al. Type II diabetes mellitus and polymorphism of insulin-receptor gene in Mexican Americans. *Diabetes*, 1989; **38**: 975–80.

125 Permutt A, McGill J, Elbein S, Province M, Bogardus C, Insulin receptor gene

polymorphisms (Rflps) in American Blacks and Pima Indians: an assessment of the use of RFLPs in evaluating a candidate locus for NIDDM. In: *Genes and Gene Products in the Development of Diabetes Mellitus* (eds J Nerup, T Mandrup-Poulsen, B Hökfelt) Elsevier, Amsterdam, 1989, pp 249–62.

126 Elbein S, Sorensen LK. Genetic variation in insulin receptor beta-chain exons among members of familial type 2 (non-insulin-dependent) diabetic pedigrees. *Diabetologia* 1991; **34**: 742–9.

127 Elbein SC, Sorensen LK, Taylor M. Linkage analysis of insulin-receptor gene in familial NIDDM. *Diabetes* 1992; **41** 648–52.

128 Elbein S, Borecki I, Corsetti L, et al. Linkage analysis of the human insulin receptor gene and maturity onset diabetes of the young. *Diabetologia* 1987; **30**: 641–7.

129 Vinik A, Cox N, Xiang K, Fajans S, Bell G. Linkage studies of maturity onset diabetes of the young—RW pedigree. *Diabetologia* 1988; **31**: 778–80.

130 Kusari J, Olefsky JM, Strahl C, McClain DA. Insulin-receptor cDNA sequence in NIDDM patient homozygous for insulin receptor gene RFLP. *Diabetes* 1991; **40**: 249–54.

131 O'Rahilly S, Krook A, Morgan R, et al. Insulin receptor and insulin-responsive glucose transporter (GLUT 4) mutations and polymorphisms in a Welsh type 2 (non-insulin-dependent) diabetic population. *Diabetologia* 1992; **35**: 486–69.

132 O'Rahilly S, Choi WH, Patel P, et al. Detection of mutations in insulin-receptor gene in NIDDM patients by analysis of single-stranded conformational polymorphisms. *Diabetes* 1991; **40**: 777–82.

133 Cocozza S, Porcellini A, Riccardi G, et al. NIDDM associated with mutation in tyrosine kinase domain of insulin receptor gene. *Diabetes* 1992; **41**: 521–6.

134 Li S, Oelbaum R, Baroni M, Stock J, Galton D. Association of genetic variant of the glucose transporter with non-insulin-dependent diabetes mellitus. *Lancet* 1988; **ii**: 368–70.

135 Kaku K, Matsutani A, Mueckler M, Permutt A. Polymorphisms of HepG2/erythrocyte glucose-transporter gene: linkage relationships and implications for genetic analysis of NIDDM. *Diabetes* 1990; **39**: 49–56.

136 Cox N, Xiang K-S, Bell G, Karam J. Glucose transporter gene and non-insulin-dependent diabetes. *Lancet* 1988; **ii**: 793–4.

137 Li S, Oelbaum R, Bouloux P, et al. Restriction site polymorphisms at the human HepG2 glucose transporter gene locus in Caucasian and West Indian subjects with non-insulin-dependent diabetes mellitus. *Hum Hered* 1990; **40**: 38–44.

138 Baroni MG, Alcolado JC, Galton DJ, Andreani D, Pozzilli P. Sib-pair analysis of the GLUT1 glucose transporter gene in type 2 (non-insulin-dependent) diabetes mellitus. *Diabetologia* 1992; **35** (Suppl 1): A72.

139 Lesage S, Vionnet N, Froguel P, et al. Non-linkage of glucose transporters genes with type 2 diabetes mellitus in 86 multiplex diabetic families. *Diabetologia* 1991; **34** (Suppl 1): A99.

140 O'Rahilly S, Patel P, Wainscoat J, Turner R. Analysis of the HepG2/erythrocyte glucose transporter locus in a family with type 2 (non-insulin-dependent) diabetes and obesity. *Diabetologia* 1989; **32**: 266–9.

141 Dohm GL, Tapscott EB, Pories WJ, et al. An in vitro human muscle preparation suitable for metabolic studies. *J Clin Invest* 1988; **82**: 486–94.

142 Matsutani A, Koranyi L, Cox N, Permutt MA. Polymorphisms of GLUT2 and GLUT4 genes: use in evaluation of genetic susceptibility to NIDDM in Blacks. *Diabetes* 1990; **39**: 1534–42.

143 Alcolado JC, Baroni MG. Restriction fragment length polymorphisms at the GLUT4 and GLUT1 gene loci in type 2 diabetes. *Diabetic Med* 1992; **9**: 58–60.

144 Weaver J, Mohan V, Kopelman P, Hitman G, Viswanathan M. Transracial study of insulin sensitive glucose transporter in type 2 (non-insulin-dependent) diabetes mellitus. *Diabetologia* 1990; **33** (Suppl 1): A13.

145 Choi WH, O'Rahilly S, Buse JB, et al. Molecular scanning of insulin-responsive glucose transporter (GLUT4) gene in NIDDM subjects. *Diabetes* 1991; **40**: 1712–18.

146 Krook A, Stratton I, O'Rahilly S. Pooled, multiplex single nucleotide primer extension (SNuPE): a novel and powerful tool for genetic studies in diabetes. *Diabetologia* 1992; **35** (Suppl 1): A71.

147 Damsbo P, Vaag A, Hother-Nielsen O, Beck-Nielsen H. Reduced glycogen synthase activity in skeletal muscle from obese patients with and without type 2 (non-insulin-dependent) diabetes mellitus. *Diabetologia* 1991; **34**: 239–45.

148 Kida Y, Esposito-del Puente A, Bogardus C, Mott DM. Insulin resistance is associated with reduced fasting and insulin-stimulated glycogen synthase phosphatase activity in human skeletal muscle. *J Clin Invest* 1990; **85**: 476–81.

149 Freymond D, Bogardus C, Okubo M, Stone K, Mott D. Impaired insulin-stimulated muscle glycogen synthase activation in vivo in man is related to low fasting glycogen synthase phosphatase activity. *J Clin Invest* 1988; **82**: 1503–9.

150 Schalin-Jäntti C, Härkönen M, Groop LC. Impaired activation of glycogen synthase in people at increased risk for developing NIDDM. *Diabetes* 1992; **41**: 598–604.

151 Groop L, Kankuri M, Schalin-Jäntti C, Lindlöf M, Kuismanen E. Restriction length fragment polymorphism (RFLP) of the human skeletal muscle glycogen synthase gene in patients with NIDDM. *Diabetes* 1991; 40 (Suppl 1): 30A.

152 Groop LC, Kankuri M, Schalin-Jäntti C. Association between polymorphism of the glycogen synthase gene and non-insulin dependent diabetes mellitus. *N Engl J Med* 1993; **328**: p 10–14.

153 Bjørbæk C, Vestergaard H, Heding LG, Cohen P, Pedersen O. Analysis of genes encoding 3 key proteins in insulin resistant glucose utilization of skeletal muscle from type 2 diabetics. *Diabetologia* 1992; **35** (Suppl 1): A72.

154 Johnson JH, Ogawa A, Chen L, et al. Underexpression of beta-cell high Km glucose transporters in non-insulin-dependent diabetes. *Science* 1990; **250**: 546–9.

155 Thorens B, Weir GC, Leahy JL, Lodish HF, Bonner-Weir S. Reduced expression of the liver/beta-cell glucose transporter isoform in glucose-insensitive pancreatic beta-cells of diabetic rats. *Proc Natl Acad Sci USA* 1990; **87**: 6492–6.

156 Unger RH, Diabetic hyperglycaemia: link to impaired glucose transport in pancreatic beta-cells. *Science* 1991; **251**: 1200–5.

157 Alcolado JC, Baroni MG, Li SR. Association between a restriction fragment length polymorphism at the liver/islet (GluT2) glucose transporter and familial type 2 (non-insulin-dependent) diabetes mellitus. *Diabetologia* 1991; **34**: 734 –6.

158 Patel P, Bell GI, Cook JTE, Turner RC, Wainscoat JS. Multiple restriction fragment length polymorphisms at the GLUT2 locus: GLUT 2 haplotypes for genetic analysis of type 2 (non-insulin-dependent) diabetes mellitus. *Diabetologia* 1991; **34**: 817–21.

159 Oelbaum RS, Li SR, Baroni MG, Alcolado JC, Galton DJ. Polymorphic pancreatic glucose transporter gene (GLUT2) in non-insulin-dependent diabetes. *Diabetic Med* 1990; **7** (Suppl 2): 22A.

160 Nishi S, Stoffel M, Xiang K, et al. Human pancreatic beta-cell glucokinase: cDNA sequence and localization of the polymorphic gene to chromosome 7, band p 13. *Diabetologia* 1992; **35**: 743–7.

161 Matsutani A, Janssen R, Donis-Keller H, Permutt MA. A polymorphic (CA)n

repeat element maps the human glucokinase gene (GCK) to chromosome 7p. *Genomics* 1992; **12**: 319–25.

162 Froguel Ph, Vaxillaire M, Sun F, et al. Close linkage of glucokinase locus on chromosome 7p to early-onset non-insulin-dependent diabetes mellitus. *Nature* 1992; **356**: 162–5.

163 Velho G, Froguel Ph. Clement K, et al. Primary pancreatic beta-cell secretory defect caused by mutations in glucokinase gene in kindreds of maturity onset diabetes of the young. *Lancet* 1992; **340**: 444–8.

164 Vionnet M, Stoffel M, Takeda J, et al. Nonsense mutation in the glucokinase gene causes early-onset non-insulin-dependent diabetes mellitus. *Nature* 1992; **356**: 721–3.

165 Froguel Ph, Zouali H, Vionnet N, et al. Familial hyperglycaemia due to mutation in glucokinase. Definition of a subtype of diabetes mellitus. *N Engl J Med* 1993; **328**: 697–702.

166 Froguel Ph, Vionnet N, Stoffel M, et al. Different phenotypic expression by three mutant alleles of glucokinase gene in MODY. *Diabetologia* 1992; **35** (Suppl 1): A63.

167 Page RCL, Hattersley AT, Barrow B, et al. Clinical characteristics of type 2 diabetes linked to the glucokinase gene. *Diabetologia* 1992; **35** (Suppl 1): A62.

168 Chiu KC, Province MA, Dowse GK, et al. A genetic marker at the glucokinase gene locus for type 2 (non-insulin-dependent) diabetes mellitus. *Diabetologia* 1992; **35**: 632–8.

169 Chiu KC, Province MA, Permutt MA. Glucokinase gene is genetic marker for NIDDM in American Blacks. *Diabetes* 1992; **41**: 843–9.

170 McCarthy MI, Hitchins M, Hitman GA, et al. Positive association in the absence of linkage suggests a minor role for the glucokinase gene in the pathogenesis of Type 2 (non-insulin-dependent) diabetes mellitus amongst South Indians. *Diabetologia* 1993, in press.

171 Saker PJ, Hattersley AT, Patel P, et al. The contribution of glucokinase to type 2 (non-insulin-dependent) diabetes: a population association study. *Diabetologia* 1992; **35** (Suppl 1): A139.

172 Cook JTE, Hattersley AT, Christopher P, et al. Linkage analysis of glucokinase gene with NIDDM in Caucasian pedigrees. *Diabetes* 1992; **41**: 1496–1500.

173 Vaxillaire M, Butal MO, Zouali H, et al. Linkage studies give evidence for genetic heterogeneity in type 2 diabetes mellitus. *Diabetologia*, 1992; **35** (Suppl 1): A62.

174 Alcolado JC, Alcolado R. Importance of maternal history of non-insulin dependent diabetic patients. *Br Med J* 1991; **302**: 1178–80.

175 Martin A, Simpson J, Ober C, Freinkel N. Frequency of diabetes mellitus in mothers of probands with gestational diabetes: possible maternal influence on the predisposition to gestational diabetes. *Am J Obstet Gynecol*, 1985; **151**: 471–5.

176 Korugan Ü, Yilmaz MT, Sipahioglu F, et al. The Istanbul family study 1: preliminary results. *Diabetologia* 1991; **34** (Suppl 1): A177.

177 Poulton J, Deadman ME, Gardiner RM. Duplications of mitochondrial DNA in mitochondrial myopathy. *Lancet* 1989; **i**: 236–40.

178 van den Ouweland JMW, Lemkes HHPJ, Maassen JA. Mutation in mitochondrial tRNA$^{Leu(UUR)}$ gene in a kindred of maternally transmitted non-insulin dependent diabetes mellitus and sensorineural hearing loss. *Diabetologia* 1992; (Suppl 1): A139.

179 Ballinger SW, Shoffner JM, Hedaya EV, et al. Maternally transmitted diabetes and deafness associated with a 10.4kb mitochondrial DNA deletion. *Nature Genet* 1992; **1**: 11–15.

180 Dowse GK, Gareeboo H, Zimmet P, et al. High prevalence of NIDDM and impaired glucose tolerance in Indian, Creole, and Chinese Mauritians. *Diabetes* 1990; **39**: 390–6.
181 Shimokata H, Muller DC, Fleg JL, et al. Age as independent determinant of glucose tolerance. *Diabetes* 1991; **40**: 44–51.
182 Manson JE, Rimm EB, Stampfer MJ, et al. Physical activity and incidence of non-insulin-dependent diabetes mellitus in women. *Lancet* 1991; **338**: 774–8.
183 Stunkard AJ, Harris JR, Pedersen NL, McClearn GE. The body-mass index of twins who have been reared apart. *N Engl J Med* 1990; **322**: 1483–7.
184 Bouchard C, Tremblay A, Després J-P, et al. The response to long-term, overfeeding in identical twins. *N Engl J Med* 1990; **322**: 1477–82.
185 van Assche FA, Aerts L. Long-term effect of diabetes and pregnancy in the rat. *Diabetes* 1985; **34** (Suppl 2): 116–18.
186 Gauguier D, Bihoreau M-T, Ktorza A, Berthault M-F, Picon L. Inheritance of diabetes mellitus as a consequence of gestational hyperglycaemia in rats. *Diabetes* 1990; **39**: 734–9.
187 Holemans K, Aerts L, van Assche FA. Evidence for an insulin resistance in the adult offspring of pregnant streptozotocin-diabetes rats. *Diabetologia* 1991; **34**: 81–5.
188 Gauguier D, Bihoreau M-T, Picon L, Ktorza A. Insulin secretion in adult rats after intrauterine exposure to mild hyperglycaemia during late gestation. *Diabetes* 1991; **40** (Suppl 2): 109–14.
189 Hales CN, Barker DJP, Clark PMS, et al. Fetal and infant growth and impaired glucose tolerance at age 64. *Br Med J* 1991; **303**: 1019–22.

Interaction of Genetic and Non-genetic Factors

Epidemiological Studies of the Causes of Non-insulin-dependent Diabetes Mellitus

William C. Knowler, David R. McCance, Dinesh K. Nagi and David J. Pettitt

Diabetes and Arthritis Epidemiology Section, National Institute of Diabetes and Digestive and Kidney Diseases, Phoenix, Arizona, USA

INTRODUCTION

Non-insulin-dependent diabetes mellitus (NIDDM) has an insidious onset and may exist for years without diagnosis. The metabolic changes leading to NIDDM have been extensively discussed and reviewed elsewhere, especially with respect to the Pima Indians[1-3]. Some risk factors, such as hyperglycaemia and hyperinsulinaemia, may be recognizable many years before the onset of NIDDM. In this chapter we review a number of risk factors for NIDDM, including obesity, physical activity, diet, socio-economic status and other metabolic abnormalities, as recognized from population-based studies.

Causes of Diabetes. Edited by R. D. G. Leslie
© 1993 John Wiley & Sons Ltd

Although family studies are described more fully in Chapter 12, we refer to family studies performed in the Pima Indians, with particular emphasis on the effects of diabetes in pregnancy. We also discuss the implications of racial differences and effects of migration on the understanding of genetic and environmental risk factors for NIDDM.

TERMINOLOGY

Fundamental to the study of the epidemiology of a disease is its definition. The National Diabetes Data Group[4] and the World Health Organization (WHO)[5] defined the terms insulin-dependent diabetes mellitus (IDDM) and NIDDM, the latter being distinguished by resistance to ketoacidosis in the absence of exogenous insulin. The 1985 WHO[6] classification also includes a third major category—malnutrition-related diabetes—which, inexplicably, is neither 'insulin-dependent' nor 'non-insulin-dependent'.

Turner et al.[7] recommended against classifying diabetes by severity or treatment, but rather by cause. In this respect the earlier terminology of type 1 and type 2 diabetes[5,8-10] is preferable, in which type 1 diabetes is caused by autoimmune or viral destruction of the pancreatic β cells, and type 2 diabetes is from any other cause. The terms type 1 and type 2 diabetes have been used interchangeably with IDDM and NIDDM, respectively. Many believe, however, that type 1 diabetes is not synonymous with IDDM, nor type 2 diabetes with NIDDM, because one classification represents suspected cause and the other clinical outcome, as reviewed by Keen[11]. The problem in equating type 1 diabetes with IDDM and type 2 diabetes with NIDDM is illustrated by the fact that many patients with NIDDM require treatment with insulin. Furthermore, some patients with NIDDM have immunological features characteristic of type 1 diabetes, and these features often predict the later requirement for insulin treatment[12-14].

As our knowledge of causation increases, the need for a subclassification of both type 1 and type 2 diabetes is increasingly recognized. In population studies—the subject of this chapter—a causal classification would be highly preferable, but with occasional exceptions, such as studies of the Pima Indians[15,16], this has not been possible. Diabetes in non-Caucasian populations and in Caucasian adults is usually NIDDM[14,17], and in keeping with the terminology of this book, we will use this term in the present chapter to describe epidemiological studies of diabetes in adults and in the Pima Indians. In some of the studies cited, an attempt was made to exclude type 1 diabetes, but in most, no immunological studies were performed.

RISK FACTORS

INSULIN RESISTANCE, HYPERINSULINAEMIA AND IMPAIRED GLUCOSE TOLERANCE

In diverse populations, hyperinsulinaemia has been recognized many years before the onset of NIDDM. Discussion has focused on the evolutionary significance of hyperinsulinaemia, insulin resistance, or both in the development of NIDDM and in particular their relation to β cell failure and hepatic dysregulation[18,19]. It remains a matter of conjecture, however, whether hyperinsulinaemia and insulin resistance should be regarded as risk factors or as manifestations of the disease process. The cellular mechanisms responsible for the alteration of insulin action are still unclear. Longitudinal studies have shown a parallel rise in glucose and insulin concentrations throughout the range of normoglycaemia and impaired glucose tolerance, before serum insulin falls with the onset of NIDDM[20,21]. From such observations, the basic underlying abnormality is perceived to be a deterioration of insulin action, resulting in progressive hyperglycaemia. Initially, compensatory hyperinsulinaemia may suffice to maintain relatively normal glycaemia (the rise or upward slope of the 'Starling curve') but, in some individuals, β cell failure and relative hypoinsulinaemia eventually ensue, resulting in worsening hyperglycaemia and NIDDM

Most evidence implicating insulin resistance in the pathogenesis of NIDDM has been indirect. Fasting hyperinsulinaemia, as a surrogate measure of insulin resistance, was predictive of subsequent NIDDM in a number of populations, including Pima Indians[2,20], Nauruans[22], Swedish women[23], French policemen[24], Mexican–Americans[25] and in Americans among the offspring of two diabetic parents[26]. Similarly, in Japanese–Americans, a high fasting plasma C-peptide was associated with the development of NIDDM[27]. Slower rates of glucose removal during an intravenous glucose tolerance test were predictive of the onset of NIDDM in the offspring of two parents with NIDDM[26], but not in Swedish women[23]. Perhaps the most direct evidence of a fundamental role for insulin resistance in the pathogenesis of NIDDM is provided by the recent results of a detailed longitudinal study of insulin action in non-diabetic Pima Indians[28]. Both insulin resistance (independent of obesity) and a low acute insulin response (controlled for the degree of insulin resistance) significantly predicted the development of NIDDM in Pima Indians. Of these two variables, insulin resistance had the predominant effect.

Obesity, which is often associated with insulin resistance, also predicts NIDDM, as described later in this chapter. However, in several studies, obesity was shown to be a weaker risk factor for NIDDM than hyperinsulinaemia or impaired insulin action[1,25,26] and it is conceivable that the effect of obesity on NIDDM is mediated by insulin resistance. Insulin resistance may therefore be a more proximate cause of NIDDM than is obesity, and it seems likely that one or both of these conditions are genetically determined[29–31]. To what extent these findings are relevant to the pathogenesis of NIDDM in lean subjects, and particularly in Caucasian populations[32], is more uncertain. In these latter populations, different genetic mechanisms may be operative.

Impaired glucose tolerance can be considered a stage in the clinical development of NIDDM. Once impaired glucose tolerance has developed, individuals with the lowest serum insulin (adjusted for other variables) at 30 minutes or 2 hours after a glucose load are most likely to develop NIDDM[1,22,24,33].

OBESITY

Obesity is a frequent concomitant of NIDDM, but in cross-sectional studies there is not always a strong association between the two conditions[34,35]. In longitudinal studies, however, obesity consistently has been a strong predictor of diabetes[34,36–42]. For example, in residents of Oslo, Norway, aged 40–49 years, a relative weight index derived from height and weight predicted the subsequent development of diabetes as diagnosed in routine clinical care. Ten-year cumulative incidence rates ranged from zero, in those with a relative weight more than 10% below normal, to 13%, in those with a relative weight $\geq 45\%$ above normal[38] (Figure 1). By contrast, among men with impaired glucose tolerance in the Whitehall Survey in England, obesity did not predict diabetes[39]. The importance of obesity, estimated by the body mass index (BMI = weight/height^2), as a risk factor for diabetes was confirmed in a longitudinal study of Pima Indians. Non-diabetic subjects were examined approximately every 2 years for the development of diabetes, as diagnosed by an oral glucose tolerance test. Incidence rates of diabetes increased almost linearly with BMI, ranging from 0.8 cases per 1000 person-years of follow-up at BMI<20 kg/m^2 to 72 cases per 1000 person-years at BMI ≥ 40 kg/m^2 [34]. A longer duration of a given level of obesity further increased the incidence of diabetes[43]. BMI also predicted the development of diabetes among Pima Indians with impaired glucose tolerance—an effect which appeared to be mediated by the association of BMI with plasma glucose and serum insulin concentrations[1]. In a cross-sectional analysis of this same population, however, there was almost no association between BMI and diabetes[34]. This apparent paradox is most likely explained by the weight loss which follows the diagnosis of diabetes[34,44]. The extent to which this phenomenon has resulted in an underestimation of the importance of obesity as a risk factor for NIDDM in other cross-sectional studies is unknown.

The calculation of BMI from measurements of weight and height is neces-

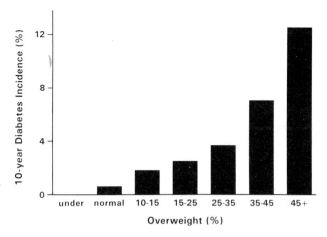

Figure 1   Ten-year age-adjusted cumulative incidence of clinically diagnosed diabetes according to degree of overweight in Norwegian men aged 40–49 years at baseline. 'Normal' includes men within 10% of normal weight for height. 'Under' includes those more than 10% below normal. (From Westlund and Nicolaysen[38], with permission)

sarily a crude estimate of obesity, which fails to distinguish among the components of body weight, such as muscle and fat. While it is possible to estimate the percentage of body fat[45], we are unaware of any reports which have compared the predictive power of percentage body fat and BMI for the subsequent development of NIDDM. Following Vague's observation that diabetic persons were more likely to have an upper, rather than lower body fat distribution[46], there has been increasing interest in the distribution of body fat as a predictor of diabetes. In a 13.5-year follow-up of non-diabetic men in Göteborg, Sweden, the development of diabetes was predicted by BMI, a sum of skinfold measurements, waist or hip circumference, and waist-to-hip ratio[47]. Twenty-one per cent of those in the upper 5% of the BMI distribution developed diabetes, compared with none of those in the lower 20% of the distribution. Controlled for BMI with multivariate analysis, either waist circumference or waist-to-hip ratio significantly predicted diabetes. Thus the combination of a high BMI and a high waist-to-hip ratio was a better predictor of NIDDM than either variable alone. In Japanese–American men living in Seattle, the best anthropometric variable predicting the development of NIDDM was the intra-abdominal body fat area determined by computed tomography[27].

The relationship of NIDDM to fat distribution has also been investigated in cross-sectional studies. In four ethnic groups in Mauritius, an island in the Indian Ocean, the prevalence of NIDDM was directly related both to BMI and to waist-to-hip ratio, and within most strata of one of these variables, the prevalence of diabetes was directly related to the other variable[48]. Similarly, among Mexican–American participants in the San Antonio Heart Study, both BMI and the waist-to-hip ratio were strongly related to NIDDM in a multiple logistic regression analysis[49]. Among residents of London of either European or southern Asian origin, waist-to-hip ratio was more strongly related to diabetes and impaired glucose tolerance than was BMI[50]. Among adult Pima Indians, diabetes was strongly related to the waist-to-thigh ratio, especially in younger adults, despite only a weak association with BMI[44]. Whether estimates of body fat distribution in Pima Indians will improve the high predictive power of BMI for future diabetes remains to be seen.

PHYSICAL INACTIVITY

Many cross-sectional and longitudinal studies have supported a causal role for physical inactivity in the development of NIDDM. These studies, however, are often limited by imprecise measures of physical activity or diabetes.

Cross-sectional Studies

Glucose and insulin concentrations, measured during an oral glucose tolerance test, were lower in 54-year-old well-trained athletic Swedish men than in randomly selected non-athletic men of similar age and body weight[51]. In other studies of healthy non-diabetic Swedish men, the amount of reported leisure physical activity was negatively related to plasma glucose concentrations[52,53]. In the Whitehall study in England, reported leisure-time physical activity was unrelated to diabetes or to blood glucose concentrations[54], whereas in Mauritius the prevalence of diabetes, determined by a glucose tolerance test, was related to current reported physical activity[48]. Melanesians and Indians living on the Pacific island of Fiji participated in a diabetes survey which included a questionnaire for occupational and sports physical activity[55]. Diabetes was determined by an oral glucose tolerance test. Age-adjusted prevalence rates of diabetes in men were much higher in the Indian than in the Melanesian populations, and within each ethnic group were more than twice as high in those classified as having sedentary or light activities than in those with moderate or heavy activities.

A physical activity questionnaire has been developed specifically for the Pima Indians, covering the occupational and leisure activities in this population[56]. Assessments of recent and past physical activities were included. In a cross-sectional study, the age–sex-adjusted prevalence of diabetes in 15–36-year-old subjects decreased linearly with the amount of reported leisure activity during the preceding year[57]. In 37–59-year-old subjects, diabetes was negatively related to reported physical activity as recalled from teenage and subsequent adult years. While such a relationship could be due to differential recall in diabetic and non-diabetic persons, these results suggest that physical inactivity preceded, rather than resulted from, diabetes.

Longitudinal Studies

A causal role for physical inactivity in the development of NIDDM is also supported by several longitudinal studies. Women who had been athletes during college were less likely than their non-athletic colleagues to report having diabetes when subsequently questioned at ages ranging from 21 to 80 years[58]. The association was stronger in older women; for example, among those aged ≥40 years, the age-adjusted risk of diabetes for non-participants was 3.4 times (95% confidence interval = 1.3–8.7) that of the former athletes. In a longitudinal study of nearly 6000 male college alumni, reported physical activity (whether expressed as total activity or vigorous sports only) was negatively related to the incidence of diabetes[41]. The relationship was approximately linear, and, in particular, there was no indication of a threshold level of activity above which further benefit was absent. The deleterious effect of inactivity was most pronounced in those men with other diabetes risk factors, such as high BMI, hypertension or parental diabetes. In the Nurses' Health Study in the USA, women were asked about their frequency of current vigorous exercise[59]. Those who exercised at least once per week had an age-adjusted incidence rate of self-reported diabetes which was 0.67 times (95% confidence interval = 0.6–0.75) that of women who exercised less frequently. Among those exercising at least once per week, there was no consistent relationship between the frequency of exercise and the incidence of diabetes. In a similar study of male physicians in the USA, the incidence of self-reported diabetes was negatively related to the self-reported frequency of vigorous exercise[42]. The age-adjusted incidence of diabetes in men exercising vigorously at least once per week was 0.64 times (95% confidence interval = 0.51–0.82) that of men exercising less than once per week. BMI also predicted diabetes, and the negative association of exercise with subsequent diabetes was greater in those subjects with the highest BMI.

Further evidence for physical inactivity as a risk factor for NIDDM is provided by a feasibility study of diet and exercise treatment in men with impaired glucose tolerance[60]. On the basis of population screening of 47–49-year-old men, 217 subjects with impaired glucose tolerance were identified, using criteria for impaired glucose tolerance similar to those of the WHO[6]. The subjects were divided into two groups: 161 who were treated with diet and exercise, and the remaining 56 who were referred to other clinics because of medical problems, such as hypertension or hyperlipidaemia, which were treated according to standard medical practice, were used as a reference group. The men receiving diet and exercise treatment were trained in physical exercise and given dietary advice to reduce sugar and fat, increase complex carbohydrate and fiber, and lose weight if they were overweight. The treated subjects, but not the reference group, experienced a significant weight loss, most of which was maintained for 5 years. By the end of the 5-year treatment period, 11% of the treated subjects and 21% of the reference group had developed diabetes according to WHO criteria. A treatment effect, however, was not definitely established because of the non-random assignment to groups and differing medical conditions of the treated and untreated groups at baseline. Nevertheless, this study supports the hypothesis that physical inactivity, obesity and a high-fat diet are risk factors for NIDDM.

DIETARY FACTORS

Evidence for a role of specific dietary components in the etiology of NIDDM is inconsistent[61-63]. Historically, evidence has been presented implicating an excessive consumption of sucrose and other refined carbohydrates[64-68], a lack of dietary fibre[67,69] and a high intake of dietary fat[70-73]. Inter-population comparisons and the study of migrant populations are hindered by the confounding of such factors as genetic susceptibility, physical activity, obesity, and changes in these variables with time[74]. Additional methodological pitfalls, including the high degree of correlation between individual dietary constituents[73,74], the unreliability of dietary recall[66,75,76] and the difficulties in distinguishing between a causal and therapeutic role for diet in cross-sectional studies[74] have been highlighted.

In 1978, West, summarizing the previous literature, was attracted by the evidence demonstrating a positive relation of fat consumption, and an inverse relation of carbohydrate consumption, to the risk of diabetes[61]. Epidemiological studies in the South Pacific[77] have shown nutrition to be one of the major changes which has accompanied evolution to a modern way of life. In these populations, a diet usually high in fibre and complex carbohydrate has been replaced by one higher in total calories, fat, refined carbohydrate and salt. Several conditions and diseases, including NIDDM, are associated with this change. Departure from a traditional lifestyle was also implicated in the high prevalence of diabetes in Japanese living in Hiroshima compared with Japanese migrants to Hawaii[78]. Calorie intake in the two groups was similar, but the Hawaiian–Japanese were more sedentary, consumed more fat, less complex and more simple carbohydrate, had a much higher frequency of obesity and approximately twice the prevalence of diabetes. As noted above these comparisons are potentially confounded by other environmental determinants.

A relationship of diabetes with total caloric intake was reported in two case-control studies from the UK. Himsworth and Marshall[79] found that, prior to the onset of symptoms, the diets of diabetic women aged 46–75 years

Reference	Subjects	Dietary assessment	Follow-up (years)	Findings
Prospective studies				
80	8688 adult Israeli men	Questionnaire	5	373 developed NIDDM; no significant association between total energy intake or any other dietary variable and incidence of NIDDM
74	187 Pima Indian women aged 24–44 years	Modified Burke interview	12	87 developed NIDDM; energy and starch intake associated with NIDDM, no relation between sugar intake and NIDDM
81	25 698 Seventh Day Adventists	Self-administered questionnaire	21	In death certificates: diabetes as contributing or cause of death in 93 men, 165 women; controlled for age and relative weight, meat consumption associated with NIDDM in men only
82	1462 Swedish women	24-hour recall	12	43 developed NIDDM; no effect of percentage energy from protein, carbohydrate, fat
68	814 Dutch men	Interview with spouse, 7-day recall	25	58 new cases of NIDDM; no significant association between intake of nutrients at baseline and risk of NIDDM
83	84 360 USA nurses aged 34–59	Semi-quantitative questionnaire	6	252 new cases; no relation between energy intake, protein, sucrose and carbohydrate; negative relation with vegetable fat, potassium, calcium and magnesium
Cross-sectional studies				
72	380 Japanese–American men	Modified Burke interview		229 cases NIDDM, 72 IGT[a], 79 NGT[b]; lower intake of animal fat and animal protein in previously undiagnosed cases than in NGT, no difference in carbohydrate; no differences between IGT and NGT
73	1317 USA subjects	24-hour dietary recall prior to OGTT[c]		70 cases undiagnosed NIDDM, 171 IGT, 1076 NGT; high-fat, low-carbohydrate diet associated with NIDDM and IGT

[a]IGT = impaired glucose tolerance; [b]NGT = normal glucose tolerance; [c]OGTT = oral glucose tolerance test.

were, in general, higher in fat and lower in carbohydrate than those of non-diabetic women. Baird[66] also observed that newly diagnosed diabetic subjects consumed more total calories than their non-diabetic siblings, but the percentage of energy derived from fat and carbohydrate were similar in the two groups. In both of these studies, the influence of current diet (and the diagnosis of diabetes) on the reporting of previous dietary practices remains unclear.

Additional studies, including those of a prospective nature, continue to report varying relationships with specific dietary components[68,80-84], and have been subject to criticism both of design and validity[73]. Some of these studies are summarized in Table 1. In the Nurses' Health Study, 702 new cases of NIDDM developed among 84 360 women during 6 years of follow-up[83]. Controlled for BMI, previous weight change and alcohol intake, the intakes of energy, protein, sucrose, carbohydrate or fibre were not associated with the risk of diabetes. In a comparison of the highest with the lowest quintiles of energy-adjusted intake, the intake of vegetable fat (relative risk, $RR = 0.61$, $p = 0.03$), potassium ($RR = 0.62$, $p = 0.008$), calcium ($RR = 0.70$, $p = 0.005$) and magnesium ($RR = 0.68$, $p = 0.02$) were inversely related to NIDDM. By contrast, it is interesting to note that several recent reports again have highlighted a relationship between a high-fat, low-carbohydrate diet and the occurrence of NIDDM[72,73,85,86]. In the San Luis Valley cross-sectional study, the age-adjusted odds ratios relating a 40 g increase in fat intake in 70 previously undiagnosed diabetic subjects and 171 subjects with impaired glucose tolerance were 1.51 (95% confidence interval = 0.85–2.67) and 1.62 (1.09–2.41) respectively compared with 1076 subjects with normal glucose tolerance[73]. An association between the consumption of saturated fat and cardiovascular disease is well known[87]. Several reports have shown a relation between fat consumption and the degree of adiposity[88,89]. There is also evidence suggesting that saturated fatty acid intake may cause insulin resistance[90,91]. Collectively these results add further significance to the epidemiological findings described earlier in this chapter, while providing another putative mechanism to explain the clustering of cardiovascular disease risk factors including dyslipidaemia and glucose intolerance. Additional prospective studies in this area are needed, along with elucidation of the possible pathophysiological relevance of specific dietary factors to glucose tolerance.

URBAN/RURAL RESIDENCE

In the National Health Interview Survey in the USA, prevalence rates of NIDDM were similar in urban and rural subjects[92]. Other studies of a single ethnic group have frequently shown a higher prevalence of diabetes in urban subjects[77,93-96]. This variation is not explained completely by differences in obesity[97,98] and would appear to be the result of additional influences of environmental factors on the expression of disease. In support of this are the persuasive findings of a recent study which examined the role of dietary intake, exercise and obesity in rural and urban populations of three Pacific island countries[99]. Urban subjects were more obese than rural ones, had a higher prevalence of diabetes and hypertension, and lower levels of physical activity. In general, energy intake was found to reflect energy expenditure[99]. The influence of environment is perhaps most clearly shown by the study of migrant populations, and by the dramatic increases in frequency of diabetes in the USA[100] and among populations such as the Pima Indians[2] and Micronesians from the South Pacific island of Nauru[101], which have recently undergone a transition from a traditional to a 'westernized' or 'modernized' society.

SOCIO-ECONOMIC STATUS

In some developing countries such as India, the wealthy are more likely to have diabetes, while in developed countries the situation is generally reversed, with socio-economic status (SES) being inversely correlated with the prevalence of NIDDM and obesity[61,102–105]. In Tecumseh, Michigan, less formal education was a risk factor for diabetes in men and women aged 20–39 years, but not in older age groups[106]. In the USA, educational attainment, annual family income and labour-force participation rates were lower in adult diabetic patients than in the general population. However, among those currently employed, the prevalence of diabetes did not vary by occupation[92].

With increasing affluence in developed societies, people may become increasingly health-conscious and may take steps to reverse some of the perceived maladaptive features of classic modernization, thereby reversing the trend towards increasing obesity and perhaps also diabetes[107]. There was only limited evidence, however, for this 'post-modernization' process or 'descending limb of the curve' in a Mexican–American population[107]. There are no data on the incidence of diabetes and SES *per se*.

OTHER PHYSIOLOGICAL AND METABOLIC ABNORMALITIES

Blood Pressure

In several epidemiological studies, systolic blood pressure was not an independent risk factor for diabetes[32,108]. By contrast, a positive association between systolic blood pressure and the subsequent incidence of diabetes was demonstrated in univariate analyses[68], and when other factors including BMI, plasma glucose and early insulin response were taken into account[40,80]. The use of thiazide diuretics and β-blocking drugs for the treatment of hypertension may also play a role[109–112]. Another study, however, has suggested that glucose intolerance antedates rather than results from hypertension[113]. Controlled for age, BMI, alcohol intake and initial blood pressure, among men in the highest third of the 1-hour plasma glucose distribution, none of whom took antihypertensive drugs at the baseline examination, the odds of having hypertension 18 years later were 1.7 times those of men in the lowest third of the distribution[113]. Among subjects followed for 8 years, fasting insulin was related to the incidence of hypertension, in univariate analysis only, and was independent of adiposity only in lean subjects[49]. As a unifying hypothesis, insulin resistance and hyperinsulinaemia have been invoked as possible common links between hypertension and glucose intolerance[114], but their relative contributions, either temporally or pathophysiologically, to the coincidence of these two conditions remain unclear[115-117] (see also Chapter 16).

Lipid Abnormalities

Many patients with hyperlipidaemia may also have glucose intolerance and obesity. Relatively few studies, however, have examined the independent relationship of serum cholesterol, very low-density lipoproteins and triglyceride levels to the subsequent development of NIDDM. Serum cholesterol was a significant multivariate risk factor in the 5-year incidence of NIDDM in 10 000 Israeli males[80] and for men in the north-east USA[118], but not in Tecumseh, Michigan[106] or in middle-aged men in Oslo, Norway[38]. Elevation of very low-density lipoproteins but not low-density lipoproteins was an independent predictor of NIDDM during 14 years of follow-up in 5000 men and women in Framingham, Massachusetts[119]. In the Paris prospective study of male civil servants, there was a greater incidence of diabetes in the highest tertile of serum triglyceride concentrations than in the lowest tertile (relative risk 3.5), but this did not persist after adjustment for blood glucose[120]. The significance of hypertriglyceridaemia as a risk factor for NIDDM, now reported in several studies, may lie in its association with hyperinsulinaemia and insulin resistance.

Other Risk Factors

Two epidemiological studies have shown an association between peripheral vascular disease and the development of NIDDM in multivariate analyses[80,108].

Both positive[68] and negative[32,80,108] associations have been reported between cigarette smoking and NIDDM. This may reflect differing degrees of precision in the quantification of cigarette consumption and the exact relationship remains unclear. Many drugs affect glucose tolerance. β-blockers and thiazide diuretics worsen insulin resistance and dyslipidaemia[112]. They may also contribute to the high incidence of diabetes among treated hypertensive patients[109-111]. Some studies have reported an increased risk in relation to elevated uric acid levels[80], resting heart rate[68], high haemoglobin levels[119] and diminished vital lung capacity[121]. Moderate alcohol intake was found not to be a risk factor for NIDDM in women[122].

In light of the association between classical cardiovascular risk factors and the incidence of diabetes, together with findings such as peripheral vascular disease antedating the development of diabetes, there is an emerging opinion which regards diabetes and atherosclerotic diseases as related disorders, possibly originating from the same metabolic environment[123–125].

FAMILIAL FACTORS

Diabetes has been found to be familial in numerous population studies. As these are described in Chapter 12, the family studies described below are largely restricted to those among the Pima Indians.

The familial transmission of diabetes in the Pimas is illustrated in Figure 2, which shows the age-specific prevalence of diabetes in 984 subjects according to parental diabetes. Each parent was classified into one of two groups: (a) diabetic with onset documented before age 55 years; or (b) non-diabetic with absence of diabetes confirmed by an oral glucose tolerance test at or after the age of 55 years. Offspring were excluded if, for either parent, the presence of diabetes at age 55 years could not be determined. These data for the offspring extend only to age 44 years, because at older ages there are few subjects both of whose parents have been examined. Parental relationships were similar among male and female offspring, so the sexes have been pooled.

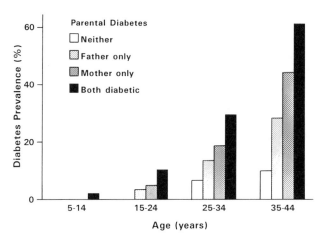

Figure 2 Age-specific prevalence of diabetes in Pima Indians (sexes combined) according to parental diabetes diagnosed by age 55 years, as described in the text

The prevalence rates were highest in offspring whose parents both developed diabetes before age 55 years. Intermediate rates were seen in the offspring of only one diabetic parent, while the lowest rates occurred in the offspring of two non-diabetic parents. Adjusted for age by the Mantel–Haenszel procedure[126], the prevalence of diabetes differed significantly among the offspring of the four groups shown in Figure 2 ($p<0.001$), but not among the two groups with only one diabetic parent.

Below 25 years of age, diabetes occurred only in persons with at least one diabetic parent. In this age range, the transmission of diabetes from parents to offspring is consistent with an autosomal dominant mode of inheritance. Among older persons, however, diabetes occurred in a number of offspring of two non-diabetic parents. This would also be consistent with a dominant mode of inheritance if some of the parents of these older offspring carried a diabetes susceptibility gene which was not penetrant. The plausibility of this hypothesis is indicated by the increasing prevalence of diabetes in this population over time[2,127], which implies that many members of the older generations carry susceptibility genes without having the disease. The familial data, however, would also be consistent with other modes of inheritance.

The severity of diabetes (as judged by the degree of hyperglycaemia[127]), insulin resistance and obesity also aggregate in Pima families. In a group of non-diabetic Pimas aged 15–35 years, insulin resistance measured by the hyperinsulinaemic, euglycaemic clamp, adjusted for age, sex and percentage body fat, had a within-sibship intraclass correlation of 0.42[29]. For the Pima population as a whole, BMI was related to parental BMI, and the within-sibship intraclass correlation of BMI, adjusted for age and sex, was 0.34[44]. These results are not unexpected given that insulin resistance[28] and BMI[34] predict diabetes. Thus some of the familial factors leading to diabetes may be manifest long before the appearance of the disease. The renal complications among Pimas with diabetes are also familial[128].

Obesity and parental diabetes are strong diabetes risk factors which interact with each other. Age-adjusted diabetes incidence rates are higher and have a stronger relationship with BMI in Pimas with diabetic parents than in those with two non-diabetic parents[2,34].

In each age group above 15 years, there was a higher prevalence of diabetes among those offspring with a diabetic mother than among those with a diabetic father (Figure 2), although this difference was not statistically significant. Such a difference would not be expected if diabetes were purely an autosomal genetic disease, and therefore suggests a non-genetic cause. This observation prompted the investigation of the effects of the diabetic pregnancy on the offspring. Since the diagnosis of diabetes in some mothers antedated the birth of their children, these offspring spent their intrauterine lives in a hyperglycaemic environment. This would not be the case for those offspring whose fathers, but not mothers, had diabetes during this period.

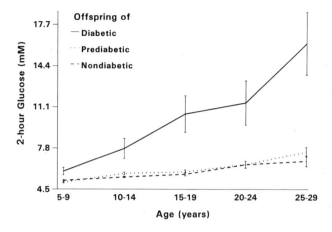

Figure 3 Mean 2-hour post-load plasma glucose concentration according to age and mother's diabetes. Ninety-five per cent confidence intervals are represented by the error bars. Diabetic women had diabetes before or during the pregnancy; prediabetic women had normal glucose tolerance until after delivery and subsequently developed diabetes; non-diabetic women have not developed diabetes to date. Offspring may be included in more than one age group. (Modified from Pettitt *et al.*[132])

This abnormal intrauterine environment appears to have long-lasting ramifications for the fetus, resulting in more frequent obesity[129,130] and diabetes[131] at young ages.

The prevalence of diabetes and obesity in the offspring during childhood and young adulthood has been examined according to the mother's glucose tolerance during the pregnancy[132]. Comparisons were made of offspring of women (a) in whom the development of diabetes occurred before the pregnancy (diabetic pregnancies), (b) after the pregnancy (prediabetic pregnancies), and (c) those who have remained non-diabetic (non-diabetic pregnancies).

Figure 3 shows the mean 2-hour plasma glucose concentration by age in offspring who were examined periodically. In each age group, the offspring of diabetic women had, on average, higher 2-hour post-load plasma glucose concentrations than the offspring of non-diabetic or prediabetic women. This difference was more marked in older age groups. The small differences between the offspring of non-diabetic and prediabetic women probably reflects genetic differences inherited from their mothers, as all of the prediabetic women subsequently developed diabetes and all of their offspring could have inherited the diabetes gene or genes. The large difference, between the offspring of diabetic and of prediabetic women, which is apparent even in the youngest age group, is probably a long-lasting effect of the intrauterine environment superimposed on a genetic predisposition.

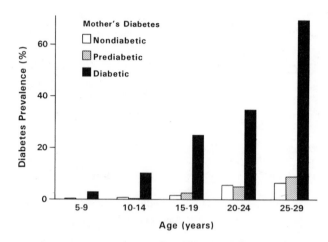

Figure 4 Prevalence of diabetes according to age and mother's diabetes. Classification of mothers is as in Figure 3. Offspring may be included in more than one age group. (Modified from Pettitt et al.[132])

Figure 4 shows the prevalence of diabetes in these three groups of offspring. Few children had diabetes before the age of 10 years, after which the prevalence of diabetes in each age group was much higher in the offspring of diabetic women than in the other two groups. By the time they reach childbearing age, one quarter to one third of the offspring of diabetic women already have developed diabetes, thus perpetuating this cycle of diabetes during pregnancy begetting diabetes in the next generation. By 25–29 years of age, seven of 10 offspring of diabetic women had diabetes.

Impaired glucose tolerance during pregnancy was associated with rates of diabetes intermediate between those offspring of women who had diabetes and those who had normal glucose tolerance during pregnancy[133,134]. Figure 5 shows the prevalence of abnormal glucose tolerance, defined as either diabetes or impaired glucose tolerance, diagnosed by the time of pregnancy in 15–24-year-old female offspring according to their mothers' 2-hour glucose concentrations during pregnancy 15–24 years earlier. There was a direct relationship between the mothers' glucose concentrations during pregnancy and the prevalence of abnormal glucose tolerance in their daughters by the time of their pregnancies[134].

Freinkel predicted that the diabetic intrauterine environment would have an effect on subsequent anthropomorphic development and metabolism[135], and initiated a longitudinal study to test this hypothesis. He and his colleagues measured amniotic fluid insulin, a reflection of the fetal response to hyperglycaemia. The offspring of diabetic women who were the most obese at age 6

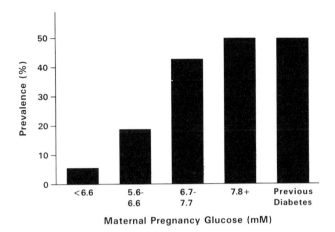

Figure 5 Prevalence of abnormal glucose tolerance (diabetes or impaired glucose tolerance) diagnosed before or during pregnancy in 15–24-year-old offspring according to their mothers' 2-hour post-load plasma glucose concentrations during pregnancy

years had had a mean amniotic fluid insulin which was significantly higher than in less obese offspring of diabetic women[136]. Although the incidence of diabetes is much lower in this population than in the Pima Indians, it would be interesting to see if these children eventually have a greater frequency of diabetes or abnormalities in insulin sensitivity than offspring of women with normal glucose tolerance during pregnancy.

The diabetic pregnancy in Pima Indians can thus lead to a vicious cycle[137]. Diabetes during pregnancy affects the genetically susceptible offspring, resulting in higher glucose concentrations and higher rates of impaired glucose tolerance and diabetes at young ages. By the time female offspring of diabetic women reach childbearing age, many already have diabetes or impaired glucose tolerance and thereby perpetuate the cycle. Thus the diabetic pregnancy must account for at least some of the increase in the prevalence of diabetes which has been observed in this population since 1965[2,138] and which has probably been occurring throughout the twentieth century[127].

Many factors, both genetic and non-genetic, can cause familial aggregation of a disease. While some familial factors result from shared environment and culture, the familial basis of several of the risk factors for diabetes appears to be, at least in part, genetic. For example, there is increasing evidence that a major portion of the predisposition to obesity is due to genotype, as reviewed by Ravussin and Swinburn[139]. Among the Pimas, there is evidence that a gene on chromosome 4 influences insulin resistance[31]. Diabetes in

Pimas is also associated with the presence of the HLA-A2 type[140]. Research on the genetics of NIDDM in general is discussed in Chapter 10.

RACIAL DIFFERENCES

Epidemiological studies of racial differences in the prevalence of NIDDM and studies of diabetes in migrant populations provide insight into the possible role of genetic and environmental influences on diabetes[125].

While diabetes is an uncommon disease in certain populations, an epidemic has occurred in some developing nations[141]. This change towards an increasing prevalence of diabetes appears to be strongly related to environmental influences resulting from changes in lifestyle and SES.

Ethnic differences in the prevalence of diabetes and studies of migrant populations and their contribution to the understanding of diabetes can be discussed under the following categories:

1. Racial differences in the worldwide prevalence of diabetes.
2. Differences in the prevalence of diabetes between different ethnic groups sharing similar environments.
3. Differences in the prevalence of diabetes in the same ethnic group living in different environments, i.e. population migration.

Worldwide Differences in Diabetes Prevalence

Table 2 shows the age-adjusted prevalence rates of abnormal glucose tolerance (diabetes and impaired glucose tolerance) in subjects aged 30–64 years in those five populations with the lowest and those five with the highest recorded prevalence rates from a compilation of many prevalence studies[141]. The prevalence of abnormal glucose tolerance in some populations, such as the Mapuche Indians of Chile, is low (2%), while at the other extreme, in the Pima Indians of Arizona, the prevalence is 66%. Similarly, diabetes is extremely prevalent in urban Hispanics in the USA[98], urban and rural Indians in Fiji[142], Nauruans[101] and in Polynesians in Western Samoa[94]. The high prevalence of diabetes in these high-risk populations is believed to be due to recent acculturation and a change from a traditional lifestyle to a more sedentary one, and cannot be explained solely by differences in prevalence of obesity[142,143]. The extent to which the high susceptibility to diabetes in these populations is due to genetic and environmental factors is incompletely understood.

The high prevalence in these populations is not merely due to increased longevity of subjects with diabetes, as a rise in incidence of diabetes has been clearly documented in Pima Indians, in whom incidence rates increased by 40% between 1965 and 1975[138]. Similar trends of an increasing incidence of diabetes are also apparent among Hispanic persons in the USA[144].

Table 2 Worldwide prevalence[a] of glucose intolerance (diabetes and impaired glucose tolerance) at ages 30–64 years in selected populations (the five lowest and five highest). From King and Rewers[141], with permission

Population	Prevalence (%)	Comment
Mapuche Indians, Chile	2	Populations which
Urban Chinese	3	have a traditional
Rural Melanesian, Papua New Guinea	3	lifestyle
Rural Polynesian, W Samoa	8	
Rural Indians, India	10	
Urban Hispanic, USA	30	Populations in which
Rural Indians, Fiji	33	rapid urbanization
Urban Indians, Fiji	35	has taken place or
Micronesians, Nauru	62	with high prevalence
Pima Indians, USA	66	of obesity

[a]Age-adjusted, both sexes combined.

Ethnic Differences in Similar Environments

Epidemiological studies have also shown that prevalence rates of diabetes vary among different ethnic groups sharing similar environments. In Singapore, the prevalence was 6.1% in the Indian population, 2.4% in the Malays and 1.6% in the Chinese[145]. The high prevalence in Indians was not due to obesity, as this ethnic group was the least obese. Similarly, in Cape Town, South Africa, the age-adjusted prevalence was higher in the Indian population (19.1%) than in the Bantus (4.2%) and Caucasians (3.6%)[146]. The age-adjusted prevalence of diabetes was higher in rural (men = 12.1%, women = 11.3%) and urban (men = 12.9%, women = 11.0%) Indians than in rural (men = 1.1%, women = 1.2%) and urban (men = 3.5%, women = 7.1%) Melanesians in Fiji[142]. In addition, the prevalence of diabetes was similar in both urban and rural Indians, in contrast to the higher prevalence in urban than in rural Melanesians. These observations suggest that the interaction of genetic and environmental risk factors varies by ethnicity. In contrast to the above findings, a recent study of a multiracial community in Mauritius found high rates of diabetes in Indians, Creoles and Chinese, but little difference in diabetes prevalence between these ethnic groups[48].

Migration

Migrant populations provide another opportunity to study the effect of environment controlled for genetic influences. Some migrant populations have higher prevalence rates of diabetes than the non-migrant populations from the same ethnic groups remaining in their countries of origin. This is

206

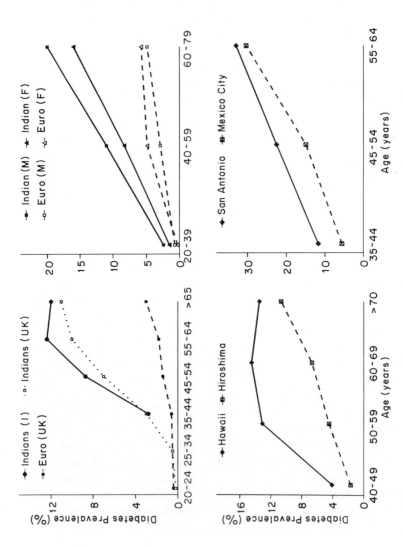

Figure 6 Diabetes prevalence in migrant populations. Upper left: prevalence of known diabetes in Indians in India (I)[148] and Indians in Southall, UK, compared with Europeans in the UK [147]. Upper right: prevalence of diabetes in male (M) and female (F) Indians and Europeans in Coventry, UK[149]. Lower left: prevalence of diabetes in Japanese–Americans in Hawaii and in Japanese in Hiroshima[78]. Lower right: prevalence of diabetes in Mexican–Americans in San Antonio and in Mexicans in Mexico City[98]

probably due to the result of affluence upon adopting a Western lifestyle. Asian Indians are perhaps the best example of migrant populations, due to their long history of migration to different parts of the world.

Figure 6 (upper left panel) shows the age-specific prevalence rates of known diabetes in Indians and Europeans in Southall, UK[147]. In subjects aged 35–64 years, diabetes prevalence was five times as high in the Indian subjects as in the Europeans. Using similar methods as in the above survey, the prevalence of known diabetes in Indians living in an affluent area of Delhi[148] was similar to that of the Indians in Southall. Similar findings of a higher prevalence of diabetes (by WHO criteria) were also reported in a population survey from Coventry, UK, where both male and female Indians had higher prevalence of diabetes than did Europeans (Figure 6, upper right panel)[149]. A high prevalence of diabetes in migrant Indians has been reported in Trinidad[150], Singapore[145], South Africa[151] and Fiji[152].

The prevalence of diabetes in subjects aged ≥16 years, as reported in a large survey in 1975 in India, was only 2.1% in the urban and 1.2% in the rural population[153]. This survey, however, used diagnostic criteria which were less stringent than those currently recommended by the WHO[6], and therefore the prevalence of diabetes was probably overestimated. However, recent studies from urban India have shown a higher prevalence both of known diabetes[148] and of diabetes as diagnosed by an oral glucose tolerance test using WHO criteria[154]. The later study showed that overall diabetes prevalence (both known and newly diagnosed) was 5%. However, the prevalence was 2% at ages <40 years and 21% in those ≥40 years of age. As the age structure of this population was younger than those reported in migrant Indian populations, these authors adjusted the diabetes prevalence to the age structure of migrant Indians in Fiji and found the age-adjusted prevalence of diabetes in southern India was 9%[154], lower than the prevalence of 13% in Fiji[142]. Thus the prevalence of diabetes in India is increasing, and may increase further given the appropriate circumstances, such as urbanization, even without emigration.

A higher diabetes prevalence in Japanese in the USA than in Hiroshima has also been reported (Figure 6, lower left panel)[78]. In another study, the effects of environmental factors such as diet, obesity and physical activity on diabetes prevalence were assessed in a study of residents of Mexico City and in Mexican–Americans in San Antonio, USA (Figure 6, lower right panel)[98]. The residents of Mexico City consumed a diet higher in carbohydrates and lower in fat, and were, on average, more physically active, and had lower BMI and higher waist-to-hip ratios. The age–sex-adjusted prevalence of diabetes was lower in Mexico City than in San Antonio. Even among non-diabetic subjects, fasting and 2-hour post-load glucose and fasting insulin concentrations were lower in Mexico City. These observations suggest that the more sedentary lifestyle and higher fat diet of subjects in San Antonio increased the diabetes prevalence in this susceptible ethnic group. Further evidence of the importance of environmental factors on diabetes was provided by a study of Australian Aborigines—an ethnic group which has developed a high prevalence of diabetes due to recent changes in lifestyle. An improvement, or complete reversion, of metabolic abnormalities associated with diabetes was observed during a temporary reversion to a traditional hunting and gathering lifestyle[155].

Thrifty Genotypes and Phenotypes

What is the difference which makes the high-risk populations more susceptible to diabetes? In 1962, Neel hypothesized a 'thrifty genotype' involving rapid insulin secretion following a meal, which provided a survival advantage during times of famine[156]. Now that food is available in abundance and on a regular basis, this genotype is detrimental, giving rise to insulin resistance, hyperinsulinaemia, and eventual β cell decompensation leading to the development of NIDDM. Whether these subjects with the so-called 'thrifty genotype' also possess a primary abnormality of β cell structure or function is unknown (see Chapter 14).

Recently, however, the concept of a 'thrifty phenotype' has been proposed by Hales and Barker[157], as described in Chapter 15. This hypothesis suggests that malnutrition during intrauterine life and soon after birth causes poor β cell development and may lead to susceptibility to NIDDM later in life.

In summary, epidemiological (including migrant) studies of NIDDM suggest:

1. Susceptibility to diabetes differs among ethnic groups.
2. This susceptibility is in part genetic and manifest as increased insulin resistance and hyperinsulinaemia.
3. The increasing prevalence of diabetes in these high-risk groups and migrant populations appears to be due to the strong influence of environmental factors unmasking an underlying susceptibility to diabetes.

CONCLUSIONS

NIDDM is usually the culmination of a process of worsening metabolic abnormalities which may have taken many years. We have hypothesized[2,3] that insulin resistance is an early metabolic defect, which is, at least in part, of genetic origin[30,31]. Hyperglycaemia (to a degree not resulting in diabetes) stimulates the β cell to secrete more insulin, resulting in partial compensation for insulin resistance. This hyperglycaemia may result in impaired glucose tolerance as recognized by an oral glucose tolerance test. The inability to maintain sufficient hyperinsulinaemia (because of 'β cell exhaustion' or an intrinsic β cell defect) may then lead to worsening hyperglycaemia, or NIDDM.

Some of the clearly identified risk factors for diabetes may operate through this sequence of worsening insulin resistance followed by deficient insulin secretion. Obesity and physical inactivity contribute to insulin resistance. Obesity also has a strong genetic component and is probably influenced by different genes than those which cause susceptibility to NIDDM. Both obesity and NIDDM share a common risk factor: high-fat diet[73,139]. The implication, which is subject to testing, is that a reduction of the fat content of the diet may be beneficial in preventing both obesity and NIDDM. Other means of reducing obesity, such as increasing physical activity, would also be expected to reduce the risk of NIDDM.

The factors initiating the pathogenic process which ultimately leads to NIDDM remain elusive, but must, in many cases, begin operating early in life. In general, serum insulin concentrations are higher in persons at high risk of NIDDM, such as American Indians[158–160], Mexican–Americans[161] and non-diabetic first-degree relatives of Caucasians with NIDDM[162]. Hyperinsulinaemia predicts the development of impaired glucose tolerance and NIDDM[3,163]. The familial aggregation of disease and the marked racial differences in susceptibility suggest an important genetic contribution, although a simple explanation for the mode of inheritance of NIDDM would seem unlikely. Some of the familial influence on risk of NIDDM may be non-genetic, for example the intrauterine environmental effects described above and the hypothesized effect of infant malnutrition (the 'thrifty phenotype') discussed elsewhere (see Chapter 15). While rapid progress is occurring in the study of the genetics of NIDDM, as discussed elsewhere in this book (see Chapter 10), a simple explanation for NIDDM throughout the world is, in our opinion, unlikely. It is probable that several different genes contribute to NIDDM, including the contribution of different genes in different families and racial groups and a role for more than one contributing gene in some individuals. These effects may be combined with those of obesity, diet, physical inactivity and socio-economic factors, not all of which are likely to have a purely genetic basis. The ability to identify persons with a high genetic risk for NIDDM, however, will lead to more precise studies of the environmental risk factors and tests of preventive measures by allowing researchers in these areas to focus on subjects with genetic susceptibility.

There is consistent evidence for risk factors with an environmental component, such as obesity and physical inactivity. Thus until genetic studies lead to the development of more precise interventions (through genetic manipulation or pharmacology based on knowledge of the basic defects causing the disorder) to prevent NIDDM, the best hope for prevention may be through lifestyle modification, which may be effective in persons of widely different genetic backgrounds.

ACKNOWLEDGEMENTS

We thank the members of the Gila River Indian Community, Arizona, USA, for participation in the studies of the Pima Indians, and Dr Peter H. Bennett for advice and support. Dr Nagi was supported in part by the BDA–ICI Transatlantic Fellowship.

REFERENCES

1 Saad MF, Knowler WC, Pettitt DJ, et al. The natural history of impaired glucose tolerance in the Pima Indians. *N Engl J Med* 1988; **319**: 1500–6.
2 Knowler WC, Pettitt DJ, Saad MF, Bennett PH. Diabetes mellitus in the Pima Indians: incidence, risk factors and pathogenesis. *Diabetes Metab Rev* 1990; **6**: 1–27.
3 Saad MF, Knowler WC, Pettitt DJ, et al. A two-step model for development of non-insulin-dependent diabetes: *Am J Med* 1991; **90**: 229–35.
4 National Diabetes Data Group. Classification and diagnosis of diabetes mellitus and other categories of glucose intolerance. *Diabetes* 1979; **28**: 1039–57.
5 WHO Expert Committee on Diabetes Mellitus, Second report. *WHO Tech Rep Ser* 1980; **646**: 9–14.
6 World Health Organization. Diabetes mellitus: report of a WHO Study Group. *Technical Report Series No 727*, WHO, Geneva, 1985.
7 Turner RC, Holman RR, Matthews DR, et al. Diabetes nomenclature: classification or grading of severity? *Diabetic Med* 1986; **3**: 216–20.
8 Cudworth AG. Aetiology of diabetes mellitus. *Br J Hosp Med* 1976; **16**: 207–216.
9 Cudworth AG. Type I diabetes mellitus. *Diabetologia* 1978; **14**: 281–91.
10 Irvine WJ. Classification of idiopathic diabetes. *Lancet* 1977; **i**: 638–42.
11 Keen H. What's in a name? IDDM/NIDDM, type 1/type 2. *Diabetic Med* 1986; **3**: 11–12.
12 Irvine WJ, McCallum CJ, Gray RS, Duncan LJP. Clinical and pathogenic significance of pancreatic-islet-cell antibodies in diabetics treated with oral hypoglycemic agents. *Lancet* 1977; **i**: 1025–7.
13 Groop L, Miettinen A, Groop P-H, et al. Organ-specific autoimmunity and HLA-DR antigens as markers for β-cell destruction in patients with type II diabetes. *Diabetes* 1988; **37**: 99–103.
14 Landin-Olsson M, Nilsson KO, Lernmark A, Sundkvist G. (1990) Islet cell antibodies and fasting C-peptide predict insulin requirement at diagnosis of diabetes mellitus. *Diabetologia* 1990; **33**: 561–8.
15 Savage PJ, Bennett PH, Senter RG, Miller M. High prevalence of diabetes in young Pima Indians. *Diabetes* 1979; **28**: 937–942.
16 Knowler WC, Bennett PH, Bottazzo GF, Doniach D. Islet cell antibodies and diabetes mellitus in Pima Indians. *Diabetologia* 1979; **17**: 161–4.
17 Melton LJ, Palumbo PJ, Chu C-P. Incidence of diabetes mellitus by clinical type. *Diabetes Care* 1983; **6**: 75–86.

18 Bogardus C, Lillioja S, Howard BV, Reaven G, Mott D. Relationship between insulin secretion, insulin action, and fasting plasma glucose concentration in nondiabetic and noninsulin-dependent diabetic subjects. *J Clin Invest* 1984; **74**: 1238–46.

19 Defronzo RA. The triumvirate: B-cell, muscle, liver. A collusion responsible for NIDDM, Lilly Lecture. *Diabetes* 1987; **37**: 667–87.

20 Saad MF, Knowler WC, Pettitt DJ, et al. Sequential changes in serum insulin concentration during development of non-insulin-dependent diabetes. *Lancet* 1989; **i**: 1356–9.

21 Lillioja S, Mott DM, Howard BV, et al. Impaired glucose tolerance as a disorder of insulin action: longitudinal and cross-sectional studies in Pima Indians. *N Engl J Med* 1988; **318**: 1217–25.

22 Sicree RFA, Zimmet PZ, King HOM. Plasma insulin response among Nauruans: prediction of deterioration in glucose intolerance over 6 yr. *Diabetes* 1987; **36**: 179–86.

23 Lundgren H, Bengtsson G, Blohmé G, Lapidus L, Waldenström J. Fasting serum insulin concentration and early insulin response as risk determinants for developing diabetes. *Diabetes Med* 1990; **7**: 407–13.

24 Charles MA, Fontbonne A, Thibult N, et al. Risk factors for NIDDM in white population. Paris Prospective Study. *Diabetes* 1991; **40**: 796–9.

25 Haffner SM, Stern MP, Mitchell BD, Hazuda HP, Patterson JK. Incidence of type II diabetes in Mexican Americans predicted by fasting insulin and glucose levels, obesity, and body-fat distribution. *Diabetes* 1990; **39**: 283–8.

26 Warram JH, Martin BC, Krolewski AS, Soeldner JS, Kahn CR. Slow glucose removal rate and hyperinsulinemia precede the development of type II diabetes in the offspring of diabetic parents. *Ann Int Med* 1990; **113**: 909–915.

27 Bergstrom RW, Newell-Morris LL, Leonetti, DL, et al. Association of elevated fasting C-peptide level and increased intra-abdominal fat distribution with development of NIDDM in Japanese–American men. *Diabetes* 1990; **39**: 104–11.

28 Lillioja S, Mott DM, Spraul M, et al. Insulin resistance, β-cell function and the risk for non-insulin dependent diabetes mellitus: longitudinal studies in Pima Indians. (Submitted for publication.)

29 Lillioja S, Mott DM, Zawadzki JK, et al. In vivo insulin action is familial characteristic in nondiabetic Pima Indians. *Diabetes* 1987; **36**: 1329–35.

30 Bogardus C, Lillioja S, Nyomba BL, et al. Distribution of in vivo insulin action in Pima Indians as a mixture of three normal distributions. *Diabetes* 1989; **38**: 1423–32.

31 Prochazka M, Lillioja S, Tait JF, et al. Linkage of chromosomal markers on 4q with a putative gene determining maximal insulin action in Pima Indians. *Diabetes* 1993; **42**: 514–19.

32 Keen H, Jarrett RJ, McCartney P. The 10 year follow up of the Bedford survey (1962–1972): glucose tolerance and diabetes. *Diabetologia* 1982; **22**: 73–8.

33 Kadowaki T, Miyake Y, Hagura R, et al. Risk factors for worsening to diabetes in subjects with impaired glucose tolerance. *Diabetologia* 1984; **26**: 44–9.

34 Knowler WC, Pettitt DJ, Savage PJ, Bennett PH. Diabetes incidence in Pima Indians: contributions of obesity and parental diabetes. *Am J Epidemiol* 1981; **113**: 144–56.

35 King H, Zimmet P, Raper LR, Balkau B. Risk factors for diabetes in three Pacific populations. *Am J Epidemiol* 1984; **119**: 396–409.

36 O'Sullivan JB, Mahan CM. Blood sugar levels, glycosuria, and body weight related to development of diabetes mellitus. *JAMA*, 1965; **194**: 587–92.

37 Kahn HA, Herman JA, Medalie JH, et al. Factors related to diabetes incidence: a multivariate analysis of two years observation on 10 000 men. *J. Chronic Dis* 1971; **23**: 617–29.
38 Westlund K, Nicolaysen R. Ten-year mortality and morbidity related to serum cholesterol: a follow-up of 3 751 men aged 40–49. *Scand J Clin Lab Invest* 1972; **30** (Suppl 127): 1–24.
39 Jarrett RJ, Keen H, Fuller JH, McCartney M. Worsening to diabetes in men with impaired glucose tolerance ('borderline diabetes'). *Diabetologia* 1979; **16**: 25–30.
40 Skarfors ET, Selinus KI, Lithell HO. Risk factors for developing non-insulin dependent diabetes: a 10 year follow up of men in Uppsala. *Br Med J* 1991; **303**: 755–60.
41 Helmrich SP, Ragland DR, Leung RW, Paffenbarger RS. Physical activity and reduced occurrence of non-insulin-dependent diabetes mellitus. *N Engl J Med* 1991; **325**: 147–152.
42 Manson JE, Nathan DM, Krolewski AS, et al. A prospective study of exercise and incidence of diabetes among US male physicians. *JAMA* 1992; **268**: 63–7.
43 Everhart JE, Pettitt DJ, Bennett PH, Knowler WC. Duration of obesity increases the incidence of non-insulin-dependent diabetes mellitus. *Diabetes* 1992; **41**: 235–40.
44 Knowler WC, Pettitt DJ, Saad MF, et al. Obesity in the Pima Indians: its magnitude and relationship with diabetes. *Am J Clin Nutr* 1991; **53**: 1543S–1551S.
45 Goldman RF, Buskirk ER. Body volume measurement by under water weighing. In: *Techniques for Measuring Body Composition* (eds J Borzek, A Henschel) National Academy of Sciences, National Research Council, Washington, DC, 1961, pp 78–106.
46 Vague J. The degree of masculine differentiation of obesities: a factor determining predisposition to diabetes, atherosclerosis, gout, and uric calculous disease. *Am J Clin Nutr* 1956; **4**: 20–34.
47 Ohlson L-O, Larsson B, Svärdsudd L, et al. The influence of body fat distribution on the incidence of diabetes mellitus: 13.5 years of follow-up of the participants in the study of men born in 1913. *Diabetes* 1985; **34**: 1055–8.
48 Dowse GK, Zimmet PZ, Gareeboo H, et al. Abdominal obesity and physical inactivity as risk factors for NIDDM and impaired glucose tolerance in Indian, Creole, and Chinese Mauritians. *Diabetes Care* 1991; **14**: 271–91.
49 Haffner SM, Mitchell BD, Stern MP, Hazuda HP, Patterson JK. Public health significance of upper body adiposity for non-insulin dependent diabetes mellitus in Mexican Americans. *Int J Obes* 1992; **16**: 177–84.
50 McKeigue PM, Pierpoint T, Ferrie JE, Marmot MG. Relationship of glucose intolerance and hyperinsulinaemia to body fat pattern in South Asians and Europeans. *Diabetologia* 1992; **35**: 785–91.
51 Björntorp P, Fahlén M, Grimby G, et al. Carbohydrate and lipid metabolism in middle-aged, physically well-trained men. *Metabolism* 1972; **21**: 1037–44.
52 Lindgärde F, Saltin B. Daily physical activity, work capacity and glucose tolerance in lean and obese normoglycaemic middle-aged men. *Diabetologia* 1981; **20**: 134–8.
53 Cederholm J, Wibell L. Glucose tolerance and physical activity in a health survey of middle-aged subjects. *Acta Med Scand* 1985; **217**: 373–8.
54 Jarrett RJ, Shipley MJ, Hunt R. Physical activity, glucose tolerance, and diabetes mellitus: the Whitehall study. *Diabetic Med* 1986; **3**: 549–51.
55 Taylor R, Ram P, Zimmet P, Raper LP, Ringrose H. Physical activity and prevalence of diabetes in Melanesian and Indian men in Fiji. *Diabetologia* 1984; **27**: 578–82.

56 Kriska AM, Knowler WC, LaPorte RE, et al. Development of questionnaire to examine relationship of physical activity and diabetes in Pima Indians. *Diabetes Care* 1990; **13**: 401–11.
57 Kriska AM, LaPorte RE, Pettitt DJ, et al. The association of physical activity with obesity, fat distribution and glucose intolerance in Pima Indians. *Diabetologia* (in press).
58 Frisch RE, Wyshak G, Albright TE, Albright NL, Schiff I. Lower prevalence of diabetes in female former college athletes compared with nonathletes. *Diabetes* 1986; **35**: 1101–5.
59 Manson JE, Rimm EB, Stampfer MJ, et al. Physical activity and incidence of non-insulin-dependent diabetes mellitus in women. *Lancet* 1991; **338**: 774–8.
60 Eriksson K-F, Lindgärde F. Prevention of type 2 (non-insulin-dependent) diabetes mellitus by diet and physical exercise: the 6-year Malmö feasibility study. *Diabetologia* 1991; **34**: 891–8.
61 West KM. *Epidemiology of Diabetes and its Vascular Complications*. Elsevier New York, 1978.
62 Zimmet P. Type 2 (non-insulin-dependent) diabetes: an epidemiological overview. *Diabetologia* 1982; **22**: 399–411.
63 Jarrett RJ. Epidemiology and public health aspects of non-insulin-dependent mellitus. *Epidemiol Rev* 1989; **11**: 151–71.
64 Yudkin J. Dietary fat and dietary sugar in relation to ischaemic heart disease and diabetes. *Lancet* 1964; **ii** 4–5.
65 Cohen AM, Teitelbaum A. Effect of different levels of protein in 'sucrose' and 'starch' diets on the glucose tolerance and growth. *Metabolism* 1966; **15**: 1034–8.
66 Baird JD. Diet and the development of clinical diabetes. *Acta Diabetol Lat* 1972; **9** (Suppl 1): 621–39.
67 Cleave T. *The Saccharine Disease*. Wright, Bristol, 1974.
68 Feskens JM, Kromhout D. Cardiovascular risk factors and the 25-year incidence of diabetes mellitus in middle-aged men. The Zutphen Study. *Am J Epidemiol* 1989; **130**: 1101–8.
69 Trowell H. Dietary-fibre hypothesis of the aetiology of diabetes mellitus. *Diabetes* 1975; **24**; 762–5.
70 Himsworth HP. Diet and the incidence of diabetes mellitus. *Clin Sci Mol Med* 1935–6; **2**: 117–48.
71 West KM, Kalbfleisch JM. Influence of nutritional factors on prevalence of diabetes. *Diabetes* 1971; **20**: 99–108.
72 Tsunehara CH, Leonetti DL, Fujimoto WY. Diet of second-generation Japanese–American men with and without non-insulin-dependent diabetes. *Am J Clin Nutr* 1990; **52**; 731–8.
73 Marshall JA, Hamman RF, Baxter J. High-fat, low-carbohydrate diet and the etiology of non-insulin-dependent diabetes mellitus: the San Luis Valley Diabetes Study. *Am J Epidemiol* 1991; **134**: 590–603.
74 Bennett PH, Knowler WC, Baird HR, et al. Diet and development of non-insulin-dependent diabetes mellitus: an epidemiological perspective. In: *Diet, Diabetes, and Atherosclerosis* (eds G Pozza, P Micossi, AL Catapano, R Paoletti) Raven Press, New York, 1984, pp 109–119.
75 Block G. A review of validations of dietary assessement methods. *Am J Epidemiol* 1982; **115**: 492–505.
76 Rohan TE, Potter JD. Retrospective assessment of dietary intake. *Am J Epidemiol* 1984; **120**: 876–7.
77 Zimmet P, Dowse G, Finch C. The epidemiology and natural history of NIDDM: lessons from the South Pacific. *Diab Metab Rev* 1990; **6**: 91–124.

78 Kawate R, Yamakido M, Nishimoto Y, et al. Diabetes mellitus and its vascular complications in Japanese migrants on the island of Hawaii. *Diabetes Care* 1979; **2**: 161–70.

79 Himsworth HP, Marshall EM. The diet of diabetics prior to the onset of the disease. *Clin Sci Mol Med* 1935–6; **2**: 95–115.

80 Medalie JH, Papier CM, Goldbourt U, Herman JB. Major factors in the development of diabetes mellitus in 10 000 men. *Arch Intern Med* 1975; **135**: 811–17.

81 Snowdon DA, Phillips RL. Does a vegetarian diet reduce the occurrence of diabetes? *Am J Public Health* 1985; **75**: 507–12.

82 Lundgren H, Bengtsson C, Blohme G, et al. Dietary habits and incidence of non-insulin-dependent diabetes mellitus in a population study of women in Gothenburg, Sweden. *Am J Clin Nutr* 1989; **49**: 708–12.

83 Colditz GA, Manson J, Stampfer MJ, et al. Diet and risk of clinical diabetes in women. *Am J Clin Nutr* 1992; **55**: 1018–23.

84 Feskens EJM, Bowles CH, Kromhout D. Carbohydrate intake and body mass index in relation to the risk of glucose in an elderly population. *Am J Clin Nutr* 1991; **54**: 136–40.

85 King H, Zimmet P, Pargeter K, Raper LR, Collins V. Ethnic differences in susceptibility to non-insulin-dependent diabetes: a comparative study of two urbanized Micronesian populations. *Diabetes* 1984; **33**: 1002–7.

86 Feskens EJM, Kronhout D. Habitual dietary intake and glucose tolerance in euglycaemic men: the Zutphen Study. *Int J Epidemiol* 1990; **19**; 953–9.

87 Stern MP. Kelly West lecture: primary prevention of type II diabetes mellitus. *Diabetes Care* 1991; **14**: 399–410.

88 Dreon DM, Frey-Hewitt B, Ellsworth N, et al. Dietary fat : carbohydrate ratio and obesity in middle-aged men. *Am J Clin Nutr* 1988; **47**: 995–1000.

89 George V, Tremblay A, Despres JP, Leblanc C, Bouchard C. Effect of dietary fat content on total and regional adiposity in men and women. *Int J Obes* 1990; **14**: 1085–94.

90 Sadur CN, Yost TJ, Eckel RH. Fat feeding decreases insulin responsiveness of adipose tissue lipoprotein lipase. *Metabolism* 1984; **33**: 1043–7.

91 Chisolm K, O'Dea K. Effect of short-term consumption of a high fat, low carbohydrate diet on metabolic control in insulin deficient diabetic rats. *Metabolism* 1987; **36**: 237–43.

92 Drury TF, Danchik KM, Harris MI. Sociodemographic characteristics of adult diabetics. In: *Diabetes in America* (eds MI Harris, RF Hamman) Diabetes Data Compiled 1984, Washington, DC, US Government Printing Office (NIH publ no 85–1468) Ch VII, pp 1–37.

93 Cruz-Vidal M, Costas P Jr, Garcia-Palmieri MR, Sorlie PD, Hertzmark E. Factors related to diabetes mellitus in Puerto Rican men. *Diabetes* 1979; **28**: 300–7.

94 Zimmet P, Faaiuso S, Ainuu J, et al. The prevalence of diabetes in the rural and urban population of Western Samoa. *Diabetes* 1981; **30**: 45–51.

95 King H, Taylor R, Zimmet P, et al. Non-insulin-dependent diabetes (NIDDM) in a newly independent Pacific nation: the Republic of Kiribati. *Diabetes Care* 1984; **7**: 409–15.

96 Martin FIR, Wyatt GB, Griew AR, Hauraheliam M, Higginbotham L. Diabetes mellitus in urban and rural Communities in Papua New Guinea: studies of prevalence and plasma insulin. *Diabetologia* 1980, **18**: 369–74.

97 Taylor RJ, Zimmet P. Obesity and diabetes in Western Samoa. *Int J Obes* 1981; **5**: 367–76.

98 Stern MP, Gonzalez C, Mitchell BD, et al. Genetic and environmental determi-
    nants of type II diabetes in Mexico City and San Antonio. *Diabetes* 1992; **41**:
    484–92.
99 Taylor R, Badcock J, King H, et al. Dietary intake, exercise, obesity and
    noncommunicable disease in rural and urban populations of three Pacific Island
    countries. *J Am Coll Nutr* 1992; **11**: 283–93.
100 Everhart J, Knowler WC, Bennett PH. Incidence and risk factors for noninsulin-
    dependent diabetes. In: *Diabetes in America* (eds MI Harris, RF Hamman)
    Diabetes Data Compiled 1984, Washington, DC, US Government Printing Office
    (NIH publ no 85–1468), Ch IV, pp 1–35.
101 Zimmet P, Taft P, Guinea A, Guthrie W, Thoma K. The high prevalence of
    diabetes mellitus on a central Pacific island. *Diabetologia* 1977; **13**: 111–15.
102 Bennett PH. Diabetes in developing countries and unusual populations. In:
    Diabetes in Epidemiological Perspective (eds JI Mann, K Pyorala, S Teuscher)
    Churchill Livingstone, New York, pp 43–57.
103 Hamman RF. Diabetes in affluent societies. In: *Diabetes in Epidemiological
    Perspective* (eds JI Mann, K Pyorala, S Teuscher) Churchill Livingstone, New
    York, pp 7–42.
104 Garn SM, Bailey SM, Cole PE, Higgins ITT. Level of education, level of income
    and level of fatness in adults. *Am J Clin Nutr* 1977; **30**: 721–52.
105 Hazuda HP, Haffner SM, Stern MP. Effects of acculturation and socioeconomic
    status on obesity and diabetes in Mexican Americans. *Am J Epidemiol* 1988; **128**:
    1289–301.
106 Butler WJ, Ostrander LD, Jr, Carman WJ, Lamphiear DE. Diabetes mellitus in
    Tecumseh, Michigan. *Am J Epidemiol* 1982; **116**: 971–80.
107 Stern MP, Knapp JA, Hazuda HP, et al. Genetic and environmental determi-
    nants of type II diabetes in Mexican Americans: is there a 'descending limb' to
    the modernization/diabetes relationship? *Diabetes Care* 1991; **14**: 649–54.
108 Wilson PWF, Anderson KM, Kannel WB. Epidemiology of diabetes mellitus in
    the elderly: the Framingham Study. *Am J Med* 1986; **80** (Suppl 5A): 3–9.
109 Bengtsson C, Blohme G, Lapidus L, et al. Do antihypertensive drugs precipitate
    diabetes? *Br Med J* 1984; **289**: 1495–7.
110 Bengtsson C, Blohme G, Lapidus L, Lundgren H. Diabetes in hypertensive
    women: an effect of antihypertensive drugs or the hypertensive state per se?
    Diabetic Med 1988; **5**: 261–4.
111 Skarfors ET, Lithell HO, Selinus I, Åberg H. Do antihypertensive drugs precipi-
    tate diabetes in predisposed men? *Br Med J* 1989; **298**: 1147–52.
112 Lithell HOL. Effect of antihypertensive drugs on insulin, glucose, and lipid
    metabolism. *Diabetes Care* 1991; **14**: 203–9.
113 Salomaa VV, Strandberg TE, Vanhanen H, et al. Glucose tolerance and blood
    pressure: longterm follow up study in middle-aged men. *Br Med J* 1991; **302**:
    493–6.
114 Modan M, Halkin H, Almog S, et al. Hyperinsulinemia: a link between hyperten-
    sion, obesity and glucose intolerance. *J Clin Invest* 1985; **75**: 809–17.
115 Donahue RP, Skyler JS, Schneiderman B, Prineas RJ. Hyperinsulinemia and
    elevated blood pressure: cause, confounder, or coincidence? *Am J Epidemiol*
    1990; **132**: 827–36.
116 Yudkin JS. Hypertension and non-insulin dependent diabetes. *Br Med J* 1991;
    303: 730–2.
117 Saad MF, Knowler WC, Pettitt DJ, et al. Insulin and hypertension: relationship
    to obesity and glucose intolerance in Pima Indians. *Diabetes* 1990; **39**: 1430–5.

118 Dunn JP, Ipsen J, Elsom KO, Ohtani M. Risk factors in coronary artery disease, hypertension and diabetes. *Am J Med Sci* 1970; **259**: 309–22.

119 Wilson PW, McGee DL, Kannel WB. Obesity, very low density lipoproteins, and glucose intolerance over fourteen years: the Framingham Study. *Am J Epidemiol* 1981; **114**; 697–704.

120 Papoz L, Eschwege E, Warnet JL, Richard JL, Claude JR. Incidence and risk factors of diabetes in the Paris prospective study (G.R.E.A.). In: *Advances in Diabetes Epidemiology* (ed E Eschwege) Elsevier, Amsterdam, 1982, pp 95–102.

121 Paffenbarger RS Jr, Wing AL. Chronic disease in former college students. XII. Early predictors of adult-onset diabetes mellitus. *Am J Epidemiol* 1973; **97**: 314–23.

122 Stampfer MJ, Colditz GA, Willett WC, et al. A prospective study of moderate alcohol drinking and risk of diabetes in women. *Am J Epidemiol* 1988; **128**: 549–58.

123 Reaven GM. Role of insulin resistance in human disease. *Diabetes* 1988; **37**: 1595–607.

124 DeFronzo, RA, Ferrannini E. Insulin resistance: a multifaceted syndrome responsible for NIDDM, obesity, hypertension, dyslipidemia, and atherosclerotic cardiovascular disease. *Diabetes Care*, 1991; **14**: 173–94.

125 Zimmet P. Kelly West Lecture 1991, challenges in diabetes epidemiology: from West to the rest. *Diabetes Care* 1992; **15**: 232–52.

126 Mantel N, Haenszel W. Statistical aspects of the analysis of data from retrospective studies of disease. *J Nat Cancer Inst* 1959; **22**: 719–48.

127 Knowler WC, Pettitt DJ, Lillioja S, Nelson RG. Genetic and environmental factors in the development of diabetes mellitus in Pima Indians. In: *Genetic Susceptibility to Environmental Factors: a Challenge for Public Intervention* (eds U Smith, S Eriksson, F Lindgärde). Almqvist & Wiksell, Stockholm, 1988, pp 67–74.

128 Pettitt DJ, Saad MF, Bennett PH, Nelson RG, Knowler WC. Familial predisposition to renal disease in two generations of Pima Indians with type 2 (non-insulin-dependent) diabetes mellitus. *Diabetologia* 1990; **33**: 438–43.

129 Pettitt DJ, Baird HR, Aleck KA, Bennett PH, Knowler WC. Excessive obesity in offspring of Pima Indian women with diabetes during pregnancy. *N Engl J Med* 1983; **308**: 242–5.

130 Pettitt DJ, Knowler WC, Bennett PH, Aleck KA, Baird HR. Obesity in offspring of diabetic Pima Indian women despite normal birthweight. *Diabetes Care* 1987; **10**: 76–80.

131 Pettitt DJ, Aleck KA, Baird HR, et al. Congenital susceptibility to NIDDM: Role of intrauterine environment. *Diabetes* 1988; **37**: 622–8.

132 Pettitt DJ, Nelson RG, Saad MF, Bennett PH, Knowler WC. Diabetes and obesity in the offspring of Pima Indian women with diabetes during pregnancy. *Diabetes Care* 1993; **16** (Suppl 1): 310–14.

133 Pettitt DJ, Bennett PH, Knowler WC, Baird HR, Aleck KA. Gestational diabetes mellitus and impaired glucose tolerance during pregnancy: long-term effects on obesity and glucose tolerance in the offspring. *Diabetes* 1985; **34**: 119–22.

134 Pettitt DJ, Bennett, PH, Saad MF, et al. Abnormal glucose tolerance during pregnancy in Pima Indian women: long-term effects on the offspring. *Diabetes* 1991; **40**: 126–30.

135 Freinkel N. The Banting Lecture 1980: of pregnancy and progeny. *Diabetes* 1980; **29**: 1023–35.

136 Metzger BE, Silverman BL, Frienkel N, et al. Amniotic fluid insulin concentration as a predictor of obesity. *Arch Dis Child* 1990; **65**: 1050–2.
137 Pettitt DJ, Knowler WC. Diabetes and obesity in the Pima Indians: a cross-generational vicious cycle. *J Obes Weight Regul* 1988; **7**: 61–75.
138 Bennett PH, Knowler WC. Increasing prevalence of diabetes in the Pima (American) Indians over a ten year period. In: *Diabetes 1979: Proceedings of the 10th Congress of the International Diabetes Federation* (ed WK Waldhäusl) Excerpta Medica, Amsterdam, 1979, pp 507–11.
139 Ravussin E, Swinburn BA. Pathophysiology of obesity. *Lancet* 1992; **340**: 404–8.
140 Williams RC, Knowler WC, Butler WJ, et al. HLA-A2 and type 2 (insulin independent) diabetes mellitus in Pima Indians: an association of allele frequency with age. *Diabetologia* 1981; **21**: 460–3.
141 King H, Rewers M. Diabetes in adults is now a Third World problem. *Bull WHO* 1991; **69**: 643–8.
142 Zimmet P, Taylor R, Ram P. Prevalence of diabetes and impaired glucose tolerance in the biracial (Melanesian and Indian) population of Fiji: a rural–urban comparison. *Am J Epidemiol* 1983; **118**: 673–88.
143 Stern MP, Gaskill SP, Hazuda HP. Does obesity explain excess prevalence of diabetes among Mexican Americans? Results of the San Antonio heart study. *Diabetologia* 1983; **24**: 272–7.
144 Haffner SM, Hazuda HP, Mitchell BD, Patterson JK, Stern MP. Increased incidence of type II diabetes mellitus in Mexican Americans. *Diabetes Care* 1991; **14**: 102–8.
145 Cheah JS, Tan BY. Diabetes among different races in a similar environment. In: *Diabetes 1979: Proceedings of the 10th Congress of the International Diabetes Federation* (ed WK Waldhäusl) Excerpta Medica, Amsterdam, 1979, pp 512–16.
146 Jackson WPU. Diabetes in South Africa. In: *Advances in Metabolic Disorders*, Vol 9 (ed R Levine, R Luft) Academic Press, New York, 1978, pp 111–46.
147 Mather HM, Keen H. The Southhall diabetes survey: prevalence of known diabetes in Asians and Europeans. *Br Med J* 1985; **291**: 1081–4.
148 Verma NPS, Mehta SP, Madhu S, Mather HM, Keen H. Prevalence of known diabetes in an urban Indian environment: the Darya Ganj diabetes survey. *Br Med J* 1986; **293**: 423–4.
149 Simmons D, Williams DRR, Powell MJ. Prevalence of diabetes in a predominantly Asian community: preliminary findings of the Coventry diabetes study. *Br Med J* 1989; **298**: 18–21.
150 Poon-King T, Henry MV, Rampersad F. Prevalence and natural history of diabetes in Trinidad. *Lancet* 1968; **i**: 155–60.
151 Marine N, Edelstein O, Jackson WPU, Vinik AI. Diabetes hyperglycaemia and glycosuria among Indians, Malays and Africans (Bantu) in Cape Town, South Africa. *Diabetes* 1969; **18**: 840–57.
152 Cassidy JT. Diabetes in Fiji. *NZ Med J* 1967; **66**: 167–72.
153 Gupta OP, Dave SH, Joshi MH. Prevalence of diabetes in India. In: *Advances in Metabolic Disorders*, Vol 9 (eds R Levine, R Luft) Academic Press, New York, 1978, pp 13–28.
154 Ramachandran A, Jali MV, Mohan V, Snehalatha C, Viswanathan M. High prevalence of diabetes in an urban population in south India. *Br Med J* 1988; **297**: 587–90.
155 O'Dea K. Marked improvement in carbohydrate and lipid metabolism in diabetic Australian Aborigines after temporary reversion to traditional lifestyle. *Diabetes* 1984; **33**: 596–603.

156 Neel JV. Diabetes mellitus: a thrifty genotype rendered detrimental by 'progress'? *Am J Hum Genet* 1962; **14**: 353–62.

157 Hales CN, Barker DJP. Type 2 (non-insulin-dependent) diabetes mellitus: the thrifty phenotype hypothesis. *Diabetologia* 1992; **35**: 595–601.

158 Aronoff SL, Bennett PH, Gorden P, Rushforth N, Miller M. Unexplained hyperinsulinemia in normal and 'prediabetic' Pima Indians compared with normal Caucasians. *Diabetes* 1977; **26**: 827–40.

159 Lillioja S, Nyomba BL, Saad MF, et al. Exaggerated early insulin release and insulin resistance in a diabetes-prone population: a metabolic comparison of Pima Indians and Caucasians. *J Clin Endocrinol Metab* 1991; **73**: 866–76.

160 Pettitt DJ, Moll PP, Knowler WC, et al. Insulinemia in children at low and high risk of non-insulin-dependent diabetes mellitus. *Diabetes Care* 1993; **16**: 608–15.

161 Haffner SM, Stern MP, Hazuda HP, et al. Hyperinsulinemia in a population at high risk for non-insulin-dependent diabetes mellitus. *N Engl J Med* 1986; **315**: 220–224.

162 Eriksson J, Franssila-Kallunki A, Ekstrand A, et al. Early metabolic defects in persons at increased risk for non-insulin-dependent diabetes mellitus. *N Engl J Med* 1989; **321**: 337–43.

163 Zimmet PZ, Collins VR, Dowse GK, Knight LT. Hyperinsulinaemia in youth is a predictor of type 2 (non-insulin-dependent) diabetes mellitus. *Diabetologia* 1992; **35**: 534–41.

Chapter Twelve

Family Studies: Perspectives on the Genetic and Environmental Determinants of Non-insulin-dependent Diabetes Mellitus

Joanne Cook and Robert Turner
John Radcliffe Infirmary, Oxford, UK

INTRODUCTION

The prevalence of diabetes in those aged in their 60s in white Caucasian populations varies from 3% to 8%, but a number of ethnic groups have prevalences of up to 35%[1,2]. These differences may in part be genetic, as evidenced by the high concordance rate for diabetes in monozygotic twins[3,4] and by the increased prevalence of the disease in the first-degree relatives of affected subjects[5]. Despite the evidence for a substantial genetic component, the mode of inheritance and the molecular basis of this inheritance are unknown[6]. The phenotypic expression is influenced by a number of environmental factors including age and obesity[7].

The discrimination of type 1 (autoimmune) diabetes from type 2 or non-insulin-dependent diabetes mellitus (NIDDM) has been an important step in

Causes of Diabetes. Edited by R. D. G. Leslie
© 1993 John Wiley & Sons Ltd

understanding the heterogeneity of diabetes[8,9]. However, progress in unravelling the aetiological basis of NIDDM has been slow. The pathophysiology of NIDDM is complex, and secondary, metabolic changes can obscure the fundamental defects. The late age of onset of a genetically determined disease and the role of environmental factors in influencing phenotypic expression introduce further complexity to the study of the inheritance of the disease[6,7].

FAMILIAL NATURE OF NIDDM

EARLY STUDIES

The hereditary basis of diabetes has been suspected for over 2000 years. The earliest reports of the familial nature of diabetes are found in the writings of the Hindu physicians Sushruta and Charaka[10]. Mention of the familial nature of the disease is made by a number of European writers from the Renaissance[10]. Early in the twentieth century several reports of familial aggregation of the disease were made. These presentations of family statistics were generally of two types: (i) the listing of genealogies in diabetic families[11,12]; (ii) the listing of diabetes incidence among relatives of diabetic patients. The statistical significance of these incidences was not tested[13,14].

A significant advance was made in 1933 when Allan[15] and Pincus and White[16] pooled groups of pedigrees and assessed whether they complied with simple genetic hypotheses. Unfortunately, in interpreting all the studies done in the next three decades, one needs to remember that a distinction between type 1 and type 2 was rarely made. Allan[15] discounted dominant inheritance as a general explanation because of the many pedigrees in which a diabetic patient reported unaffected parents, and observed that the proportions of affected to unaffected offspring from various types of matings suggested the transmission of diabetes as an autosomal recessive trait. Much of this analysis was invalidated by the use of a spuriously low estimate of the gene frequency.

Pincus and White[16] documented the family histories of 523 diabetic patients and compared them with the family histories from 153 non-diabetic control subjects. A statistically significant excess of diabetic relatives in the families of diabetic patients was documented, and approximation to Mendelian expectations for autosomal recessivity was demonstrated. Pointing out the inadequacy of family history alone, these investigators went on to perform glucose tolerance tests on a small series of relatives to identify subclinical disease[17].

Harris[18] collected familial data on a series of 1241 patients attending the King's College Hospital Diabetic Clinics. Sib–sib correlations with respect to age at onset of the disease were found. The sibs of the early-onset diabetic patients were more likely to develop the disease in early life than were the sibs of the late-onset diabetic subjects. Diabetes was considered to be heterogeneous, with the early-onset and late-onset cases being determined by different genotypes.

Steinberg and Wilder[19] observed close to the expected Mendelian ratios for recessive inheritance, and favoured this inheritance model for the majority of cases of diabetes.

A number of limitations are apparent in these early studies. Subclinical disease was not, in general, accounted for. In addition diabetes was assumed to be a discrete qualitative trait. This was shown to be inappropriate when, in the 1960s, a number of population studies and community surveys documented a unimodal distribution of glucose tolerance. Thompson[20] performed oral glucose tolerance tests on 164 case relatives and 107 control subjects. A continuous distribution of blood sugar concentrations was demonstrated with no clear-cut division into normal and abnormal values in either series.

Stimulated by this demonstration of unimodality, a number of investigators began to explore the possibility that the majority of cases of diabetes had a multifactorial basis. When the genetic contribution to a trait is thought to be multifactorial, the magnitude of the genetic contribution is expressed in terms of 'heritability', defined as the ratio of the phenotypic variation that is genetic in origin to the total phenotypic variation of the trait. The term 'threshold character' is used when the cut-off point for disease diagnosis lies on a continuum. Falconer[21] estimated the overall heritability for diabetes, disregarding age-at-onset, to be 35%. Cases with early onset were considered to be genetically different from late-onset cases. Simpson[22] estimated the heritability to range from 27% to 55%, depending on age at onset.

The inclusion of type 1 diabetic patients in the early studies described above makes their interpretation difficult. Although suspicions had previously been raised, it was not until the discrimination of juvenile-onset diabetes, termed insulin-dependent diabetes mellitus (IDDM) from NIDDM on the basis of autoimmunity and major histocompatibility complex (MHC) associations that a major source of genetic heterogeneity was effectively eliminated[8,9].

TWIN STUDIES

Since monozygotic twins share genes and in most cases early environment, concordance (i.e. both twins having the disease) is suggestive of genetic determination whereas discordance is strongly suggestive of environmental effects.

The twin studies are discussed in detail in Chapter 13. At this stage, however, we would like to raise some relevant points. Barnett et al[3]. ascertained 200 pairs of monozygotic twins with at least one member of each twin pair having diabetes. Forty-six per cent of the IDDM twins were discordant (67 out of 147 pairs), demonstrating that genetic influences cannot be the only determining factors. The NIDDM twins, on the other hand were mostly concordant (48 out of 53 pairs, 91%). This study suggested that IDDM and NIDDM were genetically independent, and that genetic factors were more influential in NIDDM than in IDDM diabetes. Concordant twins were more likely to be ascertained in this study because the authors were selecting twins with diabetes: each member of a twin pair had an additive likelihood of ascertainment, and testing of a non-diabetic co-twin was likely to have taken place once one member of a twin pair has been diagnosed. These factors may have resulted in overestimation of concordance in this study.

Newman et al.[14] excluded ascertainment bias and overestimation of concordance by investigating 176 male monozygotic twin pairs recruited without regard to the diabetic status of either twin. The twins were studied at mean age 47 years and again 10 years later. This cross-sectional study confirmed marked concordance in monozygotic twin pairs (58%) at the initial examination. However, this figure underestimated concordance since they found only one of 15 originally discordant twin pairs remained discordant at a second examination 10 years later.

The twin studies strongly suggest the importance of genetic factors in the development of NIDDM, but they tell us nothing about the mode of inheritance. The lack of complete concordance and variation in age of onset between twins indicates a non-genetic component in the aetiology of the disease.

BIMODALITY

A high prevalence of NIDDM is found in the Pima Indians, who live on a reservation by the Gila River in Arizona, and amongst the inhabitants of certain Pacific islands. These populations have undergone considerable life-style change within the past century. There has been transition from a hunter/gatherer lifestyle to a more Westernized way of life, associated with a high prevalence of obesity[23].

Bimodality of glucose tolerance has been demonstrated in the Pima Indians[24], the Nauruans[25] and the Polynesians in Western Samoa[26]. This suggested that NIDDM in these populations is not merely a quantitative deviation from normal but is a distinct disease entity. A single gene effect in these populations has been postulated on this basis. Bimodality of itself, however, does not necessarily signify a single gene effect. An alternative explanation is that a rapid rather than gradual transition from normality to disease could give an apparent discontinuum. Such a rapid transition could arise from the deleterious effects of hyperglycaemia[27]. Bimodality is not a feature of Caucasian population studies[20] but has been reported in the first-degree relatives of Caucasian subjects with NIDDM[28].

FAMILY STUDIES AND THE MODE OF INHERITANCE

The mode of inheritance of a disorder can be rigorously determined only by the segregation analysis of familial data[29]. This approach involves ascertaining probands with the disorder without regard to family history, and studying the first-degree relatives to document the pattern of inheritance.

Although it would appear obvious that segregation analysis is a necessary prerequisite for more sophisticated genetic studies, a paucity of such data has been reported since the discrimination of IDDM from NIDDM. Family studies are difficult in NIDDM. The late age of onset and the increased mortality of affected subjects result in a paucity of complete nuclear families, in which both parents of a diabetic can be studied. The major difficulty is simply that in most cases one or both parents of a subject with NIDDM are deceased, while their children are not yet old enough to express the disease. Because of the prevalence of subclinical disease, careful phenotypic assessment of all family members is essential.

The genetic hypotheses which have been entertained for NIDDM include autosomal recessivity, autosomal dominance and multifactorial inheritance.

The Autosomal Recessive Hypothesis

The moderately low reported prevalence of NIDDM in the offspring of Caucasian conjugal diabetic parents, who would in a single recessive model all develop diabetes, makes a single recessive gene an unlikely model of inheritance for the usual form of NIDDM[30–33]. The available data, however, require cautious interpretation because the majority was collected before the distinction of IDDM from NIDDM was fully elucidated. Although the majority of the parents had maturity-onset diabetes, the inclusion of IDDM patients giving genetic heterogeneity is a potential confounding variable.

Cooke et al.[30] found a prevalence of known diabetes in the offspring of conjugal diabetic parents of 4.4%. Kahn et al.[31] found a higher prevalence when they performed glucose tolerance tests. Tattersall and Fajans[32], using oral glucose tolerance tests, assessed the cumulative risk of abnormal glucose tolerance or diabetes by the age of 60 years in the offspring of conjugal diabetic parents to be approximately 60%. On the basis of 10-year follow-up of the 700 offspring of 205 conjugal diabetic parents, Ganda and Soeldner[33] have estimated that by age 85 years 33% of the offspring will have diabetes and 50% will demonstrate an abnormality of glucose tolerance. Although each of these studies has limitations, it is apparent that not all the offspring of conjugal diabetic parents develop diabetes. These results are not consistent with autosomal recessivity unless heterogeneity or a low penetrance were postulated.

The Dominant Gene Hypothesis

Other investigators have postulated that the common form of NIDDM is inherited as an autosomal dominant trait with incomplete penetrance[6]. The evidence for straightforward dominant inheritance is lacking in NIDDM. However, the dominant hypothesis has remained tenable because of the complexity of family studies in NIDDM. The high prevalence of the disease resulting in complex pedigrees, the late age of onset, the probable incomplete penetrance of the genetic predisposition, the role of age and obesity in influencing phenotypic expression, and the need to test family members to exclude subclinical disease have been regarded as the culprits, obscuring the evidence for a dominant genetic predisposition to NIDDM.

Kobberling and Tillil[5] documented the family histories of 311 subjects with NIDDM. An age correction to calculate the extrapolated prevalence at age 80 years was performed according to the modified Stromgren method. The calculated ultimate prevalences for the siblings and children of subjects with NIDDM were 38% and 32% respectively. Because of the likelihood of incomplete penetrance, these figures have been interpreted as being consistent with dominant inheritance. However, the prevalence of diabetes in the parents of subjects with NIDDM was 21%, which is lower than would be expected for a dominantly inherited disease, particularly as the parents were, by definition, considerably older than the siblings. In addition, Kobberling and Tillil showed a greater prevalence of diabetes in relatives of non-obese than obese diabetic subjects, and this suggested that a single dominant inheritance hypothesis was improbable.

The clinical subtype termed maturity-onset diabetes of the young is characterized by the presentation of diabetes in early adult life and by pedigree structures suggestive of autosomal dominant transmission[34]. A World Health Organization (WHO) study group in 1985 stated that: 'Maturity onset diabetes mellitus of the young is inherited as a dominant trait and evidence is accumulating to suggest that NIDDM susceptibility may also be conferred by a dominant gene'[35]. The academic reasons behind this statement are not known. For pragmatic reasons, linkage studies with candidate genes for NIDDM have usually been analysed assuming autosomal dominant inheritance[6,36,37].

Early-onset NIDDM

O'Rahilly et al.[38] documented a 92% prevalence of NIDDM or glucose intolerance in the available parents of 13 subjects with NIDDM presenting aged 25–40 years. The high prevalence of abnormal glucose tolerance in the parents of these subjects suggested that patients with an earlier onset of NIDDM may have a greater genetic susceptibility to diabetes, resulting from the inheritance of diabetogenic genes from both parents. An increased chance of finding diabetes in the relatives was possible in that study as six probands were ascertained through an affected family member. The data would be consistent with a co-dominant model of inheritance—the parents being heterozygous and having a relatively mild disease of late onset, and the affected children with a 'double gene dose' having a more severe form with an early age of onset. This familial pattern is also characteristic of polygenicity, where an increased prevalence of the disease occurs in the relatives as the severity of the index case increases. Severity implies a greater genetic predisposition, and in NIDDM this may be clinically manifest as an earlier age of onset.

Segregation Analysis Data

No formal segregation analysis data for NIDDM are available for Caucasian pedigrees. Cook et al.[39] documented the pattern of inheritance in the nuclear families of a consecutive series of subjects with NIDDM. The 66 first-degree relatives (parents and siblings) of 20 consecutive Caucasian subjects with NIDDM and both parents alive were studied. Seven probands had neither parent affected with diabetes or impaired glucose tolerance, 10 had one parent affected (six with diabetes and four with impaired glucose tolerance) and three had both parents affected. The probands with affected and with unaffected parents were of similar age at presentation and obesity. These findings indicate that a sizeable subgroup of subjects with NIDDM have neither parent affected with NIDDM or glucose intolerance. The assumption of autosomal dominance was not supported, although it remained possible that a dominant gene of low penetrance may play a role in some pedigrees. Oligogenic or polygenic inheritance with genetic heterogeneity would appear likely. Formal segregation analysis data are awaited.

McCarthy et al.[40] reported preliminary segregation analysis data for southern Indian pedigrees. Thirty-two pedigrees were ascertained through an affected offspring (without any bias according to the family history of diabetes) having both parents and at least one sibling available for glucose tolerance testing. A high proportion of parents studied were diabetics (46/64) and in all but one family there was at least one parent with diabetes. Twenty-seven mothers were diabetic but only 19 fathers ($X^2 = 3.8$, $p = 0.05$), indicating a maternal excess of diabetes. Segregation analysis was conducted using POINTER. Best fit for a single-locus model was obtained for a co-dominant model, however, a closer fit was obtained with a polygenic model. These results indicate that NIDDM in southern Indians could be a polygenic disease.

A number of unavoidable biases may potentially arise in segregation analysis. The need to determine accurately the affection status of living patients may lead to the preferential ascertainment of families with unaffected parents, because of the increased mortality in parents who have NIDDM. Secondly, probands with an earlier age of onset may be more likely to be ascertained in these studies because of the requirement of having living parents. In addition, families motivated to attend for testing may include an excess of those with a positive family history of NIDDM. The accumulation of further families will not overcome these potential sources of bias.

The Polygenic/Heterogeneity Hypothesis

The lack of clear evidence for a single gene has led to the suggestion that NIDDM is polygenic. Multifactorial inheritance has been a favoured hypothesis, largely because of the unimodal rather than bimodal distribution of plasma glucose concentrations in Caucasian populations. This model attributes phenotypic variation to a number of genes plus the effects of environment. An example of the interactions that might occur between different mutations is the finding that some patients with extreme insulin resistance are compound heterozygotes for different mutant alleles that impair insulin receptor function at different sites. The parents who are heterozygous carriers demonstrate only minimal insulin resistance[41]. In a similar manner it is possible that NIDDM can arise from combinations of mutations in one or more genes.

If the heterogeneity hypothesis is correct, the genetic interactions may be so complex and varied that no one specific mutation could be termed as causative. Nevertheless it remains possible that a limited number of genes contribute much of the susceptibility to NIDDM within a given population.

Both insulin resistance and insulin deficiency contribute to NIDDM. Both are likely to be governed by genetic and environmental factors. Obesity is a major determinant of diabetes and is itself known to be inherited. Each of these three fields is likely to be influenced by several mutations in different candidate genes. It is thus possible that diabetes in each person has risen from a different combination of mutations, affected in turn by different environmental influences, providing a complex polygenic and developmental pathophysiology.

PATHOPHYSIOLOGY OF NIDDM AND ITS FAMILIAL AGGREGATION

Absolute or near-absolute insulin deficiency is the prime aetiological factor in IDDM. In contrast, the metabolic derangements in NIDDM are more complex, with both impaired β cell function and reduced insulin sensitivity as recognized features.

Once diabetes has developed, the resulting hyperglycaemia has a direct effect on decreasing β cell function and impairing insulin sensitivity of muscles[27]. This makes it difficult to establish the 'primary' cause or causes of the disease. Study of first-degree relatives before frank diabetes develops provides an opportunity of assessing the pathophysiology at an early stage of development.

IMPAIRED INSULIN SENSITIVITY

The fact that a large number of patients with diabetes are 'insulin-insensitive' was first demonstrated by Himsworth[42] in 1936. Bornstein[43], using a bioassay for insulin, showed that subjects with NIDDM do not lack insulin; however, it was not until the development of the radioimmunoassay for insulin by Yalow and Berson[44] that it was proved conclusively that absolute insulin levels in subjects with NIDDM are often elevated or normal rather than depressed.

More detailed data have been provided by euglycaemic–hyperinsulinaemic clamp studies, where a fixed-rate insulin infusion is combined with a variable-rate glucose infusion adjusted to maintain precise euglycaemia; the glucose delivery required is used to derive an index of whole-body insulin sensitivity. In absolute terms, this index is reduced by 35–40% in NIDDM[45], but as the increase in glucose disposal induced by insulin in NIDDM is also subnormal, the relative impairment of insulin action is even greater[46].

Both hyperinsulinaemia and measurements of *in vivo* insulin action[47,48] show familial aggregation. Insulin resistance and hyperinsulinaemia are more prevalent among relatives of NIDDM probands than control subjects[48,49]. Schumacher et al.[50] used segregation analysis to examine fasting insulin levels in 206 family members and 65 spouses who had normal glucose tolerance tests. Segregation analysis supported a major locus determining fasting insulin levels and segregating as an autosomal recessive trait. Evidence was also found for a major locus determining 1-hour stimulated insulin levels, with co-dominant inheritance as the most likely pattern of inheritance. Individuals with impaired glucose tolerance and NIDDM were excluded from the analysis. The evidence for a major gene affecting insulin levels was detected only when the variance in insulin values attributable to body mass index (BMI) was removed. Segregation analyses of fasting insulin unadjusted for BMI yielded results almost identical to results found for BMI alone; there was no evidence for a major gene effect, and the data were best explained by the environmental model. The pedigrees in this study were ascertained for the aggregation of NIDDM cases, and this ascertainment bias may have resulted in considerable enrichment for an apparent insulin resistance gene. Bogardus et al.[51] similarly suggested inheritance of insulin resistance as an autosomal trait in the Pima Indians, based on the finding of a trimodal distribution of both fasting insulin levels and maximal insulin-stimulated glucose uptake rates. Their results were most consistent with co-dominant inheritance, although segregation analysis data are not available.

Eriksson et al.[49] measured insulin sensitivity and insulin secretion in the first-degree relatives of patients with NIDDM, and compared these subjects both with healthy control subjects and with patients with NIDDM. Impaired glucose metabolism was common in the first-degree relatives, largely accounted for by a defect in non-oxidative glucose metabolism. During hyperglycaemic clamping, the first phase insulin secretion was lacking in patients with NIDDM and was severely impaired in the first-degree relatives with impaired glucose tolerance as compared with control subjects. Insulin secretion was normal in the relatives with normal glucose tolerance. Both impaired insulin sensitivity and impaired insulin secretion were thus present in the first-degree relatives with impaired glucose tolerance.

Warram et al.[48] evaluated the 155 non-diabetic offspring of conjugal diabetic parents using the 3-hour intravenous glucose tolerance test to measure glucose clearance and insulin secretion. The offspring were followed for an average of 13 years to observe the development of NIDDM. A low glucose removal rate and hyperinsulinaemia at baseline were found to be predictors of the subsequent development of NIDDM. However, the offspring who developed diabetes were more obese than were those who remained non-diabetic, and at baseline had less efficient glucose tolerance. The apparently normal β cell responses of the offspring were probably subnormal if their raised fasting insulin were taken into account. This study thus demonstrated impaired cell function, obesity and impaired insulin sensitivity in the offspring who developed diabetes, but did not distinguish which if any of the defects is primary.

Patients with NIDDM have additional defects in the pathways through which insulin stimulates the disposal of glucose apart from activation of the insulin receptor and the transport of glucose into cells[52]. Direct measurements of enzyme activity in tissue suggest that the ability of insulin to activate pyruvate dehydrogenase[53], muscle glycogen synthase[54] and muscle glycogen synthase phosphatase[55] is impaired in NIDDM. Vaag et al.[56] found that the insulin-stimulated fractional glycogen synthase activity was decreased in the normoglycaemic first-degree relatives of subjects with NIDDM, suggesting that the defect in skeletal muscle glycogen synthase in NIDDM may be of primary origin.

These studies suggest that a component of insulin resistance is inherited, although environmental factors such as obesity, hyperglycaemia and hyperinsulinaemia are also relevant[57]. Virtually all the pleomorphic roles of insulin are affected, and it seems likely that any genetic defect might be in a key regulating mechanism, for example the phosphorylation of a key enzyme in the insulin signalling pathway such as PPIβ, or of a cyclic AMP-regulated mechanism, rather than a specific defect of one pathway such as glycogen synthase. On the other hand, there is no reason to exclude heterogeneity, and several different mechanisms may be affected in different subjects. A critical goal of future research is to identify the specific cellular defects that are responsible for insulin resistance in NIDDM.

INSULIN SECRETION

The primacy of insulin deficiency in the aetiology of IDDM is universally accepted, but the contribution of β cell dysfunction to the pathogenesis of NIDDM has been less generally acknowledged. Absolute insulin deficiency is not an early feature of NIDDM. However when β cell function is assessed with regard to the prevailing level of glycaemia and impaired insulin sensitivity, it is clear that NIDDM is characterized by β cell dysfunction manifest by relative insulin deficiency[58].

O'Rahilly et al.[59] studied 154 first-degree relatives of patients with NIDDM with a continuous infusion of glucose with model assessment to assess β cell function and insulin sensitivity. The glucose-intolerant relatives had β cell function 41% of normal and insulin sensitivity 66% of normal. The normoglycaemic relatives had β cell function 109% of normal and insulin sensitivity 86% of normal. Thus the decrease in β cell function was more marked than the impaired insulin sensitivity. When the hyperglycaemic subjects were subdivided into tertiles based on glucose responses, the glucose-intolerant relatives in each tertile had significantly impaired β cell function. Only the tertile with the greatest plasma glucose responses to the glucose infusion had significantly impaired tissue insulin sensitivity when compared with the normoglycaemic relatives. It was suggested that a β cell defect early in the course of the disease suggested a 'primary' defect.

As mentioned in the prevous section, Eriksson et al.[49] also identified impaired insulin secretion in the first-degree relatives of NIDDM at the stage of glucose intolerance.

CONCLUSIONS

Despite considerable effort, no single pathophysiological marker has clearly emerged as the earliest defect in NIDDM. The difficulty in teasing out the relative primacy of impaired insulin sensitivity and β cell dysfunction suggests that both are necessary for the development of the majority of cases of NIDDM. Subjects who are unable to compensate for reduced insulin sensitivity with increased insulin secretion may be the ones predisposed to develop hyperglycaemia. The hyperglycaemia itself may then have deleterious effects on β cell function and contribute to the establishment of continued hyperglycaemia[27,52].

Paradoxically, the question of which defect is primary cannot be answered by examining populations at an early stage of development of the disease, such as subjects with impaired glucose tolerance. A population with impaired glucose tolerance may have impaired insulin sensitivity from an environmental cause such as reduced physical activity or obesity. This may be termed primary, whereas an equally important non-apparent genetic cause could be termed secondary. The use of the term 'primary' is not helpful in a multifactorial disease where subtle interactions may occur, and the influence of any one factor is likely to be critically dependent on whether other factors are operating.

MOLECULAR GENETIC DEFECTS AND NIDDM

The ultimate test of a familial hypothesis is the identification of the genetic defects. To determine the mutations that might lead to NIDDM a direct search has been made in diabetic pedigrees for genetic markers that might indicate involvement of a specific gene abnormality. Genes that are expressed in β cells that produce insulin and in muscle, i.e a major organ responding to insulin, have been studied in an attempt to unravel the underlying molecular defects contributing to the development of hyperglycaemia. The genes that express potentially important molecules, such as hormones, receptors or enzymes, are called candidate genes. The investigation of candidate genes in NIDDM has largely involved studies of genetic markers close to the genes that can be used to identify the inheritance of genes. These include restriction fragment length polymorphisms (RFLP), in which in the population there is variation of a site for one of the many restriction endonucleases that cut up DNA. These sites are usually close to the gene or in an intron in the gene and are not in the exons of the gene that express the protein structure. The RFLP provide DNA markers which are detected as differences in the sizes of fragments produced by digesting human genomic DNA with a restriction enzyme. This is usually due to polymorphisms in non-coding regions, so that at one site only a proportion of the population has a sequence that can be cut by an enzyme. These markers can be found in all regions of the genome. More recently, microsatellite repeats, in which a variable number of repeats of a section of non-coding DNA can be identified, have been used. Microsatellite repeats also occur through the genome, and a common form of the variable number of repeats is $(CA)_n$. As with RFLP, they rarely have biological function and are used as investigative markers.

The easiest way to use these markers is in a population-based survey which assumes a major, common mutation, which contributes to diabetes occurring close to a particular RFLP or microsatellite polymorphism. This link is assumed to have persisted during evolution with few cross-overs, so that affected subjects have a greater than expected chance of having that particular polymorphism, i.e. a non-random association of that polymorphism with a putative candidate gene. Thus a candidate gene that includes a mutation which is a common cause of diabetes is likely to be in close linkage with an RFLP or CA repeat within or flanking the gene. These polymorphisms give rise to linkage disequilibrium[60] in a population association study, provided that many of the disease susceptibility genes in the population descended from a common ancestral mutation. This phenomenon is seen in other diseases such as sickle cell anaemia and thalassaemias[115]. This method is error-prone if the diabetic and control populations chosen for study happen to have different ethnic admixtures, as these can lead to apparent linkage disequilibrium that relate to their different ethnic backgrounds and not from a specific nearby mutation.

The alternative method of using these markers is in diabetic pedigrees to determine whether a specific gene accounts for the familial nature of the disease in that pedigree. Two genetic loci, e.g. the postulated diabetes mutation locus and the nearby marker locus, are said to be linked if they segregate together in pedigrees more often than expected by random chance. The co-inheritance of a genetic marker with NIDDM would indicate a possible location of a causative gene. Linkage analysis in pedigrees is a powerful tool for examining the role of candidate genes in the aetiology of inherited disease with a defined mode of transmission[62] and for practical purposes dominant inheritance is usually assumed.

Recent studies have mainly focused on the insulin gene[63,64], the liver/islet glucose transporter (GLUT2)[65], and the insulin receptor gene. The results at these loci indicate that they are unlikely to be the major genes responsible for NIDDM, but a contributory role in some patients has not been excluded.

MATURITY-ONSET DIABETES OF THE YOUNG PEDIGREES: GLUCOKINASE MUTATIONS

Maturity onset diabetes of youth (MODY) is a rare form of NIDDM that can present in the second or third decade, which can be treated with diet and has a dominant mode of inheritance[34]. As it presents at a young age, three-generation families can be available for genetic analysis. In 1992 it was shown that approximately 50% of MODY pedigrees are due to glucokinase mutations. This has been a major success for the linkage approach to defining genes that cause diabetes in specific pedigrees.

Glucokinase is expressed in liver and pancreatic β cells and plays a key role in the regulation of glucose metabolism in these tissues. It has been described as the pancreatic glucose sensor because of its role in glucose recognition and the stimulation of insulin synthesis and secretion[66]. Gluco-kinase phosphorylates glucose to produce glucose-6-phosphate in the first metabolic step for glucose within the cell. Expression of the enzyme is increased by glucose in the pancreas and by insulin in the liver.

Permutt et al.[67] identified a microsatellite, CA repeat close to the human glucokinase gene, and with this Froguel et al.[68] in France and Hattersley et al.[69] in the UK were able to show linkage with this marker of the glucokinase locus on chromosome 7 and diabetes. A nonsense mutation (codon 279 C-T, exon 7)[70] and a missense mutation (codon 299 G-C, exon 8)[71] of the gene have been identified, providing strong evidence that mutations in this gene cause the diabetes in affected family members. It seems that most MODY pedigrees each have their own specific mutation, and that there is not a common mutation causing the disease, as occurs in 65% of patients with cystic fibrosis.

The glucokinase mutations produce mild hyperglycaemia, usually 6–8 mmol/l in early adult life, which can often be treated by diet alone[69]. In later life the mutations can induce clinically presenting disease, but it continues to be diet-treated in most patients. The original MODY pedigrees described by Tattersall et al. as having 'Mason type' diabetes[34] have been shown not to be linked with a glucokinase mutation[69]. Although an early report suggested that 14 out of 17 pedigrees with MODY had the mutations of glucokinase, it seems likely that the eventual figure will be approximately 50%.

Adenosine Deaminase Gene

Bell et al.[72] did a blind linkage search with many polymorphic markers throughout the genome in a large MODY pedigree, RW. They reported linkage with the adenosine deaminase locus on chromosome 20. Parallel studies by Bowden et al.[73] found linkage on the same chromosome with a different locus. This should not necessarily be regarded as independent evidence for linkage, since Bell's and Bowden's loci were closely linked and represented the same association. In theory, the linkage could be a type 1 error, in that having investigated many markers an association by chance alone might be expected in one region. However, Bell has found that extension of the analyses to additional members of the pedigree has strengthened the LOD score, and this suggests that the linkage is real. This will be substantiated if other large pedigrees are found to be linked and if further localization of the locus and identification of causative mutations are achieved.

Many candidate genes have been excluded in specific MODY pedigrees. These include insulin gene, GLUT2, GLUT4 and the insulin receptor genes.

NIDDM DIABETIC PEDIGREES

Linkage studies in NIDDM pedigrees have not been successful in identifying mutations. This is likely to be because the candidate genes that have been studied do not have mutations that are major contributors to NIDDM. Thus many studies of insulin receptor gene and insulin gene have been fruitless. Mutations of the insulin receptor gene produce insulin resistance syndromes rather than NIDDM[74].

An equally applicable factor may be that informative NIDDM pedigrees are unusual. The late onset of the disease and the premature mortality of affected subjects means that informative two-generation 'nuclear families' (both parents of a diabetic patient are alive and available for study) are unusual[6,39]. Even when they are available, both parents are affected more often than expected by chance alone on a dominant model, and bilineal inheritance from both parents rather than the dominant inheritance may occur[38]. Thus the assumption of a dominant pattern of inheritance may not be applicable. In addition, if one has extended pedigrees, e.g. affected cousins, one cannot guarantee that they are due to the same mutation, since heterogeneity within a family may occur. Thus lack of suitable NIDDM pedigrees for study is a major obstacle.

Linkage analysis can exclude candidate genes from acting in a pedigree in a dominant fashion. Thus, to study the relationship between the glucokinase gene and NIDDM, linkage analysis has been performed in 12 Caucasian nuclear pedigrees ascertained through a proband with classic NIDDM[75]. The LINKAGE program was used under four models, including autosomal dominant and recessive, with individuals with glucose intolerance counted as either affected or of unknown status. Linkage was significantly rejected with the dominant models (LOD scores -4.65, -4.25), and was unlikely with the recessive model when glucose intolerance was considered as affected (LOD score -1.38). These findings suggest that mutations in or near the glucokinase gene are unlikely to be the major cause for the inherited predisposition to NIDDM in Caucasian pedigrees, but do not exclude a role for this locus with a polygenic model or a major role in some pedigrees.

The limitation of linkage analysis in NIDDM is shown in an NIDDM pedigree in which 10 of 15 affected members were found to have a specific glucokinase mutation on screening[71]. These members could not be distinguished phenotopically from some patients who did not have a glucokinase mutation, and linkage analysis of the pedigree with glucokinase markers gave negative LOD scores, i.e. no evidence of linkage within the whole pedigree, in spite of many members having the same mutation.

Linkage studies have been done for several candidate genes with absence of positive results. For instance, the insulin gene locus is not linked, apart from the rare instances of mutant insulins[74]. Similarly, linkage studies of the insulin receptor gene have also proved negative[76], as have studies of the islet amyloid polypeptide gene (IAPP)[77]. This latter is of interest as an abnormality of IAPP may lead to the islet amyloid formation that may be pathogenic[78].

These studies are not worthless, as they help to exclude a major, dominant role for these genes in the causation of NIDDM. Thus in a number of localized amyloidosis the synthesis of a structurally abnormal or mutant protein contributes to the formation of amyloid deposits[79,80]. The negative linkage study for IAPP is complementary to a sequencing study of Nishi et al.[81], who found no evidence for an abnormal sequence in 25 patients with NIDDM. The linkage studies provide additional information, since they make it unlikely that a mutation in the promoter region as well as in the gene itself could cause NIDDM in the pedigrees studies.

ENVIRONMENTAL FACTORS

The lack of concordance in identical twins indicates the presence of environmental factors interacting with the genotype. McGinnis[82] has suggested health status is determined by a variety of biological, behavioural, environmental and social risk factors. Biological factors are the individual's physiological and structural features, often genetic, which determine disease susceptibility or protection. Behavioural factors are the specific behaviours that may put an individual at increased or decreased risk. Environmental factors refer to the potentially hazardous or protective influences in the individual's milieu. Social factors are the exogenous influences over which the individual has little direct control, such as economic status, educational level and geographical isolation. There is considerable interaction between behavioural, environmental and social forces in determining an individual's exposure to an external risk factor, and these are generally designated as 'environmental' risk factors.

HIGH-RISK POPULATIONS

Progress towards a better understanding of the interaction of genetic and environmental factors in the aetiology of NIDDM has been made via the epidemiological study of a number of populations found to develop high prevalence rates following modernization. Examples of such populations are the Pima Indians (34% prevalence)[83] and the Micronesian Nauruans (30% prevalence)[84]:

Much valuable knowledge has been gained from:

1. Evaluating the effect of modernization in populations in a given place over a period of time.
2. Comparison of groups of the same ethnicity living relatively traditional (rural) and modern (urban) lifestyles.
3. Comparing the disease experience of migrants with that of subjects remaining at home.
4. Comparison of different ethnic groups living in the same geographic location.

A 'thrifty genotype' hypothesis, first proposed by Neel[85] (see Chapter 14), suggested that hunter/gatherer groups subject to uncertain food supplies may have had a selective advantage if they had genes that facilitated the deposition of fat during their brief times of plenty. With the advent of an assured food supply and sedentary activity patterns, this genotype may predispose to obesity, hyperinsulinaemia, insulin resistance and NIDDM. While there is no conclusive proof of the thrifty genotype hypothesis, it provides an attractive explanation for the secular changes in the frequency of the disease in high-risk populations. An alternative hypothesis is that obesity allows the expression of certain genetic variations in the population that would otherwise not be pathogenic. These variations may have no survival benefit but were not 'bred out' when the population never became obese.

The population studies emphasize that NIDDM does not exist in a vacuum, and that environmental factors are important in influencing expression of the disease. The changes that occur with urbanization and migration involve increased longevity, dietary changes, reduced physical activity and increased obesity. Age, diet, exercise and obesity are the environmental factors most frequently quoted as being important in the genesis of NIDDM.

AGE

In Caucasian populations the age-specific incidence and the prevalence of NIDDM increase with age. Prevalence represents the balance between the cumulative incidence and the excessive mortality of affected subjects. In contrast to Caucasian studies, among the Pima Indians the age-specific incidence of NIDDM peaks between 40 and 50 years of age and falls thereafter. In this population the peak age-specific incidence occurs later in the less obese, suggesting that age at onset is influenced by other factors such as obesity[86].

Less clear is the extent to which glucose tolerance deteriorates with age. One view is that deterioration of glucose tolerance is a normal physiological phenomenon; the other is that the decline in mean glucose tolerance with age is due to the gradual emergence of increasing numbers of subjects expressing their genetic predisposition for NIDDM. Evidence for the latter view comes from the US National Health Examination Surveys, which showed that the percentile blood glucose concentrations do not increase in parallel with age[87]. Barret-Connor[88] examined fasting plasma glucose levels among non-diabetic adults in a California community and found that fasting plasma glucose levels rose little with age and that the normal range was independent of both age and body mass. These data suggest that the mean rise in glucose tolerance with increasing age is primarily the result of an increase in the proportion of the population with NIDDM.

The late age at onset is a confounding variable in the analysis of genetic linkage with NIDDM, and age-dependent penetrance factors are required in order to allow for uncertainty in the exclusion of diabetes[38]. The effect of disease-specific mortality is a confounding variable in segregation analysis in NIDDM, as probands with living parents may have a reduced familial prevalence of the disorder.

The interaction of age with genetic factors is borne out by the study of O'Rahilly et al.[38], which suggests that an early age at onset of NIDDM is associated with a greater genetic predisposition to NIDDM, as evidenced by a high parental prevalence of the disorder.

Why age should be associated with an increased prevalence of NIDDM remains uncertain. It is possible that genetic susceptibility to NIDDM results in a chronic underlying disease process which remains subclinical until a critical threshold is reached. An example of this model could be a subtle abnormality of IAPP processing leading to the accumulation of islet amyloid and subsequent progressive impairment of β cell function. Alternatively, the expression of the genetic predisposition to NIDDM may be dependent upon multiple assaults with a critical threshold. If the latter is the case, in a proportion of subjects with NIDDM, the age effect on pancreatic function may be modifiable or even eliminated by the concurrent modification of other risk factors for which intervention is currently feasible.

DIET

There have been few prospective studies of the relationship between dietary intake and the risk of developing NIDDM. Over a 5-year period the Israeli heart study[89] found no effect of diet on the incidence of diabetes among men. Sartor et al.[90] examined the effects of dietary intervention on the incidence of NIDDM among subjects with impaired glucose tolerance. The incidence of diabetes among those given dietary advice (reduction of total caloric and carbohydrate intake) was significantly lower over a 10-year follow-up. The interpretation of this study is complicated by the fact that some subjects also received oral hypoglycaemic agents and these individuals were followed more closely.

Modernization from a traditional lifestyle is associated with considerable dietary change. There is, however, no evidence that moving from a high complex carbohydrate, low-fat, low-sucrose diet to the converse causes diabetes independently of changes in body weight[91]. There are no cross-sectional or prospective data available which addresses the role of diet in the development of NIDDM in pedigrees.

PHYSICAL ACTIVITY

Physical activity results in lower plasma insulin levels and increased insulin sensitivity in both normal subjects and those with NIDDM[92,93]. The mechanisms by which activity levels modulate insulin sensitivity remain to be elucidated. Studies in non-diabetic individuals suggest that the addition of exercise to dietary modification enhances weight loss, particularly of adipose tissue mass, and assists in the maintenance of reduced body weight[96].

Helmrich et al.[95] obtained questionnaire data from 5990 male US alumni. Leisure-time physical activity was inversely related to the reported incidence of NIDDM, and this association remained when the data were adjusted for obesity. Active men continued to have a reduced risk even after change in BMI since leaving college was taken into account.

Manson et al.[96] examined the association between regular vigorous exercise and the subsequent incidence of NIDDM in a prospective cohort of 87 253 US women. Women who engaged in vigorous exercise at least once a week had an age-adjusted relative risk of NIDDM of 0.67 compared with women who did not exercise weekly. The reduction in risk remained statistically significant after adjustment for body mass index.

There are no prospective or cross-sectional data documenting physical activity and its relationship to familial NIDDM. The population study evidence suggests that physical activity may have a protective effect on the development of NIDDM. Further research is needed to assess the magnitude of the benefits of exercise, and to determine the most effective programmes for reducing the incidence of NIDDM.

OBESITY

Innocent Bystander, Partner in Crime or Culprit?

Patients with NIDDM are frequently overweight, and obesity is known to be associated with insulin resistance[97]. The evidence for the association between obesity and NIDDM comes from many cross-sectional epidemiological studies in high-risk populations[98] as well as Caucasian studies[99]. Both the current weight and previous history of obesity are factors related to development of diabetes. However, the association between obesity and NIDDM remains one of the most controversial topics in diabetes epidemiology. The argument is not so much as to whether obesity is associated with NIDDM but whether it is a true determinant and, if so, to what extent.

The monozygotic twin studies cast doubt on a primary aetiological role for obesity[3]. A high concordance rate for NIDDM was observed even though the twin pairs differed considerably in body weight or were not obese. In many cases NIDDM was diagnosed earlier in the less-overweight twin. These findings indicate that environmental factors not related to obesity can play a major role. Obesity *per se* is inherited in man, as in animals[100].

Interaction of Obesity with Genetic Disease Susceptibility

Evidence of an interaction between genetic susceptibility and obesity first came from a prospective study in Oxford, Massachusetts. O'Sullivan and Mahan[101] found that the appearance of NIDDM was more frequent among the obese when there was a parental history of diabetes than when there was no parental history.

Previous Obesity and Risk of NIDDM

Several studies have documented the importance of previous obesity in the genesis of NIDDM. Kadowaki et al.[102] in Japanese subjects found previous maximal BMI to be a significant predictor of deterioration from impaired glucose tolerance to NIDDM. Modan et al.[103] examined the glucose tolerance status of 2140 members of the Israeli Jewish population aged 40–70 years. BMI was measured and compared with measurements made 10 years previously. The main determinant of the risk of NIDDM was found to be the degree of obesity 10 years earlier, while current obesity and interim weight changes had lesser effects.

Central Obesity

The metabolic implications of the distribution of body fat have recently received considerable attention. In clinical studies, body fat distribution has been estimated with the ratio of waist-to-hip circumference. Researchers in Wisconsin classified fat distribution in women on the basis of the waist-to-hip circumference ratio[104]. This ratio was found to be a significant predictor of plasma triglyceride, glucose and insulin concentrations, and correlated with an *in vivo* index of impaired insulin sensitivity[105]. Ohlson et al.[106] reported data from the 13.5 year follow-up of 792 Swedish men. Abdominal obesity, as indicated by the ratio of waist-to-hip circumference, was shown to be an important risk factor for NIDDM, even when the degree of general adiposity was accounted for.

The mechanism underlying the association between central obesity and impaired insulin sensitivity is unknown. The increased release of non-esterified fatty acids from intra-abdominal fat cells into the portal circulation may affect hepatic insulin metabolism and peripheral glucose uptake[107]. Bouchard et al.[108] documented significant similarity between monozygotic twin pairs in response to overfeeding with respect to body weight, percentage of fat, fat mass and estimated subcutaneous fat. After adjustments for the gains in fat mass, the within-pair similarity was particularly evident with respect to the changes in regional fat distribution and amount of abdominal visceral fat. Genetic factors may be important determinants of the distribution of body fat and the changes in body fat distribution with weight gain.

INTRAUTERINE ENVIRONMENT AND EARLY NUTRITION

Maternal factors have been implicated in the development of NIDDM. Among the Pima Indians NIDDM has been shown to occur more frequently in adolescence and young adulthood in the offspring of diabetic pregnancies than among the offspring of women who were non-diabetic at the time of delivery but subsequently developed the disease[109] (see Chapter 11). This may reflect a 'higher gene dose' in the offspring of mothers who were diabetic at an early age, rather than environmental factors.

Hales et al.[110] demonstrated that lower birth weight and weight at 1 year are associated with impaired glucose tolerance at age 64 years. The hypothesis that Barker and Hales have promulgated[111] (see Chapter 15) is that malnutrition during pregnancy and the postnatal period occurs at a critical stage of development of the pancreas. If a suboptimal quality of β cells develops, this could lead in later life to inadequate β cell function, impaired glucose tolerance and even diabetes. There is some evidence this hypothesis may be applicable to impaired glucose tolerance. We have examined the relationships between birth weight and β cell function and insulin sensitivity in the first-degree relatives of subjects with NIDDM[112]. Percentile birth weight correlated with the β cell function of the complete cohort ($r_s = 0.29$, $p = 0.004$) and of the non-diabetic subjects ($r_s = 0.30$, $p = 0.01$) in accord with the Hales hypothesis. However, the diabetic ($n = 27$) and the non-diabetic ($n = 74$) subjects were of similar percentile birth weight: 50% (19–91%), 53% (30–75%); although the subjects with NIDDM had significantly lower β cell function than the non-diabetic subjects: 69% (48–83%) versus 97% (86–120%), $p < 0.001$. The marked impairment of β cell function in the subjects with NIDDM could not be accounted for by low birth weight, and additional genetic or environmental factors are likely to be necessary for the development of NIDDM. Thus early malnutrition may lead to sufficiently impaired development to induce impaired glucose tolerance in later life, but it is doubtful whether this would lead to diabetes without other major influences.

REAVEN'S SYNDROME: INHERITED OR ENVIRONMENTAL?

Impaired glucose tolerance and NIDDM are often associated with a number of other cardiovascular risk factors[113] (see Chapter 16). The sharing of risk factors for NIDDM and cardiovascular disease may explain in part the increased frequency of macrovascular disease in NIDDM, since an association is found in epidemiological studies between glucose intolerance, impaired insulin sensitivity, hyperinsulinaemia, hypertension and dyslipidaemia (hypertriglyceridaemia and reduced high-density lipoprotein (HDL) cholesterol)[114].

The association of these variables may reflect genetic linkage, common environmental antecedents or a combination of these mechanisms. We have investigated the association of these variables in pedigrees, studying the 96 first-degree relatives (siblings and children) of 50 Caucasian subjects with NIDDM. The glucose-intolerant first-degree relatives had reduced insulin sensitivity but did not have other features of Reaven's syndrome. Nevertheless, in the population as a whole the associations of Reaven's syndrome occurred, in part related to obesity. These data indicate that impaired insulin sensitivity in the first-degree relatives of subjects with NIDDM is not necessarily accompanied by the other features of Reaven's syndrome. Reaven's syndrome has been described as an association of variables in populations, and does not appear to be a specific entity that is part of the inheritance of NIDDM. Obesity, rather than hyperinsulinaemia, may be its major determinant.

A genetic influence may occur, as Asian Indians have a greater prevalence of central obesity and some of the features of Reaven's syndrome than white Caucasians[115].

CONCLUSIONS

NIDDM is a disease of complex aetiology. There is evidence for genetic predisposition, with high concordance in monozygotic twins. Despite the evidence for a substantial genetic component, the mode of inheritance and the molecular basis of this inheritance remain uncertain.

The study of high-risk populations emphasizes the interplay of genetic and environmental factors in the aetiology of NIDDM. Whether the genetic susceptibility is similar in all cases of NIDDM is uncertain, and this issue will probably be resolved only when the precise gene or genes which confer susceptibility in at least some cases of NIDDM are identified. Families suitable for linkage analysis are valuable for the evaluation of candidate genes, coupled with direct genetic analysis and sequencing for the characterization of mutations. The identification of the role of glucokinase in the aetiology of MODY exemplifies this approach. In the meantime the search for other risk factors and environmental determinants continues, although whether environmental determinants alone can cause NIDDM is unknown. There is evidence that age, physical activity and obesity contribute to the expression of the genetic predisposition. Obesity may best be viewed as an independent variable resulting in impaired insulin sensitivity in both normal and diabetic individuals. The magnitude of its impact on glucose tolerance appears to vary with the duration of the obesity, the body fat distribution, and with the individual's insulin sensitivity and β cell secretory reserve prior to weight gain. There is evidence that there are genetic determinants of obesity and its distribution. The metabolic implications of the distribution of obesity may be more important than overall adiposity.

The role of environmental factors in influencing disease development offers the possibility of disease prevention. However, intervention even at the stage of minimal hyperglycaemia may not be sufficiently early to prevent the development of progressive defects. The identification of genetic markers will lead to the better understanding of the aetiological basis of NIDDM, and may permit the targeting of selected individuals for primary preventive intervention by the manipulation of environmental factors.

REFERENCES

1 King H, Zimmet P. *World Health Stat Q* 1988; **41**: 190–6.
2 Zimmet P. Type 2 (non-insulin-dependent) diabetes: an epidemiological overview. *Diabetologia* 1982; **22**: 399–411.
3 Barnett AH, Eff C, Leslie RDG, Pyke DA. Diabetes in identical twins: a study of 200 pairs. *Diabetologia* 1981; **20**: 87–93.
4 Newman B, Selby JV, King MC, et al. Concordance for type 2 (non-insulin-dependent) diabetes mellitus in male twins. *Diabetologia* 1987; **30**: 763–8.
5 Kobberling J, Tillil H. Empirical risk figures for first degree relatives of non-insulin-dependent diabetics. In: *The Genetics of Diabetes Mellitus* (eds J Kobberling, R Tattersall) Academic Press, London, 1982, pp 201–9.
6 O'Rahilly S, Wainscoat JS, Turner RC. Type 2 (non-insulin-dependent) diabetes: new genetics for old nightmares. *Diabetologia* 1988; **31**: 407–14.
7 Beaty T, Neel J, Fajans S. Identifying risk factors for diabetes in first-degree relatives of non-insulin-dependent diabetic patients. *Am J Epidemiol* 1982; **115**: 380–97.
8 Cudworth AG, Woodrow JC. HLA antigens and diabetes mellitus. *Lancet* 1974; **ii**: 1153.
9 Nerup J, Platz P, Anderson OO, et al. HLA antigens and diabetes mellitus. *Lancet* 1974; **ii**: 864–6.
10 Simpson NE. The genetics of diabetes mellitus: a review of family data. In: *The Genetics of Diabetes Mellitus* (eds W Creutzfeldt, J Kobberling, JV Neel) Springer-Verlag, Berlin, 1976, pp 12–20.

11 Buchanan JA. A consideration of the various laws of heredity and their application to conditions in man. *Am J Med Sci* 1923; **165**: 675–708.

12 Wright IS. Hereditary and familial diabetes mellitus. *Am J Med Sci* 1931; **182**: 484–97.

13 John HJ. Diabetes: a statistical study of one thousand cases. *Arch Int Med* 1927; **39**: 67–92.

14 Wendt LFC, Peck FB. Diabetes mellitus: a review of 1073 cases, 1919–1929. *Am J Med Sci* 1931; **181**: 52–65.

15 Allan W. Heredity in diabetes. *Ann Int Med* 1933; **6**: 1272.

16 Pincus G, White P. On the inheritance of diabetes mellitus. I. An analysis of 675 family histories. *Am J Med Sci* 1933; **186**: 1–14.

17 Pincus G, White P, On the inheritance of diabetes mellitus. III. The blood sugar values of the relatives of diabetics. *Am J Med Sci* 1934; **188**: 159–68.

18 Harris H. The familial distribution of diabetes mellitus: a study of the relatives of 1241 diabetic propositi. *Ann Eug* 1950; **15**: 95–116.

19 Steinberg AG, Wilder RM. A study of the genetics of diabetes mellitus. *Am J Hum Genet* 1952; **4**: 113–30.

20 Thompson GS. Genetic factors in diabetes mellitus studied by the oral glucose tolerance test. *J Med Genet* 1965; **2**: 221–6.

21 Falconer DS. The inheritance of liability to diseases with variable age of onset with particular reference to diabetes mellitus. *Ann Hum Genet* 1967; **31**: 1–20.

22 Simpson NE. Heritabilities of liability to diabetes when sex and age at onset are considered. *Ann Hum Genet* 1969; **32**: 283–303.

23 Zimmet P, Dowse G, Krista A, Serjeantson S. Current perspectives in the epidemiology of non-insulin dependent (type II) diabetes mellitus. *Diab Nutr Metab* 1990; **3** (Suppl 1): 3–15.

24 Rushforth NB, Bennett PH, Sternberg AG, Burch TA, Miller M. Diabetes in the Pima Indians: evidence of bimodality in glucose tolerance distributions. *Diabetes* 1971; **20**: 756–65.

25 Zimmet P, Whitehouse S. Bimodality of fasting and two-hour glucose tolerance distributions in a Micronesian population. *Diabetes* 1978; **27**: 793–800.

26 Raper LR, Taylor R, Zimmet P, Milne B, Balkau B. Bimodality in glucose tolerance distributions in the urban Polynesian population of Western Samoa. *Diabetes Res* 1984; **1**: 19–26.

27 Unger RH, Grundy S. Hyperglycaemia as an inducer as well as a consequence of impaired islet cell function and insulin resistance: implications for the management of diabetes. *Diabetologia* 1985; **28**: 119–21.

28 Tillil H, Richter K, Kobberling J. Bimodal distribution of the two-hour blood glucose value during OGTT among first-degree relatives of type 2 diabetics in a Caucasoid population (Abstract). *Diabetes Res Clin Pract* 1985; Suppl 1 No S460: 1462.

29 Morton NE, Lalouel JM. Segregation analysis of familial data. In: *Contributions to Epidemiology and Biostatistics. Vol. 4. Methods in Genetic Epidemiology* (eds NE Morton, DC Rao, JM Lalouel) Karger, Basel, 1983, pp 62–102.

30 Cooke AM, Fitzgerald MG, Malins JM, Pyke DA. Diabetes in children of diabetic couples. *Br Med J* 1966; **ii**: 674–6.

31 Kahn CB, Soeldner JS, Gleason RE, et al. Clinical and chemical diabetes in the offspring of diabetic couples. *N Engl J Med* 1969; **281**: 343–6.

32 Tattersall R, Fajans SS. Diabetes and carbohydrate intolerance in 199 offspring of 37 conjugal diabetic parents. *Diabetes* 1975; **24**: 452–62.

33 Ganda OP, Soeldner SS. Genetic, acquired and related factors in the aetiology of diabetes mellitus. *Arch Intern Med* 1987; **137**: 461–9.

34 Tattersall RB. Mild familial diabetes with dominant inheritance. *Q J Med* 1974; **43**: 339–57.
35 *WHO Technical Report Series* 1985, No 727, Geneva.
36 O'Rahilly S, Trembath RC, Patel P, et al. Linkage analysis of the human insulin receptor gene in type 2 (non-insulin-dependent) diabetic families and a family with maturity onset diabetes of the young. *Diabetologia* 1988; **31**: 792–7.
37 O'Rahilly S, Patel P, Wainscoat JS, Turner RC. Analysis of the HepG2/ erythrocyte glucose transporter locus in a family with type 2 (non-insulin-dependent) diabetes and obesity. *Diabetologia* 1989; **32**: 266–9.
38 O'Rahilly S, Spivey RS, Holman RR, et al. Type 2 diabetes of early onset: a distinct clinical and genetic syndrome? *Br J Med* 1987; **294**: 923–8.
39 Cook JTE, Hattersley AT, Levy JC, et al. The distribution of type 2 diabetes in nuclear families. *Diabetes* 1993; **44**: 106–12.
40 McCarthy MI, Hitman GA, Morton N, et al. Type 2 (non-insulin-dependent) diabetes mellitus in South Indians is a polygenic disease. *Diabetologia* 1992; **35** (Suppl 1): A140, No 538.
41 Kadowaki T, Kadowaki H, Rechler MM, et al. Five mutant alleles of the insulin receptor gene in patients with genetic forms of insulin resistance. *J Clin Invest* 1990; **86**: 254–64.
42 Himsworth HP. The syndrome of diabetes mellitus and its causes. *Lancet* 1936; **i**: 465–72.
43 Bornstein J, Lawrence RD. Plasma insulin in human diabetes mellitus. *Br Med J* 1951; **ii**: 1541–4.
44 Yalow RS, Berson SA. Immunoasssay of endogenous plasma insulin in man. *J Clin Invest* 1960; **39**: 1157–65.
45 DeFronzo R. The triumvirate: beta-cell, muscle, liver. A collusion responsible for NIDDM. *Diabetes* 1988; **37**: 667–75.
46 Donner CC, Fraze E, Chen Y-DI, Reaven GM. Quantification of insulin-stimulated glucose disposal in patients with non-insulin dependent diabetes mellitus. *Diabetes* 1985; **34**: 831–5.
47 Lillioja S, Mott DM, Zawadzki JK, et al. In vivo insulin action is familial characteristic in nondiabetic Pima Indians. *Diabetes* 1987; **36**: 1329–35.
48 Warram JH, Martin BC, Krolewski AS, Soeldner JS, Kahn CR. Slow glucose removal rate and hyperinsulinemia precede the development of type II diabetes in the offspring of diabetic parents. *Ann Intern Med* 1990; **113**: 909–15.
49 Eriksson J, Franssila-Kallunki A, Ekstrand A, et al. Early metabolic defects in persons at increased risk for non-insulin-dependent diabetes mellitus. *N Engl J Med* 1989; **321**: 337–43.
50 Schumacher MC, Hasstedt SJ, Hunt SC, Williams RR, Elbein SC. Major gene effect for insulin levels in familial NIDDM pedigrees. *Diabetes* 1992; **41**: 416–23.
51 Bogardus C, Lillioja S. Pima Indians as a model to study the genetics of NIDDM. *J Cell Biochem* 1992; **48**: 337–43.
52 Groop LC, Bonadonna RC, Del Prato S, et al. Glucose and free fatty acid metabolism in non-insulin-dependent diabetes mellitus: evidence for multiple sites of insulin resistance. *J Clin Invest* 1989; **84**: 205–13.
53 Mandarino LJ, Madar Z, Kolterman OG, Bell JM, Olefsky JM. Adipocyte glycogen synthase and pyruvate dehydrogenase in obese and type II diabetic subjects. *Am J Physiol* 1986; **251**: E489–E496.
54 Thorburn AW, Gumbiner B, Bulacan F, Brechtel G, Henry RR. Multiple defects in muscle glycogen synthase activity contribute to reduced glycogen synthesis in non-insulin dependent diabetes mellitus. *J Clin Invest* 1991; **87**: 489–95.
55 Kida Y, Esposito-Del Puente A, Bogardus C, Mott DM. Insulin resistance is

associated with reduced fasting and insulin-stimulated glycogen synthase phosphatase activity in human skeletal muscle. *J Clin Invest* 1990; **85**: 476–81.

56 Vaag A, Henriksen JE, Beck-Nielsen H. Defective insulin activation of glycogen synthase in skeletal muscles in first degree relatives to patients with type 2 (non-insulin-dependent) diabetes mellitus (Abstract). *Diabetologia* 1991; **34** (Suppl 2): A70.

57 Chisholm DJ, Kraegen EW. The pathogenesis of non-insulin-dependent diabetes mellitus: the role of insulin resistance. In: *Textbook of Diabetes* (eds JC Pickup, G Williams). Blackwell, London, 1991, pp 192–7.

58 Perley MJ, Kipnis DM. Plasma insulin responses to oral and intravenous glucose: studies in normal and diabetic subjects. *J Clin Invest* 1967; **46**: 1954–62.

59 O'Rahilly S, Nugent Z, Rudenski A, et al. Beta-cell dysfunction rather than insulin insensivity is the primary defect in familial type 2 diabetes. *Lancet* 1986; **ii**: 360–4.

60 Cox NJ, Bell G. Disease associations: chance, artefact or susceptibility genes. *Diabetes* 1989; **38**: 947–50.

61 Orkin SH, Kazazian HH Jr. The mutation and polymorphism of the human beta-globin gene and its surrounding DNA. *Annu Rev Genet* 1984; **18**: 131–71.

62 Ott J. *Analysis of Human Genetic Linkage*. Johns Hopkins University Press, Baltimore, 1985.

63 Dobs AS, Phillips JA III, Mallonee RL, Sandek CD, Ney RL. Pedigree analysis of the 5' flanking region of the insulin gene in familial diabetes mellitus. *Metabolism* 1986; **35**: 13–17.

64 Cox NJ, Enstein PA, Spielman RS. Linkage studies in NIDDM and the insulin and insulin-receptor genes. *Diabetes* 1989; **38**: 653–8.

65 Patel P, Lo YM, Hattersley A, et al. Linkage analysis of maturity-onset diabetes of the young with microsatellite polymorphisms: no linkage to ADA or GLUT 2 genes in two families. *Diabetes* 1992; **41**: 962–7.

66 Magnuson MA. Glucokinase gene structure: functional implications of molecular genetic studies. *Diabetes* 1990; **39**: 523–7.

67 Permutt MA, Ken CC, Tanizawa Y. A candidate gene that paid off. *Diabetes* 1992; **41**: 1367–1372.

68 Froguel PH, Vaxillaire M, Sun F, et al. Close linkage of glucokinase locus on chromosome 7p to early-onset non-insulin-dependent diabetes mellitus. *Nature* 1992; **356**: 162–4.

69 Hettersley AT, Turner RC, Permutt MA, et al. Linkage of type 2 diabetes to the glucokinase gene. *Lancet* 1992; **339**: 1307–10.

70 Vionnet N, Stoffel M, Takeda J, et al. Nonsense mutation in the glucokinase gene causes early-onset non-insulin-dependent diabetes mellitus. *Nature* 1992; **356**: 721–2.

71 Stoffel M, Patel P, Lo YM-D, et al. Missense glucokinase mutation in maturity-onset diabetes of the young (MODY) and mutation screening in late-onset diabetes. *Nature Genet* 1992; **2**: 153–6.

72 Bell GI, Xiang KS, Newman MV, et al. Gene for non-insulin-dependent diabetes mellitus (maturity-onset diabetes of the young subtype) is linked to DNA polymorphism on human chromosome 20q. *Proc Natl Acad Sci USA* 1991; **88**: 1484–8.

73 Bowden DW, Gravius TC, Akots G, Fajans SS. Identification of genetic markers flanking the locus for maturity-onset diabetes of the young on human chromosome 20. *Diabetes* 1992; **41**: 88–92.

74 Taylor SI, Kadowaki H, Accili D, Cama A, McKeon C. Mutations in insulin receptor gene in insulin resistant patients. *Diabetes Care* 1990; **13**: 257–79.

75 Cook JTE, Hattersley AT, Christopher P, Bown E, Barrow B, Patel P, Shaw JAG, Cookson WOCM, Permutt MA, Turner RC. Linkage analysis of gluco-kinase gene with NIDDM in Caucasian pedigrees. *Diabetes* 1992; **41**: 1496–1500.
76 Elbein SC. Molecular and clinical characterization of an insertional polymorph-ism of the insulin receptor gene. *Diabetes* 1989; **38**: 737–43.
77 Cook JTE, Patel P, Clark A, et al. Non-linkage of the islet amyloid polypeptide gene with type 2 diabetes. *Diabetologia* 1991; **34**: 103–8.
78 Clark A, Cooper GJS, Lewis CE, et al. Islet amyloid formed from diabetes-associated peptide may be pathogenic in type 2 diabetes. *Lancet* 1987; **ii**: 231–4.
79 Yoshioka K, Sasaki H, Yoshioka N, et al. Structure of the mutant prealbumin gene responsible for familial amyloidotic polyneuropathy. *Mol Biol Med* 1986; **3**: 319–28.
80 Ghiso J, Jensson O, Fragione B. Amyloid fibrils in hereditary cerebral haemor-rhage with amyloidosis of Icelandic type is a variant of gamma-trace basic protein (cystatin C). *Proc Natl Acad Sci USA* 1986; **83**: 2974–8.
81 Nishi M, Bell GI, Steiner DF. Islet amyloid polypeptide (amylin): no evidence of an abnormal precursor sequence in 25 type 2 (non-insulin-dependent) diabetic patients. *Diabetologia* 1990; **33**: 628–30.
82 McGinnis JM. Setting national objectives in disease prevention and health promotion: the United States experience. *Proceedings of the Annual Conference ANZSERCH/APHA*, Canberra, 1985, pp 15–46.
83 Bennett PH, Knowler WC. Increasing prevalence of diabetes in the Pima (Amer-ican) Indians over a ten-year period. In: *Diabetes 1979* (ed WK Waldhausl) Exerpta Medica, Amsterdam, 1980, pp 507–11.
84 Zimmet P, King H, Taylor R, et al. The high prevalence of diabetes mellitus, impaired glucose tolerance and diabetic retinopathy in Nauru; the 1982 survey. *Diabetes Res* 1982; **1**: 13–18.
85 Neel JV. Diabetes mellitus: a thrifty genotype rendered detrimental by 'pro-gress'? *Am J Hum Genet* 1962; **14**: 353–62.
86 Bennett PH, Knowler WC, Rushforth NB, et al. The role of obesity in the development of diabetes in the Pima Indians. In: *Diabetes and Obesity: Proceed-ings of the Vth International Meeting of Endocrinology, Marseilles* (eds J Vague, Ph Vague). Excerpta Medica, Amsterdam, 1979, pp 117–26.
87 Hadden WC, Harris MI. *Vital and Health Statistics*, Series 11, No 237. National Center for Health Statistics, Washington DC, 1987, DHHS Publication No (PHS) 87–1687.
88 Barret-Connor E. The prevalence of diabetes mellitus in an adult community as determined by history or fasting hyperglycaemia. *Am J Epidemiol* 1980; **111**: 705–12.
89 Medalie JH, Herman JB, Goldbourt U, Papier CM. Variations in incidence of diabetes among 10 000 adult Israeli males and the factors related to their develop-ment. In: *Advances in Metabolic Disorders* (eds R Levine, R Luft) Academic Press, New York, 1978, pp 93–110.
90 Sartor G, Schersten B, Carlstrom S, et al. Ten-year follow-up of subjects with impaired glucose tolerance: prevention of diabetes by tolbutamide and diet regulation. *Diabetes* 1980; **29**: 41–9.
91 Mann JI. Diabetes mellitus: some aspects of aetiology and management. In: *Refined Carbohydrate Foods, Dietary Fibre and Disease* (eds HC Trowell, D Burkett, K Heaton) Academic Press, London, 1985, pp 263–87.
92 Devlin JT, Horton ES. Effects of prior high-intensity exercise on glucose meta-bolism in normal and insulin-resistant men. *Diabetes* 1985; **34**: 973–9.

93 Krotkiewski M, Lonnroth P, Mandroukas K, et al. The effects of physical training on insulin secretion and effectiveness and on glucose metabolism in obesity and type 2 (non-insulin-dependent) diabetes mellitus. *Diabetologia* 1985; **28**: 881–90.

94 Stern JS, Titchenal CA, Johnson PR. Does exercise make a difference? In: *Recent Advances in Obesity Research* (eds EM Berry, SH Blondheim, HE Eliahov, E Shafrir) Libbey, London, 1987, pp 337–49.

95 Helmrich SP, Ragland DR, Leung RW, Paffenbarger RS. Physical activity and reduced occurrence of non-insulin-dependent diabetes mellitus. *N Engl J Med* 1991; **325**: 147–52.

96 Manson JE, Rimm EB, Stampfer MJ, et al. Physical activity and incidence of non-insulin-dependent diabetes mellitus in women. *Lancet* 1991; **338**: 774–8.

97 Bonadonna RC, Groop L, Kraemer N, et al. Obesity and insulin resistance in humans: a dose–response study. *Metabolism* 1990; **39**: 452–9.

98 Zimmet PZ, Kirk RL, Sarjeantson SW. Genetic and environmental interactions for non-insulin-dependent diabetes in high prevalence Pacific populations. In: *The Genetics of Diabetes Mellitus* (eds J Kobberling, R Tattersall) Academic Press, London, 1982, pp 211–24.

99 Baird JD. Is obesity a factor in the aetiology of non-insulin-dependent diabetes? In: *The Genetics of Diabetes Mellitus* (eds J Kobberling, R Tattersall) Academic Press, London, 1982, pp 233–41.

100 Stunkard AJ, Sorensen TIA, Hanis C, et al. An adoption study of human obesity. *N Engl J Med* 1986; **314**: 193–8.

101 O'Sullivan JB, Mahan CM. Blood sugar levels, glycosuria, and body weight related to development of diabetes mellitus. *JAMA* 1965; **194**: 587–92.

102 Kadowaki T, Miyaki Y, Hagura R, et al. Risk factors for worsening to diabetes in subjects with impaired glucose tolerance. *Diabetologia* 1984; **26**: 44–9.

103 Modan M, Karasik A, Halkin H, et al. Effect of past and concurrent body mass index on prevalence of glucose intolerance and type 2 (non-insulin-dependent) diabetes and on insulin response: the Israel study of glucose intolerance, obesity and hypertension. *Diabetologia* 1986; **29**: 82–9.

104 Evans DJ, Hoffman RG, Kalkhoff RK, Kissebah AH. Relationship of body fat topography to insulin sensitivity and metabolic profiles in premenopausal women. *Metabolism* 1984; **33**: 68–75.

105 Kalkhoff RK, Hartz AH, Rupley D, Kissebah AH, Kelber S. Relationship of body fat distribution to blood pressure, carbohydrate tolerance and plasma lipids in healthy obese women. *J Lab Clin Med* 1983; **102**: 621–7.

106 Ohlson L-O, Larsson B, Svardsudd K, et al. The influence of body fat distribution on the incidence of diabetes mellitus: 13.5 years of follow-up of the participants in the study of men born in 1913. *Diabetes* 1985; **34**: 1055–8.

107 Bolinder J, Kager L, Ostman J, Arner P. Differences at the receptor and post-receptor levels between human omental and subcutaneous adipose tissue in the action of insulin on lipolysis. *Diabetes* 1983; **32**: 117–23.

108 Bouchard C, Tremblay A, Despres J-P, et al. The response to long-term over-feeding in identical twins. *N Engl J Med* 1990; **322**: 1477–82.

109 Pettitt DJ, Aleck KA, Baird HR, et al. Congenital susceptibility to NIDDM: role of intrauterine environment. *Diabetes* 1988; **37**: 622–8.

110 Hales CN, Barker DJP, Clark PMS, et al. Fetal and infant growth and impaired glucose tolerance at age 64. *Br Med J* 1991; **303**: 1019–22.

111 Hales CN, Barker DJP. Type 2 (non-insulin-dependent) diabetes mellitus: the thrifty phenotype hypothesis. *Diabetologia* 1992; **35**: 595–601.

112 Cook JTE, Levy JC, Page RCL, Shaw JAG, Hattersley AT, Turner RC.

Association of low birthweight with β cell function in the adult first degree relatives of non-insulin dependent diabetic subject. *Br Med J* 1992; **306**: 302–6.

113 Reaven GM. Role of insulin resistance in human disease. *Diabetes* 1988; **37**: 1595–607.

114 Jarrett RJ. Type 2 (non-insulin-dependent) diabetes mellitus and coronary heart disease: chicken, egg or neither? *Diabetologia* 1984; **26**: 99–102.

115 McKeigue PM, Shah B, Marmot MG. Relation of central obesity and insulin resistance with high diabetes prevalence and cardiovascular risk in South Asians. *Lancet* 1991; **337**: 382–6.

Chapter Thirteen

Risk Factors for Non-insulin-dependent Diabetes Mellitus: Evidence from Twin Studies

B. Newman[a], E. J. Mayer[b] and J. V. Selby[b]

[a]*Department of Epidemiology, University of North Carolina at Chapel Hill, Chapel Hill, North Carolina, and* [b]*Kaiser-Permanente Division of Research, Oakland, California, USA*

Twin studies have long been cited as evidence for genetic influences on diabetes. They also have been influential in establishing the existence of disease heterogeneity by recognizing characteristic distinctions between what was previously called 'juvenile-onset' and 'maturity-onset' diabetes. Yet, despite their potential usefulness in elucidating environmental and behavioural contributions to disease, only recently have twin studies been employed for this purpose. We here review evidence from twin studies for non-genetic contributions to non-insulin-dependent diabetes mellitus (NIDDM). We proceed by posing three questions regarding: (1) the degree to which environmental and behavioural factors are important to the development of NIDDM; (2) the identity of those risk factors, both for NIDDM and for glucose and insulin levels; and (3) the similarity of the non-genetic factors with those influencing syndromes closely related to NIDDM.

Causes of Diabetes. Edited by R. D. G. Leslie
© 1993 John Wiley & Sons Ltd

Question 1. What is the Evidence that Non-genetic Factors are Important to the Development of NIDDM?

NIDDM Studies

Any review of twin studies of NIDDM is complicated by the historical evolution of the diagnostic criteria for the disease. Many twin studies of diabetes were conducted prior to the current distinction between NIDDM and insulin-dependent diabetes mellitus (IDDM)[1-6]. Even more recent studies have employed a variety of methods to determine the diabetes diagnosis, including oral glucose tolerance tests (OGTT) that differed in dose of glucose administered, times of blood sampling, and interpretation of the resultant blood glucose levels. However, all the twin studies attempt to evaluate the relative importance of genetic versus non-genetic determinants of disease by assessing the degree of similarity (measured by concordance) within *monozygotic* twin pairs, usually compared with *dizygotic* twin pairs.

Table 1 summarizes the results of two twin studies that stratified analyses by age at onset of diabetes in order to evaluate concordance separately for maturity-onset disease (typically diagnosis at age 40 or older)[3,4] and four studies that employed clinical criteria to calculate concordance specifically for NIDDM[7-10]. The concordance measure presented here uses the pairwise definition, i.e. the number of pairs in which both twins are affected (concordant pairs) divided by the number of pairs in which at least one twin is affected (concordant plus discordant pairs). Of the five studies that include both zygosities, all show excess concordance for disease among monozygotic twin pairs, who are genetically identical, relative to dizygotic twin pairs, who share on average 50% of their genes. This is generally taken as evidence for

Table 1 Twin studies of concordance for non-insulin-dependent or late-onset diabetes

	Monozygotic twin pairs		Dizygotic twin pairs		Ages (years)
	Total	Concordant	Total	Concordant	
Danish Registry[3]	47	26 (55%)	146	20 (14%)	50–90
Joslin Clinic[4]	10	7 (70%)	28	1 (4%)	49–77
UK series[7]	53	48 (91%)	None		NA
NHLBI study[8]	46	14 (41%)	421	4 (10%)[a]	52–65
Japan series[9]		37 (80%)	10	4 (40%)	18–88
Kaiser-Permanente study[10]	18	4 (22%)	22	3 (14%)	37–85

[a]Due to selective loss to follow-up of dizygotic twins with diabetes, these numbers probably represent an underestimate of concordance among dizygotic twin pairs.

an important genetic influence on NIDDM, although it also may reflect an enhanced likelihood for monozygotic co-twins to share environmental or behavioural factors as well.

Despite the consistent excess concordance for NIDDM observed among monozygotic twin pairs relative to dizygotic twin pairs, none of the studies reveal complete concordance among monozygotic twins (Table 1), which is the expectation for traits determined solely by inherited genetic susceptibility. A concordance less than 100% (i.e. the presence of discordance) among monozygotic twin pairs implies that environmental exposures or behaviours contribute to disease development. However, the data in Table 1 reveal striking variability in the level of concordance observed among monozygotic twins (22–91%), thereby compromising conclusions regarding the extent of genetic or non-genetic contributions to NIDDM. This variability may be, in part, an artefact of study design characteristics, such as the source of information regarding disease diagnosis, the ascertainment schemes used to identify study participants, or the duration of follow-up of the twins.

When disease diagnosis is made on the basis of self-report, it is difficult to predict whether concordance will be under- or overestimated. Onset of NIDDM can be insidious, and some individuals may be unaware of their diabetic status. Alternatively, co-twins of individuals with diabetes may be more likely to obtain diagnostic tests and therefore become aware of otherwise asymptomatic disease. Only the Danish study[3] relied entirely on self-report for disease diagnosis. Investigators at the Joslin Clinic[4] examined a subset of their apparently unaffected twins, and investigators of the remaining four studies[7–10] examined all twins for whom a diagnosis of diabetes had not been made. Even in the studies with complete ascertainment, a range of estimates for concordance in monozygotic twins persists.

The three studies (Joslin Clinic, UK series, Japan series) with the highest estimates of concordance among monozygotic twins all ascertained their study subjects through clinic attendance and/or referral by other clinicians and organizations catering to clinically diagnosed diabetics. With this approach, concordant pairs are more likely to come to the investigators' attention, not only because such pairs can be identified via two potential probands, but because, once identified, concordant pairs are often of greater clinical interest and therefore more readily referred to a study. Furthermore, clinic-based studies tend to identify patients with more severe disease, and as a consequence may be ascertaining twin pairs that have a stronger propensity to develop diabetes. Investigators of the UK series[7] and the Japan series[9] evaluated the representativeness of their participants, and both acknowledge that concordance is likely overestimated. Despite such bias in the estimates, none of the studies reveal 100% concordance among monozygotic twin pairs, thus suggesting that non-genetic factors are important to disease development.

This observed lack of complete concordance for NIDDM in monozygotic twins has been attributed to incomplete follow-up. Using a life-table procedure, Harvald[11] modelled the risk of developing diabetes among unaffected twin siblings of 'late-onset' diabetic subjects and determined in monozygotic twins that risk approached 100%. Furthermore, a substantial proportion of the non-diabetic co-twins of diabetic subjects had elevated glucose levels on testing, particularly among monozygotic twin pairs (Table 2). These levels were not necessarily high enough to meet the current World Health Organization (WHO) criteria for impaired glucose tolerance, but the investigators[3,4,7-10] concluded that they were above levels conventionally accepted as normal. In an early study, Then Berg[1] observed that all 35 monozygotic twin pairs in which the proband was diagnosed after age 43 were concordant when glucose intolerance as well as frank diabetes were included in the definition of affected status.

If increasing concordance for NIDDM is expected among monozygotic twin pairs as they are followed over time, the duration of discordance among pairs with one twin affected should be shorter, on average, than that experienced by pairs in which both twins are affected. When available, analyses of discordance duration reveal inconsistent results. In the UK series, Barnett et al.[7] observed that among NIDDM-discordant monozygotic twin pairs the diabetic proband had invariably been diagnosed relatively recently, and no monozygotic twin pairs remained discordant for more than 15 years. However, among monozygotic twins of the Joslin Clinic[4] and Japan[9] studies, the period of discordance was not necessarily shorter among discordant compared to concordant pairs. Thus, whether progression to diabetes is inevitable in unaffected, monozygotic co-twins of probands with NIDDM cannot be determined from existing studies of clinical endpoints alone.

Metabolic studies

Subclinical characteristics of the non-diabetic, monozygotic twin siblings of individuals with diabetes have been examined in metabolic studies that compared them to healthy controls[8-10,12-15]. Potential differences in age and weight between the twins and healthy comparison subjects were controlled through matching and/or adjustment during statistical analysis in all but two studies[9,12]. In all studies, the number of subjects was quite small, particularly when restricted to co-twins of probands with late-onset diabetes or NIDDM. In one study[14,15], it was not possible to distinguish between probands with NIDDM and IDDM, therefore results were excluded from discussion here. Because different clinical tests were utilized and investigators chose different approaches for data analysis and presentation, only a qualitative assessment of the results for glucose and insulin levels is possible.

Table 2 Proportion of non-diabetic co-twins of diabetic probands who have elevated glucose levels

	Monozygotic twin pairs	Dizygotic twin pairs
Danish Registry[3]	4/7 (57%)	1/11 (9%)
Joslin Clinic[4]	1/3 (33%)	5/11 (45%)
UK series[7]	5/7 (71%)	NA
NHLBI study[8]	13/20 (65%)	NA
Japan series[9]	6/8 (75%)	4/6 (67%)
Kaiser-Permanente study[10]	7/14 (50%)	4/19 (21%)

Four studies[8,9,12,13] reported significantly higher post-load glucose levels on average in the non-diabetic, monozygotic twin siblings of diabetic probands compared to healthy comparison subjects, although fasting levels, when available, were not always elevated. One other study[10] observed somewhat higher fasting and post-load glucose levels that were not statistically significant. Because higher glucose levels, both at fasting and following a glucose challenge, are among the strongest predictors of subsequent development of NIDDM[16,17], these findings are compatible with the notion that non-diabetic, monozygotic twin siblings of diabetic probands are at increased risk of becoming diabetic themselves. Whether this occurs for genetic or non-genetic reasons cannot be determined from these analyses.

Results comparing insulin levels of non-diabetic, monozygotic co-twins of diabetic probands with healthy comparison subjects appear more variable. Pyke et al.[13] observed significantly lower post-load insulin levels on average during a 2-hour, 50 g OGTT among monozygotic twin siblings of probands diagnosed at age 20 or older. In contrast, fasting insulin levels appeared significantly higher than that of healthy controls. Investigators of the Japan series[9] observed subnormal insulin responses during a 2-hour, 75 g OGTT in four of six tested co-twins of NIDDM probands; the remaining two had normal insulin responses. Investigators of the Kaiser-Permanente twin study[10] observed no significant difference in fasting or 2-hour, post-load (75 g) insulin levels in co-twins of NIDDM probands. Cerasi and Luft[12] observed low insulin response after a standardized glucose infusion test in three twin siblings of probands diagnosed at age 40 or older who themselves were in fact diabetic; among the three non-diabetic twin siblings of similar probands, one showed a low insulin response, another showed a normal insulin response, and the third showed a high insulin response.

Considering the small sample sizes and inconsistencies in diabetes diagnosis among probands of the twin pairs, the discrepancies in insulin findings are not surprising. Relative hyperinsulinaemia is an imperfect surrogate measure of insulin resistance because insulin levels also are determined by pancreatic secretion as well as hepatic clearance of insulin[18]. In fact, in prospective studies of both white[17] and non-white[16] populations, *higher* fasting insulin concentrations and *lower* post-load insulin concentrations were predictive of NIDDM incidence, reflecting both insulin resistance and impaired insulin secretion relative to ambient glucose levels, respectively. Two of the four studies cited above[9,13] reveal consistent patterns at least in a subset of the non-diabetic co-twins tested.

Despite our inability to resolve the question regarding the ultimate diabetic status of apparently non-diabetic, monozygotic co-twins of probands with NIDDM, twin studies provide strong evidence for the importance of both genetic and non-genetic determinants of NIDDM. The consistent excess of concordance for NIDDM among monozygotic compared to dizygotic twin pairs supports a genetic contribution to disease development. However, the obvious variation in age at onset, which is manifest as a lack of complete concordance among monozygotic twin pairs at a given point in time, suggests that non-genetic factors also are crucial. The best model available to date proposes an interaction between an underlying genetic susceptibility and subsequent exposure to specific, possibly ubiquitous, environmental or behavioural influences for development of NIDDM.

Question 2. Which Environmental Exposures or Behaviours Increase Risk of NIDDM?

Predictors of NIDDM

Because any observed differences between genetically identical co-twins must be attributed solely to non-genetic determinants, studies of NIDDM-discordant, monozygotic twin pairs can evaluate gene–environment interaction prior to the actual molecular characterization of the genetic contribution. To be especially informative, such analyses require information on specific environmental exposures and behaviours that precede development of disease. Limited longitudinal data were collected by three twin studies[7,8,10].

In the UK series, Barnett et al.[7] obtained reliable figures for weight at the time of diagnosis for a subset of their monozygotic twins. Among the five discordant pairs, the diabetic twin was heavier in two and lighter in three. Even among concordant pairs, weight at diagnosis was not predictive of NIDDM: in 12 of 21 pairs the lighter twin was the first to develop diabetes, and diabetes eventually developed in both twins whether they were overweight or not.

To avoid the possibility of changes made as a consequence of disease onset, Newman et al.[8] conducted longitudinal analyses of risk factors measured at an examination occurring up to 10 years prior to diabetes diagnosis in the

NHLBI study of male twins. Among 19 monozygotic twin pairs discordant for NIDDM, body mass at various earlier ages, education, alcohol consumption and diet (including total calories and grams of protein, fat, total carbohydrates or simple carbohydrates) were virtually identical for diabetic twins and their unaffected twin brothers. Considering the high proportion of non-diabetic twins with elevated glucose levels (65% between 11.1 and 13.8 mmol/l after a 1-hour, 50 g glucose load), this similarity may not be surprising. A comparison of these 19 non-diabetic co-twins with other non-diabetic study participants revealed that the twin brothers of diabetic twins had significantly higher mean 1-hour, post-load, glucose values (9.6 versus 8.3 mmol/l, $p < 0.05$) and were more obese (27.7 versus 25.6 kg/m^2, $p < 0.05$) 10 years earlier. Thus, it appears that body mass may be related to hyperglycaemia in these twins, but the behavioural factors studied do not explain the difference in clinical NIDDM status between discordant twin brothers.

Similar longitudinal analyses were conducted on data from the Kaiser-Permanente study of women twins[10]. Among 14 monozygotic twin pairs who became discordant for NIDDM during the 10 years between the first and second examinations, no differences between twins were observed for leisure-time physical activity, alcohol consumption, or education reported at the first examination. However, in contrast to results from the previous two studies, non-diabetic twin sisters of diabetic probands had significantly lower mean fasting glucose (95 versus 102 mg/dl, $p = 0.05$) and lower mean body mass index (BMI) (27.0 versus 29.7 kg/m^2, $p < 0.01$). Although genes are undoubtedly important contributors to both glucose levels and body mass[19], these results indicate that non-genetic influences related to fasting glycaemia and obesity may have contributed to disease development in these diabetic twins.

Analyses of monozygotic twin pairs discordant for NIDDM controls for genetic predisposition to disease and early environment, thereby providing a powerful comparison to identify non-genetic precursors of disease which potentially are amenable to modification. However, in part because of small numbers of NIDDM-discordant twin pairs and limited availability of longitudinal data, twin studies of NIDDM have provided relatively few clues to the identity of environmental and behavioural precursors of the disease. The only evidence to date points to the importance of changes in body mass and glucose levels that cannot be explained by genetic influences. These and other factors have been evaluated in analyses of the non-genetic correlates of glucose and insulin levels.

Correlates of Glucose and Insulin Levels

Considering the metabolic evidence that alterations in glucose levels and in insulin resistance and secretion predate clinical recognition of NIDDM[20], investigators have studied twins to identify determinants of glucose and insulin concentrations. The extent to which genetic factors can explain variation in glucose concentrations was evaluated in a sample of 239 monozygotic and 254 dizygotic twin pairs from the NHLBI twin study[21,22]. Based on the classic heritability estimate of twice the difference in the intraclass correlation coefficients between monozygotic and dizygotic twin pairs[23], 88% of the variation in glucose level 1 hour after a 50 g oral glucose load could be attributed to genetic influences. Using the same estimate, Bouchard et al.[24] found the heritability of fasting glucose concentration to be approximately 72% among 21 dizygotic and 23 monozygotic twin pairs. There was no evidence for genetic determination of glucose response to a carbohydrate meal in this study.

Potential genetic influences on insulin concentrations were evaluated using data collected from the women twins who participated in the second examination of the Kaiser-Permanente study[25]. Heritability of fasting insulin concentration in non-diabetic women under the age of 50 years was 38% ($p = 0.04$). These findings are consistent with other studies showing familial aggregation of relative hyperinsulinaemia[26] and insulin resistance[27], but the 62% of variation unexplained by genetic influences suggests that non-genetic factors must contribute to variation in insulin levels as well.

In a smaller twin study evaluating insulin concentrations, approximately 86% of the variation in fasting insulin level was attributable to genetic influences, but evidence for genetic effects on insulin response to a carbohydrate meal was not observed[24]. In a second study of 17 monozygotic and 18 dizygotic twin pairs from the Finnish Twin Cohort Study[28], no evidence for genetic influences on either the fasting or post-challenge insulin levels was observed. Both of these studies evaluated heritability of insulin levels after adjustment for obesity. Because obesity is itself highly heritable and strongly related to insulin resistance, such adjustment may grossly underestimate the genetic contribution to insulin levels.

The inconsistency in heritability estimates for fasting and post-load levels of glucose and insulin, and the lack of 100% heritability in any of these studies, imply that non-genetic influences are important in determining glucose and insulin concentrations. To evaluate non-genetic correlates of any continuously measured trait, matched statistical analyses that include only monozygotic twin pairs can be conducted. In these matched analyses, differences within twin pairs (Twin 1 − Twin 2) are calculated for all variables, and linear regression procedures are conducted with intrapair differences included as the dependent and independent variables. Because monozygotic twins are genetically identical, intrapair differences reflect only environmental or behavioural variability in the traits. Therefore, results of these matched regression models indicate associations between non-genetic aspects of the involved variables or chance occurrences. Since monozygotic twins reared together also share numerous early environmental exposures and behaviours, the influence of these non-genetic effects may be underestimated in the matched models. Results of the matched analyses are often compared with results of unmatched analyses that considered twins as individuals.

Intrapair differences in obesity, as measured by the BMI, were significantly, positively associated with intrapair differences in the 1-hour, post-load glucose level in matched analyses of 250 pairs of monozygotic male twins from the NHLBI twin study[29]. Moreover, weight gain during adulthood (from mean age of 20 to mean age of 48 years) was also significantly, positively associated with 1-hour, post-load glucose levels measured at middle age (42–55 years). These findings suggest that, despite genetic influences on both glucose and obesity[19,21], non-genetic variation in obesity is related to glucose concentrations and may therefore offer the possibility for prevention of elevated glucose levels and possibly of NIDDM.

In matched analyses of 230 non-diabetic, monozygotic twin pairs from the Kaiser-Permanente women twins study[30], fasting glucose concentrations were positively and significantly correlated with BMI ($p < 0.001$) and intake of alcoholic beverages as assessed by a six-point scale ($p = 0.05$). Other variables that were evaluated but were not associated with fasting glycaemia included uric acid, triglycerides, high-density lipoprotein (HDL) cholesterol, leisure-time physical activity, education, smoking, low-density lipoprotein (LDL) cholesterol and systolic blood pressure.

Fasting insulin levels were examined in 163 non-diabetic, monozygotic twin pairs attending the second clinic visit of the Kaiser-Permanente women twins study[25]. In the unmatched analyses with the women considered as individuals, BMI and waist-to-hip ratio were each signficantly, positively and independently associated with both fasting and post-load insulin concentrations[31]. As in any other sample of individuals, such analyses could be confounded by genetic influences, given the known genetic contributions to overall obesity and fat distribution[19,32]. After removal of genetic influences by matched analyses, BMI remained strongly, positively related to insulin concentrations and accounted for 21% and 9% of the non-genetic variability in fasting and 2-hour, post-load insulin levels, respectively. Interestingly, waist-to-hip ratio was no longer independently associated with either fasting or post-load insulin levels in the matched analyses. A possible explanation for this finding invokes the existence of gene(s) with pleiotropic effects on both fat distribution and insulin concentrations.

Also during the second examination of this cohort, treadmill duration was measured and was evaluated in relation to glucose and insulin levels[10]. In matched analysis of 128 monozygotic twin pairs who completed a submaximal exercise treadmill test, treadmill duration was not related to fasting glucose, but was inversely associated with the 2-hour, post-load glucose level ($p = 0.01$) and with both fasting and 2-hour, post-load insulin concentrations ($p = 0.01$ and $p = 0.002$, respectively). These associations were attenuated and were no longer statistically significant after adjustment for percentage body fat ($p = 0.09$ for post-load glucose, $p = 0.64$ for fasting insulin, and $p = 0.07$ for post-load insulin). If non-genetic variation in treadmill duration reflects the effects of physical activity, this finding may indicate that activity is related to lower glucose and insulin concentrations, and perhaps improved insulin sensitivity, via reductions in body fat. Such an interpretation is consistent with observations in non-twin populations regarding the inverse relationship of physical activity with insulin levels[33] and with incidence of NIDDM[34,35].

Two additional putative risk factors for NIDDM—alcohol intake[36] and dietary fat[37]—were examined for their associations with glucose and insulin levels, in the Kaiser-Permanente women twins study[25]. Since it was thought that genetic influences were unlikely to confound associations of these behavioural variables with glucose or insulin levels, unmatched analyses were conducted so that non-diabetic women from both monozygotic and dizygotic twin pairs could be included, thereby maximizing statistical power. Adjustment for the non-independence of the co-twins was accomplished separately for each zygosity[38]. For the second examination of the female twins, alcohol intake was assessed by food frequency methods without regard to past drinking habits. Since reasons for abstention (medical or otherwise) were not known, and since abstainers appeared less healthy than drinkers and may have been advised to stop drinking, analyses were restricted to non-diabetic twin pairs in which both members consumed alcoholic beverages ($n = 173$ twin pairs). Alcohol intake was not associated with fasting glucose level, whereas higher alcohol intake was related to lower post-load glucose level ($p = 0.02$)[36]. Similarly, alcohol intake was not related to fasting insulin concentrations but was inversely associated with post-load insulin ($p < 0.01$). All results were adjusted for BMI, waist-to-hip ratio, total daily caloric intake and family history of diabetes.

Analyses of alcohol intake and fasting glucose levels were conducted at both the first[30] and second[36] examinations of the women in the Kaiser-Permanente twin study. The apparent discrepancy in findings is difficult to resolve owing to differences in the way alcohol consumption was measured, in the subgroups of subjects included in analyses, and in the specific statistical models evaluated at the two points in time. Moreover, the generally higher alcohol intake reported at the first examination may have enabled an association to be observed that was not detectable at the somewhat lower levels of alcohol intake reported at the second examination. Finally, the original, positive association may have been statistically significant by chance given the p-value of 0.05. Indeed, data from both metabolic ward[39] and epidemiological research[40,41] are equivocal on the question of alcohol intake as a risk factor for insulin resistance and diabetes.

Since high-fat diets have been implicated in the development of glucose intolerance, cross-sectional associations between usual intake of dietary fats and insulin concentrations were evaluated among 544 non-diabetic women from monozygotic and dizygotic twin pairs who participated in the second examination of the Kaiser-Permanente women twins study[37]. Unmatched regression analyses for twin data were used as previously described. A 40 g per day higher intake of total dietary fat was related to a higher fasting insulin level both before and after adjustment for obesity (21%, $p < 0.01$, and 15.2%, $p < 0.01$, respectively). Higher intakes of saturated fat, oleic acid and linoleic acid were each positively related to higher fasting insulin values. The relation of dietary fats to fasting insulin was significantly attenuated among physically active women compared with those who were sedentary ($p = 0.04$). Only saturated fat intake was significantly associated with 2-hour, post-glucose load insulin level ($p = 0.04$).

Taken together, these studies of twins demonstrate both genetic and non-genetic influences on glucose and insulin concentrations. Although restricted to non-diabetic twins, the cross-sectional nature of most analyses precludes statements regarding the temporal sequence of relationships. However, considering the importance of both glucose and insulin levels in predicting subsequent development of NIDDM, these results arguably do identify candidate risk factors for NIDDM that operate independently of inherited genetic susceptibility. The analyses that controlled for genetic influences by use of the matched, monozygotic co-twin method were the most informative. Among the behavioural correlates studied, the most consistent finding was a positive association of body mass with both glucose and insulin levels, both for fasting and post-load values. Treadmill duration, interpreted here as a measure of conditioning through physical activity, was inversely related to post-load glucose as well as to fasting and post-load insulin levels. Among women who consumed alcohol, an inverse relation between alcohol intake and post-load values of glucose and insulin was observed. Finally, higher intake of dietary fats was associated with higher fasting insulin concentrations, particularly among sedentary women. Additional efforts have been directed towards elucidating genetic, environmental and behavioural determinants of glucose and insulin metabolism, by studying insulin resistance and its concomitant metabolic perturbations.

Question 3. Do the Same Non-genetic Influences Contribute to Syndromes Closely Related to NIDDM?

Additional metabolic derangements are known to co-occur with glucose intolerance and NIDDM[42-45]. These include centralized or abdominal obesity, an increased prevalence of hypertension, and specific lipid abnormalities, including low HDL cholesterol and high plasma triglycerides. Reaven has suggested that the common underlying defect that leads to this clustering of risk factors is insulin resistance and has labelled the constellation syndrome X[46].

Haffner et al.[47] have recently shown in longitudinal analyses that fasting hyperinsulinaemia, presumably a reflection of insulin resistance, is predictive of development of this syndrome. Cross-sectional studies confirm that each aspect of the syndrome is strongly related to insulin resistance as measured by the hyperinsulinaemic glucose clamp[48,49]. Not surprisingly, fasting hyper-insulinaemia also predicts development of NIDDM[50]. Thus, the close association of all elements of syndrome X with NIDDM suggests that these two disorders may share aetiological agents, either genetic or non-genetic. Two large studies of twins (NHLBI and Kaiser-Permanente) have examined genetic and non-genetic influences on aspects of syndrome X.

In the NHLBI twin study, Newman et al.[29] demonstrated that within white, male, monozygotic twin pairs, both BMI at age 18–25 years and subsequent weight gain were independently predictive of higher plasma triglycerides and total cholesterol, lower HDL cholesterol, higher blood pressure levels and higher 1-hour, post-load glucose levels measured in middle age (42–55 years). Thus non-genetic or behavioural aspects of adult weight gain are important determinants of these risk factor levels and, by inference, of syndrome X.

Evidence has also been demonstrated for both genetic and non-genetic influences on the occurrence of dyslipidaemic hypertension in this same population[51]. Williams et al.[52] had noted the frequent co-occurrence of dyslipidaemia (especially low HDL cholesterol and elevated triglycerides) with familial hypertension and estimated that 12% of all essential hypertension was attributable to 'familial dyslipidaemic hypertension'. Using Williams' definition of dyslipidaemic hypertension, Selby et al.[51] found excess concordance for the syndrome in monozygotic compared with dizygotic twins (Table 3). Given the overall prevalence of 6% in this sample of middle-aged, white men, the monozygotic twin brother of a proband with dyslipidaemic hypertension was seven times more likely than the average sample member to have dyslipidaemic hypertension.

Table 3 Proband concordance rates for dyslipidaemic hypertension by zygosity, NHLBI twin study, 1969–1973

	Number of pairs	Concordant[a] pairs C	Discordant pairs D	Proband concordance rate $2C/(2C + D)$
Monozygotic	236	7	18	0.44
Dizygotic	247	2	24	0.14

[a]Concordance for the presence of dyslipidaemic hypertension. Reproduced with permission from *JAMA*, 24 April 1991, volume 265, page 2081 (Copyright 1991, American Medical Association).

Twin pairs concordant for dyslipidaemic hypertension were also significantly more obese and demonstrated a higher prevalence of NIDDM and
higher post-load glucose concentrations in non-diabetics than pairs who were
concordant for absence of this syndrome. Discordant pairs were intermediate
for each measure. Thus these findings suggest that dyslipidaemic hypertension, including most if not all aspects of syndrome X, may have genetic
determinants. However, non-genetic influences shared by some pairs and not
others could produce this pattern of results as well.

Clear-cut evidence for the importance of non-genetic factors was also found
in this study[51]. Among the 18 monozygotic twin pairs discordant for dyslipidaemic hypertension, the twin with dyslipidaemic hypertension had significantly higher BMI (Figure 1). Moreover, these twins had similar body masses
at military induction when they were 18–25 years old. Thus, with identical
genes, the twin who gained more weight during adult life was at greater risk
for developing dyslipidaemic hypertension.

The Kaiser-Permanente women twins study further emphasizes involvement of non-genetic factors in development of syndrome X[53]. This study
focused primarily on the associations of LDL subclass phenotypes with
aspects of syndrome X. LDL subclass phenotypes are based on the particle
diameter of the predominant LDL subclass, as determined by non-denaturing

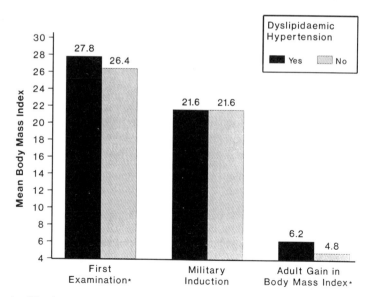

Figure 1 Obesity and adult weight gain in 18 monozygotic twin pairs discordant for
dyslipidaemic hypertension, NHLBI twin study, 1969–1973; $*p = 0.01$. (Reproduced
with permission from *JAMA*, 24 April 1991, vol. 265, p. 2082. Copyright 1991,
American Medical Association)

gradient gel electrophoresis, and consist of two patterns: subclass phenotype A is characterized by a predominance of larger, more buoyant LDL; subclass phenotype B by smaller, denser LDL[54,55]. Family studies[56,57] have suggested that subclass pattern B represents the phenotypic expression of a single major gene, with a dominant mode of inheritance but incomplete penetrance in premenopausal women and men below age 20. Recently, evidence for linkage between phenotype B and the LDL receptor locus on chromosome 19 has been presented[58].

Phenotype B, or small, dense LDL, has been associated with both ischaemic heart disease[59] and NIDDM[60]. Among the female twins[53], subclass phenotype B was closely linked to each aspect of syndrome X, including higher plasma insulin, glucose, blood pressure and waist-to-hip ratio. As in previous studies, subclass phenotype B was most closely related to higher plasma triglycerides and lower HDL cholesterol levels. These associations were so strong as to suggest a central role for LDL subclass phenotype or LDL particle size in syndrome X. Within the 25 monozygotic twin pairs discordant for LDL subclass phenotype, the twin with phenotype B had significantly higher levels of BMI and waist-to-hip ratio (Table 4). Thus non-genetic variation in obesity and fat distribution is important in expression of LDL subclass phenotype.

Some evidence was found that physical activity may be an additional determinant of LDL subclass and other aspects of syndrome X. Within 136 identical twin pairs who completed a treadmill exercise test, the co-twin difference in exercise duration—a measure of fitness—was significantly related to lower HDL cholesterol level and higher levels of waist-to-hip ratio, systolic blood pressure and LDL particle size after adjustment for differences in body fat. In addition, in the 17 twin pairs who were discordant for phenotype B and completed the treadmill test, the twin with phenotype B had a shorter treadmill duration by a mean of 70.1 seconds than the twin with phenotype A ($p = 0.004$). This analysis in twins confirms data from a non-twin study[61]. Thus non-genetic differences in fitness, presumably related to

Table 4 Means and intrapair differences in risk factor levels in 25 monozygotic twin pairs discordant for LDL subclass phenotype, Kaiser-Permanente women twins study, 1989–1990

	Twin with subclass B	Twin with subclass A	Mean difference	p-value
Triglycerides (mg/dl)	182.7	111.9	70.88	0.0002
HDL cholesterol (mg/dl)	49.0	55.9	−6.92	0.002
Body mass index (kg/m²)	28.7	26.1	2.50	<0.01
Waist-to-hip ratio	0.88	0.81	0.07	0.02

differences in physical activity, influence LDL subclass phenotype and other aspects of syndrome X.

The emphasis of these twin studies has been to identify non-genetic influences on the various manifestations of syndrome X. They provide very strong and clear-cut evidence that non-genetic aspects of adult weight gain and possibly physical activity are important to the expression of this syndrome. When considered along with studies in other populations, these findings help to confirm and explain the role of weight gain and physical inactivity as risk factors for development of NIDDM. Whether additional factors, either genetic or non-genetic, are necessary for development of NIDDM, remains unclear.

CONCLUSIONS

In summary, we have reviewed the evidence from twin studies for genetic and non-genetic determinants of NIDDM, including correlates of glucose and insulin concentrations and risk factors for syndromes related to NIDDM. Studies of concordance for NIDDM in twin pairs suggest strong genetic effects, as do heritability analyses of glucose levels. The importance of genetic influences is also supported by heritability analyses of insulin concentrations and concordance among twins for dyslipidaemic hypertension, a condition related to syndrome X and NIDDM. However, environmental and/or behavioural influences are also important to the development of NIDDM, as indicated by disease discordance in monozygotic twin pairs, in some cases lasting many years. Even if development of NIDDM is inevitable in genetically susceptible individuals, identification of the non-genetic influences that delay or hasten disease onset can play a crucial role in minimizing subsequent complications.

To date, twin studies of NIDDM have had limited success in identifying disease risk factors. Some indication that non-genetic variation in body mass may contribute to development of NIDDM has been reported. The potential importance to NIDDM of adult weight gain is further supported by analyses revealing higher levels of fasting and post-load glucose and insulin levels as well as adverse profiles in various components of syndrome X among the heavier co-twins within monozygotic twin pairs. The remainder of the evidence from twin studies regarding non-genetic risk factors for NIDDM relies heavily on analyses of glucose, insulin and components of syndrome X, which may reflect underlying insulin resistance. Studies of self-reported exercise information from monozygotic twin pairs discordant for NIDDM have not revealed meaningful associations. However, analyses within monozygotic twin pairs demonstrate that non-genetic variation in treadmill duration, presumably related to differences in physical activity, are associated with post-load glucose, fasting and post-load insulin, and key elements of syndrome X. Low levels of alcohol intake and high levels of dietary fat consumption also may be related to NIDDM risk through their observed relationship with insulin levels.

The causes of NIDDM are clearly complex, requiring some interaction between genetic and non-genetic factors to explain disease development. Prior to molecular characterization of the gene(s) conferring increased risk of NIDDM, analyses of disease-discordant monozygotic twin pairs theoretically provide an important means for identifying potentially modifiable, non-genetic influences. However, in practice, small sample sizes, limited longitudinal information and incompatible data across studies have hindered the successful application of this approach. The most compelling alternative is to focus on subclinical measures that predict NIDDM. More direct measures of insulin resistance, insulin secretion and other determinants of glucose homeostasis, such as hepatic glucose production, in the context of twin studies would yield valuable information regarding genetic and non-genetic influences on the development of NIDDM.

REFERENCES

1 Then Berg H. The genetic aspect of diabetes mellitus (Foreign letter). *JAMA* 1939; **112**: 1091.
2 White P. Evidence in favor of the theory that diabetes is inherited. In: *The Treatment of Diabetes Mellitus* (eds EP Joslin, HF Root, P White, A Marble) Lea & Febiger, Philadelphia, 1959, pp 48–63.
3 Harvald B, Hauge M. Selection in diabetes in modern society. *Acta Med Scand* 1963; **173**: 459–65.
4 Gottlieb MS, Root HF. Diabetes mellitus in twins. *Diabetes* 1968; **17**: 693–704.
5 Pollin W, Allen MG, Hoffer A, Stabenau JR, Hrubec Z. Psychopathology in 15,909 pairs of veteran twins: evidence for a genetic factor in the pathogenesis of schizophrenia and its relative absence in psychoneurosis. *Am J Psychiatry* 1969; **126**: 597–610.
6 Tattersall RB, Pyke DA. Diabetes in identical twins. *Lancet* 1972; **ii**: 1120–5.
7 Barnett AH, Eff C, Leslie RDG, Pyke DA. Diabetes in identical twins: a study of 200 pairs. *Diabetologia* 1981; **20**: 87–93.
8 Newman B, Selby JV, King M-C, et al. Concordance for type 2 (non-insulin-dependent) diabetes mellitus in male twins. *Diabetologia* 1987; **30**: 763–8.
9 Committee on Diabetic Twins, Japan Diabetes Study. Diabetes mellitus in twins: a cooperative study in Japan. *Diabetes Res Clin Pract* 1988; **5**: 271–80.
10 Mayer E, Newman B, Selby JV. Previously unpublished data from the Kaiser-Permanente women twins study, 1992.
11 Harvald B. Genetic perspectives in diabetes mellitus. *Acta Med Scand* 1967; Suppl 476: 17–27.
12 Cerasi E, Luft R. Insulin response to glucose infusion in diabetic and non-diabetic monozygotic twin pairs: genetic control of insulin response? *Acta Endocrinol* 1967; **55**: 330–45.

13 Pyke DA, Cassar J, Todd J, Taylor KW. Glucose tolerance and serum insulin in identical twins of diabetics. *Br Med J* 1970; **4**: 649–51.
14 Gottlieb MS, Soeldner JS, Kyner JL, Gleason RE. Oral glucose-stimulated insulin release in nondiabetic twin siblings of diabetic twins. *Diabetes* 1974; **23**: 684–92.
15 Gottlieb MS, Soeldner JS, Gleason RE. Evidence of increased oral glucose-stimulated insulin release in nondiabetic twin siblings of diabetic twins (Abstract). *Diabetes* 1969; **18** (Suppl 1): 357.
16 Saad MF, Knowler WC, Pettitt DJ, et al. The natural history of impaired glucose intolerance in the Pima Indians. *N Engl J Med* 1988; **319**: 1500–6.
17 Charles MA, Fontbonne A, Thibult N, et al. Risk factors for NIDDM in a white population: the Paris Prospective Study. *Diabetes* 1991; **40**: 796–9.
18 Bergman RN, Finegood DT, Ader M. Assessment of insulin sensitivity in vivo. *Endocrinol Rev* 1985; **6**: 45–86.
19 Austin MA, King M-C, Bawol RD, Hulley SB, Friedman GD. Risk factors for coronary heart disease in adult female twins: genetic heritability and shared environmental influence. *Am J Epidemiol* 1987; **125**: 308–18.
20 DeFronzo RA, Bonadonna RC, Ferrannini E. Pathogenesis of NIDDM: a balanced overview. *Diabetes Care* 1992; **15**: 318–68.
21 Feinleib M, Garrison RJ, Fabsitz R, et al. The NHLBI twin study of cardiovascular disease risk factors: methodology and summary of results. *Am J Epidemiol* 1977; **106**: 284–95.
22 Havlik R, Garrison R, Fabsitz R, Feinleib M. Genetic variability of clinical chemical values. *Clin Chem* 1977; **23**: 659–62.
23 Cavalli-Sforza LL, Bodmer WF. *The Genetics of Human Populations.* Freeman, San Francisco, 1971.
24 Bouchard C, Tremblay A, Nadeau A, et al. Genetic effect in resting and exercise metabolic rates. *Metabolism* 1989; **38**: 364–70.
25 Mayer EJ. *Genetic and Behavioral Determinants of Insulin Concentrations in Healthy Twins*, Doctoral Dissertation, University of California, Berkeley, 1992.
26 Haffner SM, Stern MP, Hazuda HP, Mitchell BD, Patterson JP. Increased insulin concentrations in non-diabetic offspring of diabetic parents. *N Engl J Med* 1988; **319**: 1297–301.
27 Laws A, Stefanick ML, Reaven GM. Insulin resistance and hypertriglyceridemia in nondiabetic relatives of patients with noninsulin-dependent diabetes mellitus. *J Clin Endocrinol Metab* 1989; **69**: 343–7.
28 Kesaniemi YA, Koskenvuo M, Miettinen TA. Responses of blood glucose and serum insulin to peroral glucose load in normoglycemic twins. *Acta Genet Med Gemellol (Roma)* 1984; **33**: 467–74.
29 Newman B, Selby JV, Quesenberry CP, et al. Nongenetic influences of obesity on other cardiovascular disease risk factors: an analysis of identical twin pairs. *Am J Public Health* 1990; **80**: 675–8.
30 Selby JV, Newman B, King M-C, Friedman GD. Environmental and behavioral determinants of fasting plasma glucose in women: a matched co-twin analysis. *Am J Epidemiol* 1987; **125**: 979–88.
31 Mayer EJ, Newman B, King M-C, Selby JV. Genetic susceptibility and associations of obesity and fat patterning with insulin concentrations in identical twins (Abstract). *Am J Epidemiol* 1992; **136**: 983.
32 Selby JV, Newman B, Quesenberry CP, et al. Genetic and behavioral influences on body fat distribution. *Int. J. Obesity* 1990; **14**: 593–602.
33 Regensteiner JR, Mayer EJ, Shetterly SM, et al. Relationship between habitual physical activity and insulin levels among non-diabetic men and women: the San Luis Valley Diabetes Study. *Diabetes Care* 1992; **14**: 1066–74.

34 Manson JE, Rimm EB, Stampfer JJ, et al. Physical activity and incidence of non-insulin-dependent diabetes mellitus in women. *Lancet* 1991; **338**: 774–8.

35 Helmrich SP, Ragland DR, Leung RQ, Paffenbarger RS. Physical activity and reduced occurrence of non-insulin-dependent diabetes mellitus. *N Engl J Med* 1991; **325**: 147–52.

36 Mayer EJ, Newman B, Quesenberry CP, Friedman GD, Selby JV. Alcohol consumption and insulin concentrations: the role of insulin in associations of alcohol intake with HDL-cholesterol and triglyceride. *Circulation* 1993 (in press).

37 Mayer EJ, Newman B, Quesenberry CP, Selby JV. Usual dietary fat intake and insulin concentrations in healthy women twins. *Diabetes Care* 1993 (in press).

38 Fabsitz R, Feinleib M, Hubert H. Regression analysis with correlated errors: an example from the NHLBI twin study. *J Chronic Dis* 1985; **38**: 165–70.

39 Yki-Jarvinen H, Koivisto VA, Ylikahui R, Taskinen M-R. Acute effects of ethanol and acetate on glucose kinetics in normal subjects. *Am J Physiol* 1988; **254**: E175–80.

40 Stampfer MJ, Colditz GA, Willett WC, et al. A prospective study of moderate alcohol drinking and risk of diabetes in women. *Am J Epidemiol* 1988; **128**: 549–58.

41 Holbrook TL, Barrett-Conner E, Wingard DL. A prospective population-based study of alcohol use and non-insulin dependent diabetes mellitus. *Am J Epidemiol* 1990; **132**: 902–9.

42 Fuh MM-I, Shieh S-M, Wu D-A, Chen Y-DI, Reaven GM. Abnormalities of carbohydrate and lipid metabolism in patients with hypertension. *Arch Intern Med* 1987; **147**: 1035–8.

43 Criqui MH, Barrett-Connor E, Holbrook MJ, Austin M, Turner JD. Clustering of cardiovascular disease risk factors. *Prev. Med* 1980; **9**: 525–33.

44 Ohlson LO, Larsson B, Svardsudd K, et al. The influence of body fat distribution on the incidence of diabetes mellitus. *Diabetes* 1985; **34**: 1055–8.

45 Modan M, Halkin H, Almog S, et al. Hyperinsulinemia: a link between hypertension, obesity and glucose intolerance. *J Clin Invest* 1985; **75**: 807–17.

46 Reaven GM. Role of insulin resistance in human disease. *Diabetes* 1988; **37**: 1595–607.

47 Haffner SM, Valdez RA, Hazuda HP, et al. Prospective analysis of the insulin-resistance syndrome (syndrome X). *Diabetes* 1992; **41**: 715–22.

48 Ferrannini E, Buzzigoli G, Bonadonna, R, et al. Insulin resistance in essential hypertension. *N. Engl J Med* 1987; **317**: 350–7.

49 Laakso M, Sarlund H, Mykkanen L. Insulin resistance is associated with lipid and lipoprotein abnormalities in subjects with varying degrees of glucose tolerance. *Arteriosclerosis* 1990; **10**: 223–31.

50 Haffner SM, Stern MP, Mitchell BND, Hazuda HP, Paterson JK. Incidence of type II diabetes mellitus in Mexican Americans predicted by fasting insulin and glucose levels, obesity, and body fat distribution. *Diabetes* 1990; **39**: 283–9.

51 Selby JV, Newman B, Quiroga Jr, et al. Concordance for dyslipidemic hypertension in male twins. *JAMA* 1991; **265**: 2079–84.

52 Williams RR, Hunt SC, Hopkins PN, et al. Familial dyslipidemic hypertension: evidence from 58 Utah families for a syndrome present in aproximately 12% of patients with essential hypertension. *JAMA* 1988; **259**: 3579–86.

53 Selby JV, Austin MA, Newman B, Mayer EJ, Krauss RM. LDL subclass phenotypes, insulin, hypertension and obesity in women (Abstract). *Circulation* 1991; **84** (Suppl II): II-547.

54 Shen MMS, Krauss RM, Lindgren FT, Forte TM. Heterogeneity of serum low density lipoproteins in normal human subjects. *J Lipid Res* 1981; **22**: 236–44.

55 Krauss RM, Burke DJ. Identification of multiple subclasses of plasma low density lipoproteins in normal humans. *J Lipid Res* 1982; **23**: 97–104.

56 Austin MA, King MC, Vranizan KM, Newman B, Krauss RM. Inheritance of low density lipoprotein subclass patterns: results of complex segregation analysis. *Am J Hum Genet* 1988; **43**: 838–46.

57 Austin MA, Brunzell JD, Fitch WL, Krauss RM. Inheritance of low density lipoprotein subclass patterns in familial combined hyperlipidemia. *Arteriosclerosis* 1990; **10**: 520–30.

58 Nishina PM, Johnson JP, Naggert KJ, Krauss RM. Linkage of atherogenic lipoprotein phenotype to the low density lipoprotein receptor locus on the short arm of chromosome 19. *Proc Natl Acad Sci USA* 1992; **89**: 708–12.

59 Austin MA, Breslow JL, Hennekens CH, et al. Low density lipoprotein subclass patterns and risk of myocardial infarction. *JAMA* 1988; **260**: 1917–21.

60 Bakarat HA, Carpenter JW, McLendon VD, et al. Influence of obesity, impaired glucose tolerance, and NIDDM on LDL structure and composition: possible link between hyperinsulinemia and atherosclerosis. *Diabetes* 1990; **39**: 1527–33.

61 Williams PT, Krauss RM, Vranizan KM, Wood PDS. Changes in lipoprotein subfractions during diet-induced and exercise-induced weight loss in moderately overweight men. *Circulation* 1990; **81**: 1293–304.

Two additional references of potential interest to readers were omitted because they did not appear in the published literature or associated databases until after completion of the chapter:

Kaprio J, Tuomilehto J, Koskenvuo M, et al. Concordance for type 1 (insulin-dependent) and type 2 (non-insulin-dependent) diabetes mellitus in a population-based cohort of twins in Finland. *Diabetologia* 1992; **35**: 1060–7.

Lo SSS, Tun RYM, Hawa M, Leslie RDG. Studies of diabetic twins. *Diabetes/Metabolism Rev* 1991; **7**: 223–38.

Chapter Fourteen

Thrifty Genotypes

P. Zimmet and K. O'Dea
International Diabetes Institute and Department of Human Nutrition, Deakin University, Victoria, Australia

INTRODUCTION

During the last century, there has been a dramatic change in the epidemiological profile of diseases in developed countries and many developing countries[1]. Until the latter part of the nineteenth century, epidemics of infectious diseases such as typhoid, cholera, diphtheria, smallpox and influenza were the main causes of morbidity and mortality in developed nations. The Industrial Revolution heralded major changes in society, including major improvements in public health. Thus progress in housing, sanitation, water supply and nutrition all played important roles, along with the later developments of immunization and antibiotics, in reducing the morbidity and mortality from infectious diseases.

As a result, non-communicable disorders such as cardiovascular diseases (CVD), cancers, non-insulin-dependent diabetes mellitus (NIDDM) and strokes rank amongst the main causes of ill health and death in developed nations, and the same picture is occurring in many developing countries[1,2]. Today, the highest rates of NIDDM are seen in populations that have been subjected to rapid lifestyle change such as the American Indians, Pacific

Causes of Diabetes. Edited by R. D. G. Leslie
© 1993 John Wiley & Sons Ltd

islanders, Australian Aborigines and certain migrant populations such as Asian Indians[1,3-5]. As NIDDM provides a good example of the concept of the 'thrifty genotype', this review will focus on it. However, as glucose intolerance is a major CVD risk factor, and it and other CVD risk factors such as hyperinsulinaemia, dyslipidaemia and hypertension appear to be interrelated[3], they will also be discussed in the context of their possible common pathogenesis.

THE EVOLUTION OF THE 'THRIFTY GENOTYPE' HYPOTHESIS

Thirty years ago, the American geneticist James Neel raised the question of why a disease such as diabetes, which is associated with significant morbidity and mortality, had reached such a high prevalence in populations such as the American Indians[6]. After all, for the now lethal genotype to survive into this century, it must have conveyed some advantage in terms of natural selection.

Neel suggested that under the conditions of feast and famine which brought about fluctuating and often sparse food supplies—a situation not uncommon throughout human history—people with a 'thrifty gene' were better able to store food as fat during the feast periods[6]. He proposed that they had a 'quick insulin trigger' which facilitated this process. The Pacific islanders were subjected to periodic and regular food deprivation associated with long migratory canoe voyages, and the droughts and hurricanes encountered as natural phenomena. The possession of the 'thrifty gene' would have allowed them to survive bouts of starvation. Diabetes would only develop under the modern scenario of constantly available high-caloric, low-energy density foods along with sedentary physical activity patterns. Thus the genotype became disadvantageous in this situation and manifests as obesity, hyperinsulinaemia and insulin resistance. These lead ultimately to pancreatic β cell decompensation and NIDDM[3].

There are animal models of NIDDM which appear to fit the 'thrifty genotype' scenario. The Israeli sand rat (*Pasammomus obesus*) and the spiny mouse (*Acomys caharinis*), originating in the desert regions of North Africa and the Middle East, mirror the pattern of development of NIDDM seen in highly susceptible human populations in response to Westernization[7]. In the wild state, a physically active lifestyle and a diet of saltbush ensure that they remain lean and free of diabetes. However, when these animals are brought into the laboratory, the sedentary life in captivity and the diet of laboratory chow (not usually considered typical of the affluent Western diet!) result in a significant proportion of these rats becoming obese and diabetic. They develop the cluster of metabolic abnormalities seen in susceptible human populations when exposed to rapid Westernization: obesity, hyperinsulinaemia, impaired glucose tolerance, insulin resistance and frank diabetes. Like the human populations, they exhibit a wide range of responses to Westernization, with a minority retaining normal glucose tolerance and normal insulin levels, and the remainder exhibiting varying degrees of impaired glucose tolerance and hyperinsulinaemia through to frank diabetes and hypoinsulinaemia (β cell exhaustion)[7,8].

AN ANTHROPOLOGICAL PERSPECTIVE OF THE 'THRIFTY GENOTYPE'

As far as the American Indians are concerned, Wendorf has suggested that this genotype representing susceptibility to obesity and NIDDM arose from natural selection during the peopling of North America south of the continental glaciers[9]. This selection may have happened during a period of alternating feast and famine as early Paleo-Indian hunter/gatherers from an unusual mid-latitude tundra environment (the 'ice-free' corridor) adapted to more typical mid-latitude environments. This occurred at least 20 000 years ago. These populations relied on big game causing frequent but short-lived food shortages, and a 'thrifty gene' could have allowed a survival advantage during these alternating periods of feast and famine. In contrast to the Pima Indians, who today share the world's highest NIDDM prevalence[3,10], certain American Indian groups including the Athapaskans, Aleuts and Eskimos do not exhibit these high rates[9]. They either remained in high latitudes or migrated south after the glaciers had retreated and did not experience the sudden changes in environment that confronted the Paleo-Indians. As Wendorf points out, in these other groups, the 'thrifty gene' metabolism would not have conveyed as much survival advantage as in the Paleo-Indians. This could have resulted in one form of the 'thrifty genotype'.

Yet another form of the 'thrifty genotype' could have evolved in the Pacific region. There is abundant evidence that Micronesians, Polynesians and Austronesian (AN)–Melanesians have a heightened genetic susceptibility to NIDDM which appears to be unmasked by change in their way of life[1–3]. Dietary change, obesity, reduced physical activity and other factors have been invoked as possible determinants[1]. The 'thrifty genotype' hypothesis would seem to explain how NIDDM has attained such a high prevalence with rates in excess of 30% in Micronesian Nauruans[11] and AN–Melanesians of Papua New Guinea[12].

The story of migration into the Pacific may provide an explanation for this[2]. It appears that there have been three major migrations from South-East Asia, and there is archaeological evidence that suggests that New Guinea was first settled over 50 000 years ago by Australoid populations. Some 10 000 years ago, Papuan-speaking migrants reached New Guinea from the west and then spread further east to Fiji. Between 3500 and 5000 years ago, Austronesian speakers arrived in New Guinea and intermarried with the Australoids who were living in the coastal areas. The Austronesians—the people who subsequently went on to populate the rest of the Pacific—did not penetrate into the New Guinea highlands. The highlanders are the survivors of the earlier migrations and are referred to as non-Austronesian (NAN)–Melanesians. The Austronesian speakers moved on and intermarried with the coastal people of New Britain, New Hebrides (Vanuatu) and New Caledonia, and by 3000 years ago had moved on to Fiji. They later continued their migration in canoes, moving further east into Polynesia, colonizing Samoa, Tahiti and then other parts of Polynesia.

The New Guinea highlands have not been subjected to the vagaries of food supplies and weather as have the coastal regions of New Guinea and most of the rest of the Pacific islands. Thus the populations there have lived settled lives for many thousands of years, with well-developed agriculture taking advantage of high rainfalls and fertile soils[13]. In this situation, there was no need for a 'thrifty gene'. Even now, the prevalence of NIDDM is still quite low in highland communities[1]. On the other hand, the AN–Melanesians from the coast, and the Austronesians who populated Polynesia and probably parts of Micronesia, have been subjected to the cycle of feast and famine through their long canoe voyages and droughts and hurricanes which have affected food productivity on their often barren coral atoll soils[13]. In these situations, the acquisition of a 'thrifty gene' would clearly provide a survival advantage.

Recently, we have reported that the AN–Melanesians of Papua New Guinea have soared into the prevalence range of NIDDM in excess of 30%[12]—a range that was only shared by the American Pima Indians and the Nauruans previously. These two latter populations have been invoked as excellent examples of the 'thrifty gene' in operation. Not only this, but many other Pacific island populations of Austronesian origin have developed high prevalence of NIDDM with modernization[1-3].

The same or yet another variation of the 'thrifty gene' may exist in the Australian Aboriginal community. When the Australian Aborigines make the transition from a traditional hunter/gatherer lifestyle to that of urban Australia, they develop high prevalence rates of obesity (with an android pattern of fat distribution), NIDDM and CVD[4]. The crude prevalence of diabetes has been reported to be two to six times as high as that in Australians of European descent. However, because of the lower life expectancy and earlier age of onset of diabetes in Aborigines, these figures do not reflect the true severity of the problem. In the 20–50-year age group, diabetes is about 10 times more prevalent in Aborigines than in Australians of European descent[4,5].

There is no evidence that Australian Aborigines experienced these non-communicable diseases when they lived as hunter/gatherers[4]. There is paucity of quantitative data on the health of Aborigines with little or no European contact. However, early reports describe them as being lean and apparently physically fit. In the most remote areas of Australia, small groups of Aborigines continued to live traditionally until relatively recently. Data from such groups indicate that they were extremely lean (body mass index (BMI) usually below 20 kg/m^2), with low blood pressure (usually below 110/70 mmHg), and no increase of body weight or blood pressure with age[4]. More recent observations in traditionally orientated groups indicate low fasting glucose and cholesterol levels, but higher than expected fasting insulin and triglyceride levels (in view of their leanness and regular physical activity)[14]. This latter observation is consistent with the possibility of insulin resistance preceding Westernization.

We argue below that this may have been important to the survival of Aborigines when they lived traditionally by allowing them to efficiently convert any excess energy to fat in times of food abundance, but that it becomes a disadvantage following Westernization by facilitating excessive weight gain and eventually NIDDM[4,15].

Wendorf has suggested that the high prevalence of NIDDM that we have reported in migrant Asian Indians, Creoles and Chinese in Mauritius[16] may be due to a slightly different 'thrifty gene' (M. Wendorf, personal communication). He points out that the population of Mauritius is not obese and there was not a period of adaptation to new environments similar to that in the American Indians, Pacific islanders and Australian Aborigines. In fact, Mauritius has only been populated by these groups within the last 300 years[16].

HYPERINSULINAEMIA AND INSULIN RESISTANCE: THE PHENOTYPIC EXPRESSION OF THE THRIFTY GENE?

The 'thrifty genotype' hypothesis provides a plausible basis for the high prevalence of NIDDM in the Pima Indians, Nauruans and Australian Aborigines[1,3,4,6]. The central feature of this hypothesis is the existence of hyperinsulinaemia. In fact, both Neel[17] and Szathmary[18] suggested that the hypothesis can best be tested through longitudinal studies in children. Szathmary suggested that obesity and small increases in insulin levels should become manifest in individuals with 'thrifty genes', and follow-up studies should document the role these factors play in the development of NIDDM[18]. In this context, we have recently reported that hyperinsulinaemia in the presence of normal glucose tolerance is already evident in young people in Nauru and Tuvalu[19]—populations where the prevalence of NIDDM is high[1] (Figure 1). Even in youth elevated fasting and 2-hour post-glucose load

274

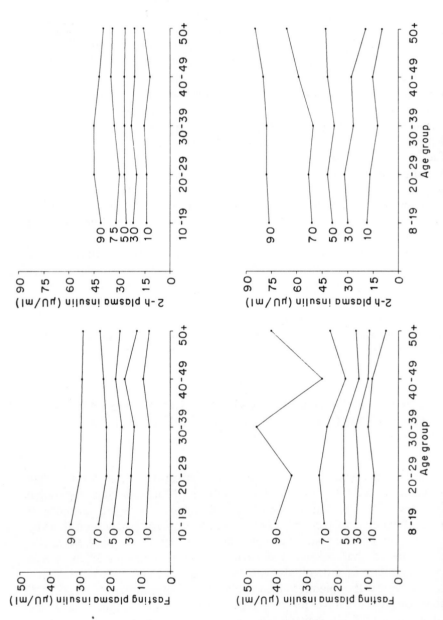

Figure 1 Percentile values for fasting and 2-hour plasma insulin according to age group for Nauruans (lower figures) and Tuvaluans (upper figures) with normal glucose tolerance. (Reproduced by permission of *Diabetologia* from Zimmet *et al.*[19])

insulin concentrations are predictive of subsequent development of NIDDM in these populations[19].

It seems relevant to discuss the contemporary view of the role of hyperinsulinaemia and insulin resistance in the aetiology of NIDDM before discussing the possible biochemical mechanisms that could explain how the 'thrifty gene' operates.

HYPERINSULINAEMIA AND/OR INSULIN RESISTANCE: THE CHARACTERISTIC METABOLIC ABNORMALITY IN NIDDM?

Controversy has centred around whether NIDDM is caused by β cell dysfunction (characterized by hypoinsulinaemia) or insulin resistance (characterized by hyperinsulinaemia) or a combination of the two[19-21]. Further confusion has resulted because at different times in the natural history of NIDDM both islet cell dysfunction and insulin resistance can occur and, in fact, can coexist[21,22]. Furthermore, vigorous debate continues as to whether hyperinsulinaemia precedes insulin resistance in the natural history of NIDDM[3]. In their original report on the development of a radioimmunoassay for insulin, Yalow and Berson noted that plasma insulin concentrations after oral glucose exceeded normal in patients with maturity-onset diabetes (now termed NIDDM) and suggested insulin was unable to exert its full effect[23]. Hales and Randle reported 'supranormal' concentrations of plasma insulin in this form of diabetes[24], and extended the concept of insulin resistance. They proposed that an abnormality of triglyceride metabolism led to increased release of free fatty acids (FFA) in adipose tissue and muscle and suggested that this would cause resistance to the hypoglycaemic action of insulin. What is now named the 'pancreatic exhaustion' hypothesis for the aetiology of NIDDM can be found in their paper, i.e. that increased insulin resistance would result in a rise in plasma glucose and insulin with eventual exhaustion of the pancreatic β cells.

The case for hyperinsulinaemia as the primary defect in NIDDM was further supported by numerous studies over the next few years[25-32]. Rimoin demonstrated hyperinsulinaemia in Navajo Indians and found a three-fold difference in plasma insulin response between the Navajos and the Pennsylvania Amish[27]. This ethnic variability in plasma insulin responses was subsequently confirmed in Pima Indians[34], Micronesians and Polynesians[35], Australian Aborigines[32], Asian Indians[36,37], Chinese and Creoles[37].

There was a fundamental understanding of the natural history of NIDDM over 20 years ago and there was a strong case made for hyperinsulinaemia as the most likely and possibly primary characteristic feature. The Hales and Randle proposal[24] that increased FFA concentrations cause insulin resistance

(Randle's cycle) has resurfaced more recently and the evidence has been reviewed in detail elsewhere by Reaven[38]. Circulating FFA concentration is suppressed quickly by insulin in normal subjects. However, persons with NIDDM have a reduced capacity to suppress FFAs, thereby increasing hepatic glucose output and contributing to hyperglycaemia in these subjects. This could further exacerbate hyperinsulinaemia and insulin resistance. However, contemporary opinion is that this mechanism does not play a major role in the insulin resistance of NIDDM although such an effect can be induced acutely[39].

The confusion as to whether hypoinsulinaemia or hyperinsulinaemia is the fundamental defect in NIDDM can, in part, be explained because of possible heterogeneity and also at what point in the natural history of NIDDM that glucose tolerance is studied[3]. Hyperinsulinaemia is a well-documented feature of impaired glucose tolerance (IGT)[40–42], and in longitudinal studies in a number of ethnic groups it clearly precedes decompensation to diabetes[19,40–43]. Studies in subjects with well-established NIDDM will often demonstrate hypoinsulinaemia due to the natural history of the disorder[43]. Reaven and his colleagues demonstrated clearly that the discrepant results were due to the stage of glucose intolerance that existed when the studies were made[44,45]. The typical inverted 'U'-shaped pattern of insulin secretion that they demonstrated was subsequently confirmed in another group of Europids[46], Pima Indians[34], and Micronesians and Polynesians[35] (Figure 2), and this phenomenon has more recently been labelled the Starling curve of the pancreas[22].

There is now a firm basis for the current position that the predominant and initial abnormality in the natural history of NIDDM is hyperinsulinaemia.

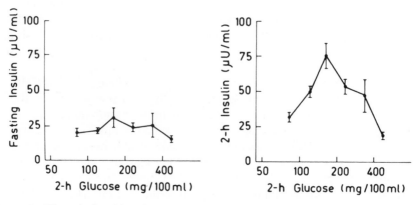

Figure 2 The relationship of mean logarithmic 2-hour plasma glucose with 2-hour plasma glucose insulin response (±SEM) in Micronesian Nauruans showing the typical inverted 'U'-shaped curve

There may also be a smaller subgroup of NIDDM subjects where hypoinsulinaemia causing deficient insulin secretion could play a role.

HYPERINSULINAEMIA: THE TELEOLOGICAL RELATIONSHIP TO THE DEVELOPMENT OF NIDDM

Convincing data exist from numerous epidemiological studies to indicate an important aetiological role for hyperinsulinaemia in the development of NIDDM[3]. Hyperinsulinaemia is a characteristic feature of populations with a high prevalence of NIDDM such as American Indians[27,34], Micronesian Nauruans and Polynesians[35], Mexican–Americans[42], Australian Aborigines[32,47], Asian Indians[3] and American blacks[48]. As most of these studies were cross-sectional, only limited inference can be made from them regarding the aetiological role of hyperinsulinaemia. However, longitudinal studies provide a more substantive basis to permit the conclusion that hyperinsulinaemia has an important role in the natural history of glucose intolerance[3]. Hyperinsulinaemia predates the onset of both IGT and NIDDM by many years, as is well documented in Micronesian Nauruans, Pima Indians, Mexican–Americans and Europids[19,40–43]. Figure 3 shows that Nauruans with hyperinsulinaemia, i.e. those in the higher quartiles of baseline 2-hour plasma insulin, were more likely to develop both IGT and NIDDM over time.

Somewhat surprisingly at first sight, but quite compatible with the concept of pancreatic β cell exhaustion, was the fact that progression from IGT to

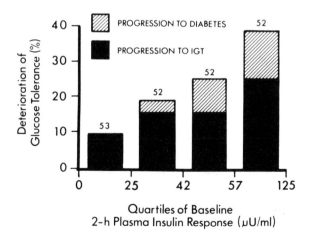

Figure 3 The percentage of Nauruan subjects progressing to impaired glucose tolerance and NIDDM in relation to quartile of baseline 2-hour plasma insulin. (Reproduced by permission of *Diabetes* from Sicree *et al.*[40])

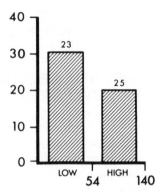

Baseline 2-h Plasma Insulin Response
(µU/ml)

Figure 4 Percentage of Nauruans developing NIDDM from IGT according to baseline 2-hour insulin response. Value above each bar represents the number of people in that category. (Reproduced by permission of *Diabetes* from Sicree *et al.*[40])

NIDDM could be predicted by lower (but still high relative to normal) basal post-glucose load insulin response (Figure 4). This apparent paradox has been confirmed in other populations[41–43,49]. It certainly provides a basis for a better understanding of the natural history of the progression from normal to abnormal glucose tolerance.

De Fronzo has suggested that the major site of insulin resistance may be muscle and/or adipose tissue[22]. While it has been previously accepted that the hyperinsulinaemia is secondary to insulin resistance, this is still a question of debate. There are data to support this[3], but only a very careful long-term prospective study could prove which of hyperinsulinaemia or insulin resistance is the primary defect, albeit that there is evidence from animal models that hyperinsulinaemia is the primary event[50–52].

Hyperinsulinaemia predates insulin resistance in both rodent[50] and monkey models[51] of NIDDM. In a longitudinal study of onset of NIDDM in monkeys (*Macaca mulatta*) hyperinsulinaemia appeared to precede insulin resistance by several years[51]. In the progression from normal glucose tolerance to diabetes, the earliest change that was noted was a slight and progressive increase in fasting plasma insulin concentration. This event preceded any change in the fasting plasma glucose concentration or glucose disappearance during an intravenous glucose tolerance test. Furthermore, based on 7 years' surveillance, Hansen and Bodkin[52] have suggested a primary defect in β cell control or sensitivity in these monkeys. The evidence for this is the initial increase in insulin release in response to glucose, and a slight and subsequent significant increase in fasting plasma insulin—abnormalities that precede the fasting plasma glucose elevations followed by a decrease in plasma insulin and insulin response and the development of glucose intolerance. There are also studies in humans that support the contention that hyperinsulinaemia *per se* can cause insulin resistance[53,54].

That NIDDM develops in a progressive fashion is suggested by the combined experimental data from animals, and human epidemiological and clinical research data[3]. In subjects with genetic susceptibility to NIDDM, whatever the initial defect, i.e. hyperinsulinaemia or insulin resistance, a vicious cycle appears to develop between hyperinsulinaemia and insulin resistance in an attempt to maintain normal glucose homeostasis. However, pancreatic secretion of insulin eventually begins to fall, resulting in deterioration of glucose tolerance with increasing hyperglycaemia through IGT to diabetes. If the hyperinsulinaemia is primary, it could be the result of increased central nervous system sympathetic activity or a primary β cell phenomenon or a combination of the two. While insulin receptor molecular defects have been shown in rare instances, it is most unlikely that these or an abnormal insulin gene play a role in a wider sense[55,56]. Reduced hepatic clearance of insulin as the cause of hyperinsulinaemia cannot be discounted and needs to be further investigated.

HYPERINSULINAEMIA AND THE 'THRIFTY GENOTYPE' HYPOTHESIS: A UNITARIAN EXPLANATION FOR NIDDM AND CVD

While we have discussed the relationship of hyperinsulinaemia to the development of diabetes in isolation, there are possibly other metabolic abnormalities, including dyslipidaemia, that may also occur, as well as hypertension and upper body obesity. NIDDM is a disorder with multiple metabolic defects[57–59], and the major cause of mortality in NIDDM is coronary artery disease[60], so it is possible that the major CVD risk factors share a common aetiology.

How might the suggested role of hyperinsulinaemia in the aetiology of upper body obesity, atherosclerosis and hypertension as well as glucose intolerance be explained? It has been suggested that there may be an anthropological basis for this association. As discussed earlier, Neel hypothesized that hunter/gatherers who relied on the feast and famine cycle of food sources and availability developed a 'thrifty genotype'[6]. This provided a selective advantage during periods of variable food supply in earlier times in history. With lifestyle change (constant and abundant food supply and physical inactivity of our contemporary society), many previously hunter/gatherer or peasant agriculturist populations now exhibit a high prevalence of NIDDM. Neel suggested that the 'thrifty genotype' has become a disadvantage, and has contributed to the high frequency of NIDDM. Wendorf and Goldfine have recently suggested that insulin resistance may be the phenotypic expression of this genotype[9]. While this hypothesis may explain the high prevalence of glucose intolerance now seen in certain populations, how does the 'thrifty genotype' explain the other components of the CVD risk factor cluster, and is there evidence for the link?

O'Dea demonstrated striking improvements in all of the metabolic abnormalities of NIDDM and reduction in other CVD risk factors[15,61], in a study in which 10 diabetic Australian Aborigines reverted to their traditional hunter/gatherer lifestyle for 7 weeks (Table 1). Although insulin sensitivity was not measured directly, there were marked reductions in both fasting glucose and fasting insulin concentrations, consistent with improved insulin sensitivity. The pronounced reduction in hypertriglyceridaemia and the fall in blood pressure were also consistent with reduced insulin resistance. Hyperinsulinaemia and insulin resistance have been demonstrated in both diabetic and non-diabetic Australian Aborigines[4,32,47], and the effect of traditional lifestyle—either dietary factors, regular physical activity or a combination of both—on reducing the hyperinsulinaemia and insulin resistance may have played a role in the improvement in the CVD risk factor profile. The fact that these improvements occurred simultaneously lend support to their linkage and the possible central aetiological role of hyperinsulinaemia.

A better understanding of how the 'thrifty genotype' operates in a survival mode and in contemporary society is required, and we suggest here how it

Table 1 Summary of major changes in the metabolic abnormalities of diabetes and other risk factors for cardiovascular disease in a group of diabetic Aborigines in response to 7 weeks' reversion to a traditional hunter/gatherer lifestyle (mean ± SEM, $n = 10$)

	Before	After 7 weeks	
Body weight (kg)	81.9 ± 3.4	73.8 ± 2.8	$p < 0.001$
BMI (kg/m²)	27.2 ± 1.1	24.5 ± 0.8	$p < 0.001$
Fasting glucose (mmol/l)	11.6 ± 1.2	6.6 ± 0.5	$p < 0.001$
Glucose 2 hours after 75 g OGTT[a]	18.5 ± 1.3	11.9 ± 0.9	$p < 0.001$
Fasting insulin (mU/l)	23 ± 3	12 ± 1	$p < 0.001$
Insulin 2 hours after 75 g OGTT	49 ± 9	59 ± 11	n.a.
Fasting triglycerides (mmol/l)	4.02 ± 0.46	1.15 ± 0.10	$p < 0.001$
Fasting cholesterol (mmol/l)	5.65 ± 0.23	4.98 ± 0.34	n.s.
Blood pressure: systolic (mmHg)	121 ± 5	114	$p < 0.08$
diastolic	80 ± 2	72 ± 2	$p < 0.02$
Bleeding time (min)	4.1 ± 0.4	5.9 ± 0.4	$p < 0.01$

[a]OGTT = oral glucose tolerance test.
Data summarized from references 15 and 61.

might operate (Figure 5). For the greater part of their history, humans lived as hunter/gatherers. Even agriculture can be viewed as a relatively recent development[62], occurring only in the last 10 000 years—and the Western lifestyle a very recent development. It has been argued that the human genetic constitution is tailored to our hunter/gatherer past[62]. By studying the diet and lifestyle of those few hunter/gatherer societies which have survived into the twentieth century, it is possible to gain insight into what may well represent our original 'natural state'—a background and benchmark against which our current lifestyle and associated health problems can be studied. As a result of our work with one such population—Australian Aborigines—we have developed a 'working model' of how the 'thrifty genotype' may have operated to favour survival under one set of circumstances (hunter/gatherer lifestyle) but could promote the development of obesity, NIDDM and associated conditions under a different set of circumstances (Western lifestyle)[4].

The energy intake of Aboriginal hunter/gatherers varied greatly from day to day and seasonally, depending on food availability (a feast-and-famine pattern of food intake). A metabolism which could efficiently convert excess energy intake into depot fat would allow an individual to benefit maximally from feasts and thereby confer survival advantage. As hunter/gatherers,

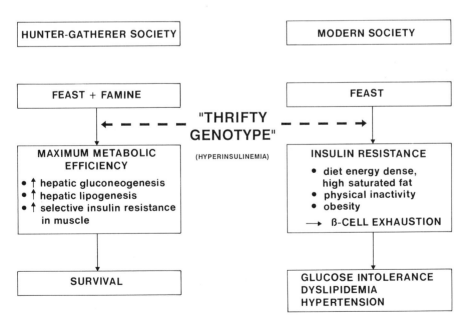

Figure 5 The proposed mechanisms for the operation of the 'thrifty genotype' in the aetiology of glucose intolerance and other key cardiovascular disease risk factors in former hunter/gatherer populations

Australian Aborigines were omnivorous, consuming a wide variety of wild animals and plant foods[63]. Their feasts were often provided by large animals (terrestrial or marine). In general, wild animals have low carcass fat contents[64] in marked contrast to domesticated meat animals such as beef cattle and sheep[65]. Thus the feasts may often have been high in protein and relatively low in fat and carbohydrate.

We have hypothesized that selective insulin resistance would have been advantageous to survival under these circumstances[3,4]. An efficient system for converting dietary protein into glucose and fat as readily available forms of energy could be achieved by a high capacity for hepatic gluconeogenesis, which was not sensitive to suppression by insulin, coupled with a high capacity for hepatic lipogenesis, which was sensitive to stimulation by insulin. Furthermore, an efficient system for fat accumulation to take advantage of 'feasts' could be achieved under conditions of hyperinsulinaemia in which there was resistance to the hypoglycaemic actions of insulin but normal sensitivity to those actions of insulin involved in fat deposition.

This concept of selective insulin resistance is not new[8,66–68] and is consistent with available data on insulin-resistant states such as obesity, impaired glucose tolerance and NIDDM. There is a great deal of evidence from studies in humans and animals demonstrating that in such insulin-resistant states, the glucoregulatory actions of insulin are impaired (suppression of hepatic glucose output, stimulation of peripheral glucose uptake and of glucose oxidation, and non-oxidative glucose utilization[59,69]. In contrast, those actions of insulin involving fat deposition (stimulation of hepatic lipogenesis, very low-density lipoprotein (VLDL) output and adipose tissue lipoprotein lipase activity, and inhibition of adipose tissue lipolysis) exhibit normal or near-normal activity[8,66–68,70,71].

Under the conditions of the hunter/gatherer lifestyle, this selective insulin resistance would have had the beneficial effect of facilitating the supply of energy from protein which was abundant in the diet, by providing a mechanism for the efficient conversion of amino acids to carbohydrate and fat[4].

However, the changes in diet and lifestyle associated with Westernization exacerbate insulin resistance in numerous ways[3]. Reduced physical activity produces insulin resistance in skeletal muscle[72] and reduction in skeletal muscle lipoprotein lipase activity[73], thereby compromising the ability of this tissue to take up glucose and triglyceride from the bloodstream. Excess energy intake and diets high in fat and/or sucrose are associated with increased insulin resistance[74–76], as is body fat accumulation (particularly in the abdominal region)[77]. The increased insulin resistance described above is selective, at least in the early stages, applying primarily to the glucoregulatory actions of insulin. The net result of this selective insulin resistance is to favour those pathways in which insulin is functioning normally—including triglyceride and VLDL synthesis in the liver and hepatic VLDL secretion—and thereby facilitating fat accumulation in adipose tissue (adipose tissue lipoprotein lipase activity).

This would initiate a vicious cycle with a cascade effect of exaggerated hyperinsulinaemia, insulin resistance and dyslipidaemia (with hypertriglyceridaemia and lower high-density lipoprotein (HDL) cholesterol), upper body obesity and hypertension, and this would result in increased risk of CVD. Thus the components of the 'thrifty gene' that favoured survival of the hunter/gatherers became the 'risk factors' for coronary artery disease and other forms of CVD risk in modern humans[3,4].

If insulin has a role as a survival hormone, as may be inferred from the above discussion, then the presence of hyperinsulinaemia predating the onset of NIDDM by many years in certain populations may also explain the presence of hyperinsulinaemia in Papua New Guinea, Nauruan and Tuvaluan, Australian Aboriginal and Pima Indian children[19]. These are all populations where high rates of NIDDM have been reported when modernization of lifestyle has taken place[1,4,11]. This finding is of potential importance in relation to the primary prevention of NIDDM, as it appears that the cascade of risk factors for NIDDM and associated CVD could commence in childhood[19]. There is clearly a need for more detailed studies of this possibility.

'THRIFTY GENOTYPE': FACT OR CONJECTURE?

Are there data to support the 'thrifty genotype' hypothesis? The rodent models, such as the Israeli sand rat[7], fulfil the conditions that might be imposed to validate this hypothesis. Shafrir has provided strong supportive data by demonstrating that, with increasing severity of hyperinsulinaemia and insulin resistance in the 'Westernized' Israeli sand rat, there is evidence of selective insulin resistance in the liver[8]: key enzymes in the control of gluconeogenesis (phosphoenopyruvate carboxykinase and glucose-6-phosphatase) became resistant to insulin suppression, while key enzymes in lipogenesis (acetyl coenzyme A carboxylase, nicotinamide adenine dinucleotide phosphate malate dehydrogenase and pyruvate kinase) retain their sensitivity to insulin stimulation. The outcome of this selective insulin resistance is that elevations in both gluconeogenesis and lipogenesis occur simultaneously, consistent with fat accumulation in the face of insulin resistance and impaired glucose tolerance. In this model, insulin resistance of muscle precedes insulin resistance in enlarged adipocytes. In a further parallel with susceptible human populations, Shafrir[7] has demonstrated that food restriction can lead to a reversal of the hyperinsulinaemia and associated metabolic abnormalities, analogous to the consequences of temporary reversion to traditional hunter/gatherer lifestyle in overweight urbanized Australian Aborigines[15].

Table 2 Changes in the incidence and natural history of glucose intolerance in Nauruans between 1975/6–1982 and 1982–1987 (sexes combined). Reproduced by permission of the American Journal of Epidemiology from Dowse et al.[11]

Category and period	Person-years	Incident cases (n)	Crude incidence rate (cases per 1000 person-years)	Age-standardized incidence rate (cases per 1000 person-years)	Incidence rate ratio[a]	95% CI[b]	X^2_1
Normal							
IGT[b]							
1975/6–1982	876	32	36.5	41.4	0.55	(0.36–0.84)	7.5**
1982–1987	3299	64	19.4	21.6			
Normal							
NIDDM							
1975/6–1982	876	15	17.2	17.1	0.46	(0.24–0.85)	6.0*
1982–1987	3299	27	8.2	7.4			
IGT							
NIDDM							
1975/6–1982	390	22	58.3	35.2	1.23	(0.72–2.10)	0.6
1982–1987	959	58	60.5	56.1			
IGT							
Normal							
1975/6–1982	390	23	59.0	69.8	1.28	(0.80–2.04)	1.0
1982–1987	959	77	80.3	88.1			
All							
NIDDM							
1975/6–1982	1266	37	29.2	26.2	0.77	(0.52–1.16)	1.5
1982–1987	4258	85	20.0	22.5			

*$p < 0.05$; **$pp < 0.01$.
[a]Mantel–Haenszel incidence density rate ratio and test-based confidence interval[19].
[b]CI, confidence interval; IGT, impaired glucose tolerance.

Recently, we have reported a decline in the incidence of epidemic glucose intolerance in Nauruans[11] and related this to the 'thrifty genotype'. We studied changes in the prevalence and incidence and natural history of impaired glucose tolerance and NIDDM in Nauruans between 1975/6–1982 and 1982–1987. Based on World Health Organization criteria, the age-standardized prevalence of NIDDM remained relatively constant (24.0% in 1987), but the prevalence of impaired glucose tolerance decreased significantly from 21.1% in 1975/6 to 8.7% (95% confidence interval 7.1–10.3) in 1987. Between the periods 1975/6–1982 and 1982–1987, the incidence of progression from normal glucose tolerance to either impaired glucose tolerance (incidence ratio (IRR) = 0.55, $p<0.01$) or NIDDM (IRR = 0.46, $p<0.05$) has decreased dramatically, while progression from impaired glucose tolerance to NIDDM has increased (IRR = 1.23) (Table 2) The overall age-standardized incidence of NIDDM declined from 26.2 cases per 1000 person-years in 1975/6–1982 to 22.5 cases per 1000 person-years in 1982–1987[11].

These data suggest that the NIDDM epidemic in Nauru is on the decline. This was not due to a decline in the environmental risk factors as their prevalence did not change significantly during the years of the study[11]. A likely explanation is that the epidemic has hit most of the Nauruans who were genetically susceptible, and the remaining genetic pool will have more NIDDM-resistant individuals.

NIDDM has an early age of onset in highly susceptible populations such as Nauruans (with a prevalence of 10–30% through much of the reproductive phase). The young diabetic patients experience the full range of disease sequelae, including retinopathy, renal failure and obstetric complications, compared with non-diabetics. There is evidence that both impaired glucose tolerance and NIDDM in young Nauruan women are strongly associated with stillbirth occurrence. Diabetic Nauruan women of all age groups have a lower number of live births than do their non-diabetic peers[11]. Of more importance appears to be the fact that the longitudinal data suggest that the fertility deficit is pronounced in women with an early onset (and possibly therefore those with the more adverse genotype).

This combination of circumstances implies that the 'thrifty (non-diabetic) genotype' will be transmitted with decreasing frequency in future generations, as the wheel has come full circle on this formerly advantageous genotype. An analogous situation has been observed in diabetes-susceptible rat species, where the tendency to hyperglycaemia decreases in successive generations of laboratory-raised animals[7].

It is unclear whether the 'thrifty genotype' ever occurred in the ancestors of developed European populations with frequencies of a magnitude similar to those now seen in Pacific islanders, American Indians, Australian Aborigines and other developing populations. If it was common at some time in the past, then it may well have been selected against until the gene(s) reached

286 ———————————————————————————— P. Zimmet and K. O'Dea

a relatively low potency and constant population frequency, consistent with the currently observed pattern of disease onset in middle and older age, following completion of the reproductive phase[11]. While the existence of the 'thrifty genotype' as a true entity has not been proven, the concept provides a reasonable explanation of the phenomenon of epidemic levels of NIDDM in certain ethnic groups. Certainly, there are animal models which behave in a manner consistent with the hypothesis and show biochemical features that fit the picture. The concept of selective insulin resistance with switch-on/switch-off features as part of the feast and famine scenario does provide a reasonable explanation of how the 'thrifty genotype/s' might operate.

REFERENCES

1 Zimmet P, Dowse G, Serjeantson S, Finch C, King H. The epidemiology and natural history of NIDDM: lessons from the South Pacific. *Diabetes Metab Rev* 1990; **6**: 91–124.
2 Zimmet P. Diabetes and other non-communicable diseases in Paradise: the evolutionary and genetic connection. *Med J Aust* 1987; **146**: 457–8.
3 Zimmet P. Kelly West Lecture 1991. Challenges in diabetes epidemiology: from West to the rest. *Diabetes Care* 1992; **15**: 232–52.
4 O'Dea K. Westernisation, insulin resistance, and diabetes in Australian Aborigines. *Med J Aust* 1991; **155**: 258–64.
5 Guest CS, O'Dea K, Hopper JL, Nankervis AJ, Larkins RG. The prevalence of glucose intolerance in Aborigines and Europids or south-eastern Australia. *Diabetes Res Clin Pract* 1992; **15**: 227–35.
6 Neel JV. Diabetes mellitus: a thrifty genotype rendered detrimental by 'progress'? *Am J Hum Genet* 1962; **14**: 353–62.
7 Shafrir E. Animals with diabetes: progress in the understanding of diabetes through study of its pathogenesis in animal models. In: *The Diabetes Annual/6* (eds KGMM Alberti, LP Krall) Elsevier, Amsterdam, 1991, pp 634–63.
8 Shafrir E. Nonrecognition of insulin as gluconeogenesis suppressant: a manifestation of selective hepatic insulin resistance in several animal species with type II diabetes: sand rats, spiny mice and *db/db* mice. In: *Frontiers in Diabetes Research. Lessons from Animal Diabetes II* (eds E Shafrir, AE Reynold) Libbey, London, pp 304–15.
9 Wendorf M, Goldfine ID. Archeology of NIDDM: excavation of the 'thrifty' genotype. *Diabetes* 1991; **40**: 161–5.
10 Bennett PH, Bogardus C, Zimmet P, Tuomilehto J. The epidemiology of non-insulin dependent diabetes: non-obese and obese. In: *International Textbook of Diabetes Mellitus* (eds H Keen, R DeFronzo, KGMM Alberti, P Zimmet) Wiley, Chichester, 1992, pp 147–76.
11 Dowse GK, Zimmet PZ, Finch CF, Collins V. Decline in incidence of epidemic glucose intolerance in Nauruans: implications for the 'thrifty genotype'. *Am J Epidemiol* 1991; **133**: 1093–104.
12 Dowse GK, Spark RA, Hodge AM, et al. Epidemic type 2 (non-insulin-dependent) diabetes and bimodal plasma glucose distribution in Wanigela people of Papua New Guinea. *Diabetologia* 1992; **35** (Suppl 1): A132.

13 Zimmet P, Serjeantson S, Dowse G, Finch C, Collins V. Diabetes mellitus and cardiovascular disease in developing populations: hunter-gatherers in the fast lane. In: *Sugars in Nutrition* (eds M Gracey, N Kretchmer, E Rossi) Nestlé Nutrition Workshop Series Vol 25. Nestec, and Vevey/Raven Press, New York, 1991, pp 197–209.

14 O'Dea K, White NG, Sinclair AJ. An investigation of nutrition-related risk factors in an isolated Aboriginal community in northern Australia: advantages of a traditionally-oriented lifestyle. *Med J Aust* 1986; **148**: 177–180.

15 O'Dea K. Marked improvement in carbohydrate and lipid metabolism in diabetic Australian Aborigines after temporary reversion to traditional lifestyle. *Diabetes* 1984; **33**: 596–603.

16 Dowse GK, Gareeboo H, Zimmet PZ, et al. High prevalence of NIDDM and impaired glucose intolerance in Indian, Creole and Chinese Mauritians. *Diabetes* 1990; **39**: 390–6.

17 Neel JV. The thrifty genotype revisited. In: *The Genetics of Diabetes Mellitus* (eds J Kobberling, R Tattersall) Proceedings of the Serono Symposium. Academic Press, London, 1982, pp 283–93.

18 Szathmary EJE. Diabetes in Arctic and Subartic populations undergoing acculturation. *Collegium Antropologicum* 1986; **10**: 145–58.

19 Zimmet PZ, Collins VR, Dowse GK, Knight LT. Hyperinsulinaemia in youth is a predictor of non-insulin-dependent diabetes mellitus. *Diabetologia* **35**: 534–41.

20 Gerich JE. Role of insulin-resistance in the pathogenesis of type 2 (non-insulin-dependent) diabetes mellitus. *Baillière's Clin Endocrinol Metab* **2**: 307–26.

21 Leahy JL. Natural history of β-cell dysfunction in NIDDM. *Diabetes Care* 1990; **13**: 992–1010.

22 De Fronzo RA. Lilly Lecture 1987. The triumvirate: β-cell, muscle, liver: a collusion responsible for NIDDM. *Diabetes* 1987; **37**: 667–87.

23 Yalow RS, Berson SA. Plasma insulin concentrations in non-diabetic and early diabetic subjects. *Diabetes* 1960; **9**: 254–60.

24 Hales CN, Randle PJ. Effects of low carbohydrate diet and diabetes mellitus on plasma concentrations of glucose, nonesterified fatty acid, and insulin during oral glucose tolerance tests. *Lancet* 1963; **i**: 790–4.

25 Ricketts HT, Cherry RA, Kirsteins L. Biochemical studies of 'prediabetes'. *Diabetes* 1966; **15**: 880–8.

26 Reaven G, Miller R. Study of the relationship between glucose and insulin responses to an oral glucose load in man. *Diabetes* 1968; **17**: 560–9.

27 Rimoin DL. Ethnic variability in glucose tolerance and insulin secretion. *Arch Intern Med* 1969; **124**: 695–700.

28 Frohman LA, Doeblin TD, Emerling FG. Diabetes in the Seneca Indians: plasma insulin responses to oral carbohydrate. *Diabetes* 1969; **18**: 38–43.

29 McKiddie MT, Buchanan KD. Plasma insulin studies in two hundred patients with diabetes mellitus. *Q J Med* 1969; **38**: 445–65.

30 Chiles R, Tzagournis M. Excessive serum insulin response to oral glucose in obesity and mild diabetes. *Diabetes* 1970; **19**: 458–64.

31 Jackson WPU, Van Mieghem W, Keller P. Insulin excess as the initial lesion in diabetes. *Lancet* 1972; **i**: 1040–4.

32 Wise PH, Edwards FM, Craig RJ, et al. Diabetes and associated variables in the South Australian aboriginal. *Aust NZ J Med* 1976; **6**: 191–6.

33 Rimoin DL, Saiki JH. Diabetes mellitus among the Navajo. II. Plasma glucose and insulin responses. *Arch Intern Med* 1968; **122**: 6–9.

34 Aronoff SL, Bennett PH, Gordon P, Rushforth N, Miller M. Unexplained hyperinsulinemia in normal and 'pre-diabetic' Pima Indians compared with normal

Caucasians: an example of racial differences in insulin secretion. *Diabetes* 1977; **26**: 827–40.

35 Zimmet P, Whitehouse S, Kiss J. Ethnic variability in the plasma insulin response to oral glucose in Polynesian and Micronesian subjects. *Diabetes* 1979; **28**: 624–8.

36 Snehalatha C, Mohan V, Ramachandran A, Jayashree R, Viswanathan M. Pancreatic beta cell function in offspring on conjugal diabetic parents: assessment by IRI and C-peptide ratio. *Horm Metab Res* 1984; **16** (Suppl): 142–4.

37 Dowse GK, Zimmet PZ, Brigham L, Gareeboo H, Finch CF. Reproducibility of the relationship between serum insulin and plasma glucose levels in Mauritians of four ethnic groups. *Diabetes* 1990; **39** (Suppl): 74A.

38 Reaven GM. Insulin resistance, hyperinsulinemia, hypertriglyceridemia and hypertension: parallels between human disease and rodent models. *Diabetes Care* 1991; **14**: 195–202.

39 Bevilacqua S, Buzzigoli G, Bonadonna R, et al. Operation of Randle's cycle in patients with NIDDM. *Diabetes* 1990; **39**: 383–9.

40 Sicree RA, Zimmet PZ, King HOM, Coventry JS. Plasma insulin response among Nauruans: prediction of deterioration in glucose tolerance over 6 yrs. *Diabetes* 1987; **36**: 179–86.

41 Saad MF, Knowler WC, Pettitt DJ, et al. The natural history of impaired glucose tolerance in the Pima Indians. *N Engl J Med* 1988; **319**: 1500–6.

42 Haffner SM, Stern MP, Mitchell BD, Hazuda HP, Patterson JK. Incidence of type II diabetes in Mexican Americans predicted by fasting insulin and glucose levels, obesity and body-fat distribution. *Diabetes* 1990; **39**: 283–8.

43 Charles MA, Fontbonne A, Thilbult N, et al. Risk factors for NIDDM in white population: Paris Prospective Study. *Diabetes* 1991; **40**: 796–9.

44 Reaven GM, Shen SW, Silvers A, Farquhar JW. Is there a delay in the plasma insulin response of patients with chemical diabetes? *Diabetes* 1971; **20**: 416–23.

45 Reaven GM, Olefsky J, Farquhar JW. Does hyperglycaemia or hyperinsulinaemia characterize the patient with chemical diabetes? *Lancet* 1972; **i**: 1247–9.

46 Welborn TA, Breckenridge A, Rubinstein AH, Dollery CT, Fraser TR. Serum insulin in essential hypertension and in peripheral vascular disease. *Lancet* 1966; **i**: 1336–7.

47 O'Dea K, Traianides K, Hopper JL, Larkins RG. Impaired glucose tolerance, hyperinsulinemia, and hypertriglyceridemia in Australian Aborigines from the desert. *Diabetes Care* 1988; **11**: 23–9.

48 Saad MF, Lillioja S, Nyomba BL, et al. Racial differences in the relation between blood pressure and insulin resistance. *N Engl J Med* 1991; **324**: 733–9.

49 Kadowaki T, Miyake Y, Hagura R. Risk factors for worsening to diabetes in subjects with impaired glucose tolerance. *Diabetologia* 1984; **26**: 44–9.

50 Jeanrenaud B, Halimi S, Van de Werve G. Neuro-endocrine disorders seen as triggers of the triad: obesity–insulin resistance–abnormal glucose tolerance. *Diabetes Metab Rev* 1985; **1**: 261–91.

51 Hansen BC, Bodkin HL. Heterogeneity of insulin responses: phases leading to type 2 (non-insulin-dependent) diabetes mellitus in the rhesus monkey. *Diabetologia* 1986; **29**: 713–19.

52 Hansen BC, Bodkin NL. β-Cell hyper-responsiveness: earliest event in development of diabetes in monkeys. *Am J Physiol (Regulatory)* 1990; **259**: R612–17.

53 Rizza RA, Mandarino LJ, Genest J, Baker BA, Gerich JE. Production of insulin resistance by hyperinsulinaemia in man. *Diabetologia* 1985; **28**: 70–5.

54 Marangou AG, Weber KM, Boston RC, et al. Metabolic consequences of pro-

longed hyperinsulinemia in humans: evidence for induction of insulin insensitivity. *Diabetes* 1986; **35**: 1383–9.

55 Bell GI. Lilly Lecture 1990. Molecular defects in diabetes mellitus. *Diabetes* 1991; **40**: 413–22.

56 Raben N, Barnetti F, Cama A, et al. Normal coding sequence of insulin gene in Pima Indians and Nauruans, two groups with highest prevalence of type II diabetes. *Diabetes* 1991; **40**: 118–22.

57 Reaven GM. Role of insulin resistance in human disease. *Diabetes* 1988; **37**: 1595–607.

58 Zimmet P. Non-insulin-dependent (type 2) diabetes mellitus: does it really exist? *Diabetic Med* 1989; **6**: 728–35.

59 De Fronzo RA, Ferrannini E. Insulin resistance: a multifaceted syndrome responsible for NIDDM, obesity, hypertension, dyslipidemia and atherosclerotic cardiovascular disease. *Diabetes Care* 1991; **14**: 173–94.

60 Finch CF, Zimmet PZ. Mortality from diabetes. In: *The Diabetes Annual/4* (eds KGMM Alberti, LP Krall) Elsevier, Amsterdam, 1988, pp 1–16.

61 O'Dea K, Sinclair AJ. The effects of low fat diets rich in arachidonic acid on the composition of plasma fatty acids and bleeding time in Australian Aborigines. *Int J Nutr Vitaminol* 1985; **33**: 441–53.

62 Eaton SB, Konner M. Paleolithic nutrition: a considering of its nature and current implications. *N Engl J Med* 1985; **312**: 283–98.

63 O'Dea K. Traditional diet and food preferences of Australian Aboriginal hunter-gatherers. *Phil Trans R S B* 1991; **334** (1270): 233–41.

64 Naughton JM, O'Dea K, Sinclair AJ. Animal foods in traditional Aboriginal diets: polyunsaturated and low in fat. *Lipids* 1986; **21**: 684–90.

65 Sinclair AJ, Slattery WJ, O'Dea K. The analysis of polyunsaturated fatty acids in meat by capillary gas liquid chromatography. *J Sci Food Agric* 1982; **33**: 771–6.

66 Nagulesparan M, Savage PJ, Knowler WC, Johnson GC, Bennett PH. Increased in vivo insulin resistance in non-diabetic Pima Indians compared with Caucasians. *Diabetes* 1982; **31**: 952–6.

67 Howard BV, Klimes I, Vasquez B, et al. The antilipolytic action of insulin in obese subjects with resistance to its glucoregulatory action. *J Clin Endocrinol Metab* 1984; **58**: 544–8.

68 Assimacopoulos-Jeannet F, Singh A, Le Marchand Y, Loten EG, Jeanrenaud B. Abnormalities in lipogenesis and triglyceride secretion by perfused livers of obese–hyperglycemic (ob/ob) mice: relationship with hyperinsulinemia. *Diabetologia* 1974; **10**: 155–62.

69 Thorburn AW, Gumbiner B, Bulacan F, Brechtel G, Henry RR. Multiple defects in muscle glycogen synthase activity contribute to reduced glycogen synthesis in non-insulin dependent diabetes mellitus. *J Clin Invest* 1991; **87**: 489–95.

70 Reitman JS, Kosmakos FC, Howard BV, et al. Characterisation of lipase activities in obese Pima Indians. *J Clin Invest* 1982; **70**: 791–7.

71 Ginsberg HN. Very low density lipoprotein metabolism in diabetes mellitus. *Diabetes Metab Rev* 1987; **2**: 571–89.

72 James DE, Kraeger EW, Chisholm DJ. Effects of exercise training on in vivo insulin action in individual tissues to the rat. *J Clin Invest* 1985; **76**: 657–60.

73 Svedenbag J, Lithell H, Jublin-Dannfelt A, Hendriksson J. Increase in skeletal muscle lipoprotein lipase following endurance training in man. *Atherosclerosis* 1983; **49**: 203–7.

74 Himsworth HP. The dietetic factor determining the glucose tolerance and sensitivity to insulin of healthy men. *Clin Sci* 1935; **2**: 67–94.

75 Storlein LH, James DE, Burleigh KM, Chisholm DJ, Kraegen EW. Fat feeding causes widespread *in vivo* insulin resistance, decreased energy expenditure and obesity in the rat. *Am J Physiol* 1986; **251**: E576–83.
76 Wright DW, Hansen RI, Mandon CE, Reaven GM. Sucrose-induced insulin resistance in the rat: modulation by exercise and diet. *Am J Clin Nutr* 1983; **38**: 879–83.
77 Bjorntorp, P. Metabolic implications of body fat distribution. *Diabetes Care* 1991; **14**: 1132–43.

Chapter Fifteen

The Thrifty Phenotype Hypothesis

D. I. W. Phillips and D. J. P. Barker

*MRC Environmental Epidemiology Unit, Southampton General Hospital,
Southampton, UK*

INTRODUCTION

Investigations into the aetiology of non-insulin-dependent diabetes mellitus
(NIDDM) have led to inconclusive and sometimes contradictory results.
Although a sedentary lifestyle and the development of obesity are important,
they seem to lead to diabetes only in predisposed individuals. Family and
twin studies have suggested that the predisposition has a strong genetic basis.
However, the search for genetic markers has been unrewarding. In this
chapter we describe a new hypothesis concerning the aetiology of NIDDM.
The concept underlying the hypothesis is that poor fetal and infant development has long-term consequences on carbohydrate metabolism. These consequences may include impaired function of the endocrine pancreas and an
increased resistance to the action of insulin, leading in turn to the development of NIDDM. According to the hypothesis the disease is the result of
early adaptations to an adverse environment. Poor nutrition is thought to be
one of the important adverse influences, in adapting to which the fetus and
infant have to be nutritionally 'thrifty'. If poor nutrition continues throughout
life, these adaptations are not detrimental. However, if nutrition in adult life

Causes of Diabetes. Edited by R. D. G. Leslie
© 1993 John Wiley & Sons Ltd

becomes abundant the ability of the pancreas to maintain glucose homeostasis is overstretched and diabetes follows. The 'thrifty phenotype' hypothesis demands a reinterpretation of some data and explains other observations which at present are not easy to understand.

FETAL AND INFANT GROWTH AND NIDDM

Suspicion that cardiovascular disease (CVD), and its associated conditions, NIDDM and hypertension, originated in fetal life and infancy came from geographical studies. Differences in death rates from CVD in different areas of England and Wales are closely related to differences in neonatal mortality (deaths before 1 month of age) 70 or more years ago[1,2]. At that time most neonatal deaths were associated with low birth weight. These findings suggested that cardiovascular disease is linked to impaired fetal growth.

The link was subsequently established by a series of studies of individual men and women whose fetal growth had been recorded. The first such study was carried out in the county of Hertfordshire where, since 1911, all babies have been weighed at birth by the midwife and details of feeding, illnesses and weight in infancy recorded by health visitors. These records were found and in 71% of the men it was possible to determine whether they were alive or dead, and if dead, from what cause[3]. Among 6500 men born in eight districts during 1911–1930, the death rate from ischaemic heart disease fell with increasing birth weight and weight at 1 year (Table 1). In contrast, there was no trend among the non-circulatory diseases. These findings supported the conclusions from geographical studies, suggesting that factors which determine fetal and infant weight gain are related to the later risk of ischaemic heart disease. CVD may therefore be a 'programmed' effect of interference with early growth and development. Programming is a permanent or long-term change in structure or metabolism resulting from a stimulus or adverse influence acting at a critical period of early life[4]. The studies in Hertfordshire were confirmed by one in Sheffield. Among 1585 men born during 1907–1924, those who had low birth weight, were thin at birth and had a small head circumference had the highest death rates from CVD[5]. These findings posed the question of what processes link lower fetal and infant growth rates with CVD. Subsequent studies in Hertfordshire and in the city of Preston, Lancashire, showed that lower birth weight, especially if associated with disproportionately high placental weight, is linked with raised blood pressure in adult life[6]. The known associations of NIDDM and impaired glucose tolerance with ischaemic heart disease and hypertension suggested that impaired glucose tolerance might be another outcome of early growth restraint. To investigate this a full 75 g oral glucose tolerance test was carried out on 370 men who were born at Hertfordshire and still live there.

Table 1 Standardized mortality ratios for ischaemic heart disease, according to weight at 1 year, in 6500 men born during 1911–1930 (numbers of deaths in parentheses)

Weight at 1 year (lb)	Ischaemic heart disease	All non-circulatory disease
≤18	100 (36)	74 (39)
−20	84 (90)	99 (157)
−22	92 (180)	74 (215)
−24	70 (109)	67 (155)
−26	55 (44)	84 (99)
≥27	34 (10)	72 (31)
All	78 (469)	78 (696)

Of these men 66 had impaired glucose tolerance and 27 had diabetes[7]. Compared with the 277 normoglycaemic men, they had been an average of 0.5 lb lighter at birth and 1.0 lb lighter at 1 year. The percentage of men with impaired glucose tolerance or NIDDM fell progressively with increasing birth weight and weight at 1 year (Table 2). Two-hour plasma glucose concentrations of 7.8 mmol/l or over were found in 43% (10/23) of men who had the lowest weights at 1 year compared with 13% (3/24) among men with the highest weights. If an adjustment for current body mass index (BMI) is made, there is an eight-fold increase in the risk of having 2-hour glucose ≥7.8 mol/l among men with lowest weights at 1 year compared with men with the highest weights. Although birth weight and the weight at 1 year are

Table 2 Proportions of men aged 64 with impaired glucose tolerance or diabetes, according to weight at one year

Weight at 1 year (lb)	No. of men	No. (%) of men with 2-hour glucose (mmol/l) of:			Odds ratio (95% confidence interval)[a]
		7.8–11.0	≥11.1	≥7.8	
≤18	23	6 (26)	4 (17)	10 (43)	8.2 (1.8–38)
−20	63	13 (21)	7 (11)	20 (32)	4.8 (1.2–19)
−22	107	24 (22)	8 (7)	32 (30)	4.2 (1.1–16)
−24	105	14 (13)	5 (5)	19 (18)	2.1 (0.5–7.9)
−26	48	6 (13)	3 (6)	9 (19)	2.1 (0.5–9.0)
≥27	24	3 (13)	0	3 (13)	1.0 –
Total	370	66 (18)	27 (7)	93 (25)	

[a]Ods ratio for 2-hour glucose of ≥7.8 mmol/l adjusted for body mass index (χ^2 for trend = 14.9, $p < 0.001$).

Table 3 Geometric mean plasma glucose concentration (mmol/l) 2 hours after a 75 g oral glucose load, according to weight at 1 year and adult BMI (numbers of men given in brackets)

Adult body mass index (kg/m²)	Weight at 1 year (lb)			
	≤21.5	–23.5	>23.5	Total
≤25.4	6.6 [45]	6.1 [39]	5.8 [36]	6.2 [120]
–28	6.7 [47]	6.9 [44]	5.9 [36]	6.5 [127]
>28	7.7 [39]	7.4 [43]	6.6 [41]	7.2 [123]
Total	7.0 [131]	6.8 [126]	6.1 [113]	6.6 [370]

Geometric standard deviation of plasma glucose = 1.4.

highly correlated, the relationship with weight at 1 year has a component which is independent of birth weight. Some infants with heavier birth weights were possibly the outcome of pregnancies complicated by gestational diabetes. Such babies would have been proportionately few, however, and their survival 60 or more years ago would probably have been poor. Although there is evidence that gestational diabetes predisposes to diabetes in the offspring, this would not explain our finding that the largest babies are those least likely to develop diabetes.

Analysis of the effects of obesity, measured as BMI (weight/height²), shows that its diabetogenic effect adds to that of poor early growth (Table 3). The mean 2-hour glucose concentration ranged from 5.8 mmol/l in men who had been above the highest tertile of weight at 1 year but were at or below the lowest tertile of current BMI (≤25.4) to 7.7 mmol/l in men below the lowest tertile of weight at 1 year and above the highest tertile of current BMI (>28). Weight at 1 year is not importantly related to fatness in adult life, but is strongly related to height. This suggests that babies with high weights at 1 year were long rather than fat.

It could be argued that lower birth and infant weights merely indicate an adverse early environment, and that people born into an adverse environment tend to remain in one. Associations with early growth could therefore reflect influences acting in later life. However, the associations of impaired glucose tolerance and NIDDM with early weight were found within each social class, defined currently or at birth, and were independent of possible confounding variables such as cigarette smoking and alcohol consumption. The associations were subsequently confirmed in women in Hertfordshire, among men and women aged 50 years in Preston, and among young men[8,9]. We studied 42 young men aged 18–25 years who were given glucose tolerance tests. Details of their early growth was obtained from their mothers' antenatal and delivery records. The results (Table 4) show that the 30-minute plasma

Table 4 Mean plasma glucose, insulin and proinsulin concentrations, BMI and systolic blood pressure according to birth weight in 21-year-old men

Birth weight (g)	n	Plasma glucose (mmol/l)	Plasma insulin[a] (pmol/l)	Plasma proinsulin[a] (pmol/l)	BMI (kg/m²)	Systolic blood pressure (mmHg)
–3204	14	8.8	244	4.3	22.5	145
–3572	13	8.2	314	5.3	24.6	149
>3572	13	7.3	241	4.7	23.3	144
All	40	8.1	264	4.7	23.4	146
Standard deviation		1.4	1.7	1.8	2.6	14

[a]Geometric means and standard deviations.

glucose concentrations were highest in those with the lowest birth weights. The inverse association was such that an increase of 1500 g in birth weight corresponded to a decrease of 1.5 mmol/l in 30-minute glucose. This trend was independent of gestational age and current body mass, height and social class.

FETAL AND INFANT GROWTH AND THE PATHOGENESIS OF DIABETES

Controversy concerning the relative roles of insulin deficiency and insulin resistance in the pathogenesis of NIDDM continues unresolved. The correlation of low birth weight and weight at 1 year with impaired glucose tolerance suggests a single influence acting prenatally and during infancy which reduces early weight gain. The mechanism linking low early growth with adult glucose tolerance is still a matter for speculation. We know that much of the development of the islets of Langerhans occurs in utero[10,11]. The exact timing of islet formation differs among species. In rats the numbers of islets increase rapidly in the last 4–6 days of intrauterine life. In humans β cell mass increases more than 130-fold between the 12th intrauterine week and the fifth postnatal month. There is a body of evidence both in men and in experimental animals that defective β cell growth and function can result from undernutrition in early life. In rats weaned onto a low-protein diet the insulin response to glucose was permanently impaired[12]. James and Coore studied malnourished children and suggested that they showed a permanent reduction of insulin response to glucose[13]. The same observation was also reported by Milner[14], who even questioned whether this might predispose to adult

Table 5 Mean BMI; geometric mean plasma glucose and insulin concentrations in fasting blood samples and following a 75 g oral glucose tolerance test according to weight at 1 year

	Weight at 1 year (lb)							
	≤18	−20	−22	−24	−26	≥27	All	Trend test[a]
Fasting blood samples								
No. of men	28	75	143	132	63	27	468	
BMI (kg/m^2)	26.2	26.4	26.9	26.9	26.9	28.3	26.9	
Glucose (mmol/l)	6.0	6.1	6.1	6.1	6.0	5.8	6.1	0.2
Insulin (pmol/l)	34	49	43	38	42	43	42	0.11
Glucose tolerance tests								
No. of men	23	63	107	105	48	24	370	
Glucose (mmol/l): 30 min	9.7	9.7	9.8	9.4	9.0	8.7	9.5	0.004
2 h	7.9	7.0	6.7	6.5	6.3	6.0	6.6	0.0006
Insulin (pmol/l): 30 min	220	286	290	279	253	238	273	0.16
2 h	153	201	156	138	129	144	153	0.002

[a]p-Value adjusted for BMI.

diabetes. These two studies were of postnatally malnourished children. Other evidence suggests a major effect of intrauterine malnutrition. Growth-retarded newborn infants have reduced numbers of β cells and reduced insulin secretion[15]. Studies in experimental animals also show clearly that these changes can be reproduced by subjecting either fetal or early postnatal animals to protein energy malnutrition or even protein deficiency alone[12,16].

The data from Hertfordshire show that birth weight and weight at 1 year correlate with the post-glucose load insulin or glucose concentrations rather than the fasting levels (Table 5). This suggests that early events affect the response to a metabolic challenge rather than altering fasting homeostasis. Because fasting insulin levels correlate with insulin resistance, while the post-glucose load insulin response reflects β cell function, it is tempting to speculate that the defect in people who were growth-retarded babies is at the level of the β cell. As a working hypothesis, therefore, it seems reasonable to propose that nutritional and other factors determining fetal and infant growth influence the size and functions of the adult pancreatic β cell complement. Whether and when NIDDM supervenes will be determined by the rate of attrition of β cells with ageing and by the development of insulin resistance, of which the most important determinant is obesity.

An alternative explanation is that the association between reduced early weight gain and adult NIDDM reflects pancreatic changes secondary to insulin resistance. This possibility is encouraged by the observation that reduced fetal growth is associated with a tendency to store fat abdominally known to be a marker of insulin resistance[17]. However, insulin deficiency and resistance are not mutually exclusive and it may be that both are the result of reduced early growth. A possible link between insulin resistance and impaired β cell function could lie in abnormalities of blood vessel development. If the capillary density in peripheral tissues, especially muscle, were reduced as a result of impaired fetal development, this would impair the sensitivity of the tissues to insulin[18,19]. Coexisting capillary abnormalities in the pancreas would also impair islet cell function. The animal experiments showing that insulin secretion was reduced by early protein–energy malnutrition also demonstrated a reduction in islet vascularization[12]. As a result the degree of loss of insulin secretion was more severe than would have been expected from the degree of reduction of islet volume. This is reminiscent of the situation in NIDDM and suggests that poor insulin secretion may be due not only to fewer β cells but also to abnormal islet structure and vascularization. Poor vascularization may in turn lead to poor clearance of insoluble peptides which could be the basis for islet cell amyloid production. This would, of course, have an accelerating effect on the underlying pathology.

NIDDM, HYPERTENSION AND HYPERLIPIDAEMIA (SYNDROME X): AN ALTERNATIVE EXPLANATION

NIDDM and hypertension tend to occur in the same patients. People with both disorders often have other abnormalities, including high plasma insulin concentrations, high serum triglyceride concentrations, low serum high-density lipoprotein concentrations and high body mass indices (BMI) and waist-to-hip ratios. This combination of abnormalities is called syndrome X and is associated with raised death rates from ischaemic heart disease. Reaven has suggested that the primary defect in syndrome X is insulin resistance and consequent hyperinsulinaemia[20]. The associations of both NIDDM and hypertension with reduced fetal growth have, however, raised the possibility that these and the other components of syndrome X may have a common origin in suboptimal development at a particular stage of intrauterine life.

In the study in Hertfordshire 56 of the 407 men had syndrome X, defined as a 2-hour plasma glucose concentration of 7.8 mmol/l or more, a systolic blood pressure of 160 mmHg or more or currently receiving antihypertensive treatment, and a serum triglyceride concentration equal to or above the median value of 1.4 mmol/l. They also had the other abnormalities associated with syndrome X. The percentage of men with syndrome X fell progressively from 30% in those who had birth weights of less than 5.5 lb (Table 6). The corresponding odds ratios, adjusted for BMI, fell from 18 to 1[21]. A similar analysis of men and women with syndrome X in Preston suggests that they are not only characterized by low birth weight, independently of duration of gestation, but also by a small head circumference and low ponderal index at birth. In a previous analysis of data from Preston, we have shown that there

Table 6 Percentages of men in Hertfordshire with syndrome X according to birth weight

Birth weight (lb)	Total no. of men	No. (%) with syndrome X	Odds ratio[a] (95% confidence interval)
≤5.5	20	6 (30)	18 (2.6–118)
–6.5	54	10 (19)	8.4 (1.5–49)
–7.5	114	19 (17)	8.5 (1.5–46)
–8.5	123	15 (12)	4.9 (0.9–27)
–9.5	64	4 (6)	2.2 (0.3–14)
>9.5	32	2 (6)	1.0
Total	407	56 (14)	

[a]Odds ratio adjusted for BMI (χ^2 for trend = 16.0, $p < 0.001$).

are two groups of babies who, as adults, develop high blood pressure[6]. One group have below average birth weight and head circumference and are thin at birth. These babies, it seems, are also liable to develop syndrome X. The other group have above average birth weight and head circumference but are short. These babies do not appear to develop syndrome X, though they develop other abnormalities, including raised fibrinogen concentrations. Our finding that syndrome X is associated with reduced head circumference as well as birth weight suggests that the influences which cause it may act early in gestation.

RELATIONSHIP OF THE HYPOTHESIS TO CURRENT CONCEPTS OF THE EPIDEMIOLOGY AND AETIOLOGY OF NIDDM

GEOGRAPHICAL VARIATIONS AND MIGRANT STUDIES

The prevalence of NIDDM varies in different countries and in different parts of the same country. Rates tend to be lower in places that have retained a traditional lifestyle, for example rural Africa, where the prevalence in adults is between 1% and 2%, or the highlands of Papua New Guinea, where there was a complete absence of diabetes in one survey[22,23]. Rates in European populations are typically around 5% of the adult population[24]. In developing countries where there has been rapid Westernization the prevalence is considerably higher than that in European populations. The highest prevalences of NIDDM are found in certain indigenous North American and western Pacific societies where up to one third of the adult population may be affected. The best studied of these are the Pima Indians and Nauruan islanders[25,26].

The proposal that the disease is the outcome of reduced early growth is consistent with these geographical variations. If growth restraint during fetal life and infancy results in impaired growth and function of the β cells of the islets of Langerhans, a sudden change to relative overnutrition may expose this reduced function and lead to diabetes. The effect of a rapid transition from subsistence to overnutrition could explain the high diabetes rate in the Nauruan islanders. The population suffered severe nutritional deficiency up to the Second World War. Thereafter they became affluent from phosphate mining, and diabetes on the island became epidemic. A similar situation was shown recently in the Ethiopian Jews transported to Israel, among whom a high prevalence of diabetes was observed[27].

SECULAR TRENDS

An increase in the incidence of NIDDM has been documented in several developing countries. It remains uncertain, however, whether there has been any change in prevalence in the Western world[28]. A consequence of the hypothesis is that the advent of good nutrition should lead to a rise and then a fall in the prevalence of diabetes. The prevalence of the disease may depend on two environmental factors: one acting through childhood and associated with poor living standards; the other acting in later life and associated with overnutrition. A rise in diabetes results from an increase in the latter, and a fall from a reduction in the former. Evidence in support of this has come from the most recent survey of the Nauruan islands, which has shown a marked reduction in the prevalence of impaired glucose tolerance and diabetes[29]. There had been no change in the prevalence of obesity or other risk factors and the speed of the change makes a eugenic effect of reduced fertility in diabetes unlikely. As the reduction in prevalence was seen in those born after 1945 we suggest that it was due to the improvement in fetal and infant nutrition consequent on postwar affluence. A further prediction of the hypothesis is that the improvements in maternal and infant nutrition that have occurred in the Western world over the past 50 years should lead to a reduction in the prevalence of NIDDM in future generations.

TWIN AND FAMILY STUDIES

Evidence for a genetic aetiology of NIDDM comes from twin studies and study of family pedigrees. Three studies—two in the USA and one in the UK[30,31,33]—of monozygotic twin pairs found a much higher concordance rate when the age of onset of the proband was more than 40 years, i.e. the diabetes was non-insulin-dependent. Although two of these studies are likely to have been affected by serious ascertainment bias, the most recent study was carried out using a population-based sample of twins identified from military records[30]. Twin pairs were examined twice, at a mean age of 47 years and then at 57 years. At the first examination when the prevalence was 5.7%, there was no difference in concordance rates. Ten years later, however, the disease prevalence was 13% and the concordance rate in monozygotic twins, 58.3% compared with 17.4% in dizygotic twins.

In a large study of 3117 NIDDM subjects carried out in Canada, the risk of NIDDM was increased between two- and four-fold in the siblings of probands with the disease[33]. Similar findings were observed in the Whitehall survey of civil servants[34]. In populations with a higher prevalence of glucose intolerance the familial clustering of the disease is more marked. Thus in the Nauruan islanders glucose intolerance develops in approximately 40% of offspring of two diabetic parents, in 6% of offspring if one parent is diabetic and in no children if the parents have normal glucose tolerance[35].

Although it has been suggested that glucose intolerance in these populations is governed by a single autosomal dominant gene, there has been no agreement as to the mode of inheritance of NIDDM in Western populations.

The evidence which we have presented raises a question about the interpretation of family and twin data. Because maternal physique and nutrition have such a strong influence on fetal and infant growth, the reason for the familial clustering of NIDDM may be that family members share a similar early environment. Likewise, a genetic interpretation of high concordance rates in monozygous twins may not be justifiable as identical twins share a common early environment.

CONCLUSION

The observations of familial clustering of diabetes, a high concordance rate in twins and the high prevalence rate in communities which had abandoned their traditional lifestyle and adopted a Western diet led Neel to suggest the 'thrifty genotype' hypothesis[36]. He proposed that genes existed which gave a survival advantage in harsh conditions when food was scarce. In times of plenty, however, the same genes were detrimental, leading to obesity and glucose intolerance.

We suggest that a 'thrifty phenotype' hypothesis offers a more satisfactory explanation of the epidemiology of NIDDM including recent observations on the associations with reduced early growth (Figure 1). The essence of this

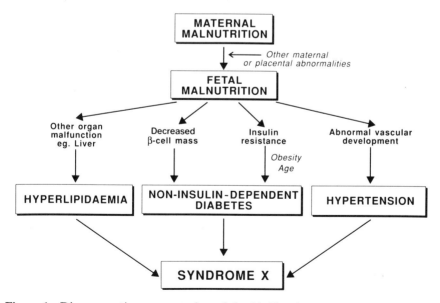

Figure 1   Diagrammatic representation of the 'thrifty phenotype' hypothesis of the aetiology of NIDDM. Also outlined is the suggestion that the features of syndrome X have closely related origins in failure of early development

hypothesis is that poor nutrition in fetal and early infant life is detrimental to the mechanisms maintaining carbohydrate tolerance. It may affect the structure and function of the β cells of the islets of Langerhans, perhaps by interfering with the more complex features of islet anatomy, such as the vasculature or innervation. Alternatively, poor nutrition in fetal life may affect the tissues, primarily muscle, that respond to insulin and as a consequence lead to insulin resistance. Although these early changes determine susceptibility, additional factors such as obesity, ageing and physical inactivity leading to insulin resistance must also play a part in determining the time of onset and severity of NIDDM. The 'thrifty phenotype' hypothesis also explains the clustering of several metabolic abnormalities such as hypertension and hyperlipidaemia with NIDDM (syndrome X). It suggests that these abnormalities are associated because they have a common origin in suboptimal development at a particular stage of intrauterine life.

REFERENCES

1 Barker DJP, Osmond C. Infant mortality, childhood nutrition, and ischaemic heart disease in England and Wales. *Lancet* 1986; **i**: 1077–81.
2 Barker DJP, Osmond C, Law C. Intra-uterine and early postnatal origins of cardiovascular disease and chronic bronchitis. *J Epidemiol Community Health* 1989; **43**: 237–40.
3 Barker DJP. Intra-uterine origins of cardiovascular and obstructive lung disease in adult life. *JR Coll Phys Lond* 1991; **25**: 129–33.
4 DJP Barker (ed.). *Fetal and Infant Origins of Adult Disease*. British Medical Journal, London, 1992.
5 Barker DJP, Osmond C, Simmonds SJ, Wield GA. The relation of head circumference and thinness at birth to death from cardiovascular disease in adult life. *Br Med J* 1993; **306**: 422–6.
6 Barker DJP, Bull AR, Osmond C, Simmonds SJ. Fetal and placental size and risk of hypertension in adult life. *Br Med J* 1990; **301**: 259–62.
7 Hales CN, Barker DJP, Clark PMS, et al. Fetal and infant growth and impaired glucose tolerance at age 64. *Br Med J* 1991; **303**: 1019–22.
8 Phipps K, Barker DJP, Hales CN, et al. Fetal growth and impaired glucose tolerance in men and women. *Diabetologia* 1993; **36**: 225–8.
9 Robinson S, Walton RJ, Clark PM, et al. The relation of fetal growth to plasma glucose in young men. *Diabetologia* 1992; **35**: 444–6.
10 Rahier J, Wallon J, Henquin JC. Cell populations in the endocrine pancreas of human neonates and infants. *Diabetologia* 1981; **20**: 540–6.
11 Bonner-Weir S. Anatomy of the islet of Langerhans. In: *The Endocrine Pancreas* (ed E Samols) Raven Press, New York, 1991, pp.15–27.
12 Snoeck A, Remacle C, Reusens B, Hoet JJ. Effect of a low protein diet during pregnancy on the fetal rat endocrine pancreas. *Biol Neonate* 1990; **5**: 107–18.
13 James WPT, Coore HG. Persistent impairment of insulin secretion and glucose tolerance after malnutrition. *Am J Clin Nutr* 1970; **23**: 386–9.
14 Milner RDG. Metabolic and hormonal responses to glucose and glucagon in patients with infantile malnutrition. *Pediatr Res* 1971; **5**: 33–9.

15 Van Assche FA, Aerts L. The fetal endocrine pancreas. *Contrib Gynecol Obstet* 1979; **5**: 44–57.

16 Weinkove C, Weinkove EA, Pimstone BL. Insulin release and pancreatic islet volume in malnourished rats. *S Afr Med J* 1974; **48**: 1888.

17 Law CM, Barker DJP, Osmond C, Fall CHD. Early growth and abdominal fatness in adult life. *J Epidemiol Community Health* 1992; **46**: 184–6.

18 Lithell H, Lindgarde F, Hellsing K, et al. Body weight, skeletal muscle morphology and enzyme activities in relation to fasting serum insulin concentration and glucose tolerance in 48 year old men. *Diabetes* 1981; **30**: 19–25.

19 Lillioja S, Young AA, Cutler CL, et al. Skeletal muscle capillary density and fiber type are possible determinants of in vivo insulin resistance in man. *J Clin Invest* 1987; **80**: 415–24.

20 Reaven GM. Role of insulin resistance in human disease. *Diabetes* 1988; **37**: 1595–607.

21 Barker DJP, Hales CN, Fall CHD, et al. Type 2 (non-insulin dependent) diabetes mellitus, hypertension and hyperlipidaemia (syndrome X): relation to reduced fetal growth. *Diabetologia* 1993; **36**: 62–7.

22 McLarty DG, Kitange HM, Mtinangi BL, et al. Prevalence of diabetes and impaired glucose tolerance in rural Tanzania. *Lancet* 1989; **i**: 871–4.

23 King H, Heywood P, Zimmet P, et al. Glucose tolerance in a highland population in Papua New Guinea. *Diabetes Res* 1984; **1**: 45–51.

24 Butler WJ, Ostrander LD, Carman WJ, et al. Diabetes mellitus in Tecumseh, Michigan: prevalence, incidence, and associated conditions. *Am J Epidemiol* 1982; **116**: 971–80.

25 Knowler WC, Bennett PH, Hamman RF, Miller M. Diabetes incidence in the Pima Indians: a 19-fold greater incidence than in Rochester, Minnesota. *Am J Epidemiol* 1978; **108**: 497–504.

26 Zimmet P, King H, Taylor R, et al. The high prevalence of diabetes mellitus, impaired glucose tolerance and diabetic retinopathy in Nauru: the 1982 survey. *Diabetes Res* 1984; **1**: 13–18.

27 Cohen MP, Stern E, Rusecki Y, Zeidler A. High prevalence of diabetes in young adult Ethiopian immigrants to Israel. *Diabetes* 1988; **37**: 824–8.

28 Jarrett RJ. Epidemiology and public health aspects of non-insulin dependent diabetes mellitus. *Epidemiol Rev* 1989; **11**: 151–71.

29 Dowse GK, Zimmet P, Finch CF, Collins VR. Decline in incidence of epidemic glucose intolerance in Nauruans: implications for the 'thrifty genotype'. *Am J Epidemiol* 1991; **133**: 1093–104.

30 Newman B, Selby JV, King MC, et al. Concordance for type 2 (non-insulin dependent) diabetes mellitus in male twins. *Diabetologia* 1987; **30**: 763–8.

31 Barnett AH, Eff C, Leslie RDG, Pyke DA. Diabetes in identical twins: a study of 200 pairs. *Diabetologia* 1981; **20**: 87–93.

32 Gottlieb MS, Root HF. Diabetes mellitus in twins. *Diabetes* 1968; **17**: 693–704.

33 Simpson NR. Diabetes in the families of diabetics. *Can Med Assoc J* 1968; **98**: 427–32.

34 Keen H, Jarrett RJ. Environmental factors and genetic interactions. In: *The Genetics of Diabetes Mellitus* (eds W Creutzfeldt, J Köbberling, JV Neel) Springer-Verlag, Berlin, 1976, pp 115–24.

35 Serjeantson SW, Zimmet P. Diabetes in the Pacific: evidence for a major gene. In: *Diabetes Mellitus: Recent Knowledge on Aetiology, Complications and Treatment* (eds S Baba, M Gould, P Zimmet) Academic Press, Sydney, 1984, pp 23–30.

36 Neel JV. Diabetes mellitus: a 'thrifty' genotype rendered detrimental by progress? *Am J Hum Genet* 1962; **14**: 353–62.

Syndrome X

M. Walker and K. G. M. M. Alberti
The Medical School, University of Newcastle upon Tyne, UK

INTRODUCTION

The clustering of certain cardiovascular risk factors within individuals was first described over 25 years ago[1]. The initial description reported an association between hyperlipidaemia, obesity and glucose intolerance in the form of non-insulin-dependent diabetes mellitus (NIDDM). At this early stage, it was proposed that the different factors might be aetiologically linked, as it was noted that dietary treatment led to an improvement in each of the three risk factors. A link with hypertension and ischaemic heart disease was also proposed. The concept was later developed and culminated with the description of syndrome X by Reaven[2], now also known as the 'metabolic syndrome'. Six components were described (Table 1) which tended to cluster within an individual and were associated with an increased risk of coronary artery disease (CAD)[2]. Central obesity was added at a later date[3], although an association between this and certain cardiovascular risk factors had been recognized many years ago[4].

Causes of Diabetes. Edited by R. D. G. Leslie

Table 1 Principal features of syndrome X

Hypertension
Abnormal glucose tolerance
Increased VLDL triglyceride levels
Decreased HDL cholesterol levels
Obesity
Hyperinsulinaemia/insulin insensitivity

IS SYNDROME X A GENUINE ENTITY?

Several population studies have shown associations between the cardiovascular risk factors that comprise syndrome X[5-7]. However, more compelling evidence that the features of syndrome X do indeed cluster within individuals comes from the study of Ferrannini and colleagues[8]. They determined the prevalence rates for obesity, NIDDM, elevated triglyceride (and cholesterol) levels, impaired glucose tolerance (IGT) and hypertension in 2930 subjects recruited into the San Antonio heart study. The major finding was that a combination of three or more factors was much more prevalent than the presence of each risk factor in isolation, and even more prevalent than any combination of just two of the factors. Moreover, hyperinsulinaemia was the common factor linked with each of the six risk factors and, as hyperinsulinaemia is thought to reflect decreased insulin sensitivity, suggested a potential and unifying aetiology. We have found similar clustering in recent studies in Mauritius (Zimmet, Dowse, Tuomilehto, Alberti et al., unpublished observations).

It has been proposed that syndrome X is simply an alternative description of NIDDM, where the association with excess cardiovascular risk has long been known. Hypertension, elevated triglyceride and low high-density lipoprotein (HDL) levels[9,10] are more common in NIDDM compared with healthy control populations, but there is still a significant proportion of NIDDM patients without any of these features. This probably reflects the increasingly apparent heterogeneity of NIDDM. Thus NIDDM and syndrome X may represent separate conditions but which have an important and significant area of overlap.

The mechanism(s) underlying the development of syndrome X have yet to be properly defined. However, the favoured explanation proposes a central role for hyperinsulinaemia. As Reaven described in detail[2], there is evidence for a direct causal role for hyperinsulinaemia in initiating and maintaining the cardinal features of syndrome X, as well as making a direct contribution to the increased risk of coronary artery disease. As outlined above, there is also epidemiological evidence that provides strong evidence for a pivotal role of hyperinsulinaemia[8]. The evidence for a role for hyperinsulinaemia in the development of the individual features of syndrome X will be considered below.

HYPERTENSION

Hypertension is a key feature of syndrome X, and is a well established risk factor for the development of coronary heart disease in the general population[11]. The aetiological mechanism(s) for the development of hypertension in syndrome X have yet to be properly defined, although the initial description of the condition favoured a central role for hyperinsulinaemia[2].

A series of cross-sectional epidemiological studies has found a positive association between hyperinsulinaemia and hypertension[12–14], and several different mechanisms have been proposed whereby the hyperinsulinaemia might increase blood pressure[2,15]. Thus there is evidence that hyperinsulinaemia can increase sympathetic neural activity and, as a consequence, blood pressure. In man, increased insulin levels have been associated with increased circulating catecholamine concentrations[16], while sucrose feeding in spontaneously hypertensive rats increased both sympathetic activity and blood pressure values following an associated increase in insulin concentration[17,18]. An alternative mechanism involves the action of insulin at the proximal renal tubule, leading to an increased sodium absorption[19], which would be expected to increase circulating blood volume and blood pressure.

There is also, however, a large body of evidence that argues against the role of hyperinsulinaemia as an independent factor in the initiation and maintenance of hypertension. Epidemiological surveys conducted in the Pima Indians[20], Mauritians[21] and a large population based in California[22] failed to identify a significant correlation between hyperinsulinaemia and hypertension. Further evidence, albeit indirect, comes from the observation that the isolated hyperinsulinaemia that characterizes insulinoma is not accompanied by hypertension[23]. Thus the association between hypertension and hyperinsulinaemia may well be anomalous and the result of the associations of the latter with other common variables such as obesity and insulin insensitivity[24].

Insulin insensitivity was demonstrated in a group of untreated, white, non-obese patients with essential hypertension[25], the primary defect invoking peripheral glucose disposal. Similar observations were made in black African subjects with untreated hypertension[26]. Further work, however, would suggest that hypertension is not the cause of insulin insensitivity, as anti-hypertensive treatment has not been shown to improve the insulin insensitivity[27]. Similarly, in a group of hypertensive subjects it was found that insulin insensitivity was only detected in a subgroup defined in terms of an elevated sodium–lithium countertransport activity[28]. We have also found insulin insensitivity to be associated with elevated countertransport activity in a group of normotensive IDDM[29]. The link between altered sodium–lithium countertransport activity and insulin insensitivity remains unclear, but it is possible that the disturbed transporter activity is a consequence of the latter. Thus, the sodium–proton transporter, which is thought to be the physiological equivalent of the sodium–lithium transporter[30], is insulin-responsive, so that the insulin insensitivity and hyperinsulinaemia in syndrome X would be expected to stimulate transporter activity and the influx of sodium into the cells[15]. Based on previous observations, it would be predicted that an increased intracellular sodium concentration in vascular smooth muscle would exaggerate the response to certain potent pressor agents, in particular angiotensin 2^{31}. It is also conceivable that both insulin insensitivity and raised sodium–proton transporter activity arise independently from a common cell membrane defect. Overall, it is unlikely that hyperinsulinaemia alone is the cause of hypertension in syndrome X, but it could play a role in conjunction with other factors, including those associated with insulin insensitivity.

DYSLIPIDAEMIA

Increased very low-density lipoprotein (VLDL) triglyceride and decreased HDL cholesterol concentrations are features that are shared by syndrome X (Table 1) and NIDDM[10]. Moreover, there is epidemiological evidence indicating that these lipid abnormalities may act as independent risk factors for the development of ischaemic heart disease. Elevated plasma triglyceride levels have been shown in prospective studies to be an independent risk factor for death from coronary artery disease in both healthy[32] and impaired glucose tolerance[33] subjects. Similarly, a low HDL cholesterol level has been identified as an independent risk factor for coronary artery disease in a non-diabetic population[34], while a low HDL cholesterol expressed in the form of an elevated LDL/HDL ratio has also shown to be predictive of CAD in diabetic subjects[35]. Although not proven, it is probable that the identical dyslipidaemias in syndrome X and NIDDM result from the operation of common mechanisms. As many of the studies in this field have been conducted in the context of NIDDM, these data will be considered as a basis for the potential mechanisms occurring in syndrome X.

It has been demonstrated that the increase in VLDL triglyceride levels in NIDDM is primarily due to an increase in hepatic synthesis[10,36]. VLDL triglyceride production rates were shown to be closely correlated with insulin levels following an oral glucose tolerance test in non-obese healthy subjects[37], suggesting a potential role for insulin in the stimulation of VLDL triglyceride production. A wealth of *in vitro* and *in vivo* data has subsequently defined a direct stimulatory effect of insulin on hepatic VLDL triglyceride synthesis, and this has been considered in a detailed review[38]. However, it is the rate of hepatic VLDL triglyceride secretion rather than the production rate that is the more important determinant of the circulating triglyceride levels. The balance of evidence favours an inhibitory effect of insulin on hepatic VLDL triglyceride secretion[38]. Thus insulin modulates the supply of VLDL triglyceride to the peripheral tissues depending upon the nutritional state. Under conditions of feeding the elevated insulin levels promote the synthesis and storage of VLDL triglyceride, while the decreased insulin levels during a fast allow the stored VLDL triglyceride to be secreted. Therefore, while the hyperinsulinaemia in syndrome X would be expected to stimulate hepatic VLDL triglyceride production, the inhibitory effect on secretion would limit its contribution to the circulating levels. However, this argument assumes that the normal hepatic sensitivity to insulin persists in syndrome X. Abbott and colleagues[39] have shown that elevated VLDL triglyceride levels in a group of obese Pima Indians with normal glucose tolerance were strongly correlated with the degree of whole-body insulin resistance. Thus it is possible that a combination of both hyperinsulinaemia and decreased insulin sensitivity, particularly at the liver, is required for the sustained increase in circulating VLDL triglyceride levels to develop in syndrome X. Impaired adipose tissue insulin sensitivity in NIDDM and the increased adipose tissue mass in obesity are responsible for the increase in circulating non-esterified fatty acid levels in these conditions[40,41], and this in turn increases the supply of substrate for hepatic VLDL triglyceride synthesis[38].

An additional determinant of VLDL triglyceride levels is the activity of lipoprotein lipase, which is the principal enzyme involved with the catabolism of VLDL triglyceride. The balance of evidence supports a deficiency in lipoprotein lipase in NIDDM[10], although the cause remains unclear.

The decreased circulating HDL cholesterol levels in NIDDM are due to an increased rate of clearance[42], primarily mediated by hepatic lipase[10]. Fasting insulin levels correlate with the rate of HDL cholesterol clearance[42], and there is a strong inverse correlation between circulating HDL cholesterol levels and whole body insulin resistance[39]. It remains to be determined whether these observations point to a possible cause for the decreased HDL cholesterol levels and whether they apply to syndrome X.

The association of hypertriglyceridaemia with insulin insensitivity is a two-way process. Thus acute elevation of triglyceride levels can induce insulin insensitivity[43], while both acute and chronic lowering of triglyceride levels with agents such as acipimox, a nicotinic acid analogue, and bezafibrate improves insulin sensitivity and glucose tolerance[44,45]. In all cases, circulating non-esterified fatty acid (NEFA) and triglyceride levels change in the same direction and this may point to the underlying mechanism. Thus an increase in circulating NEFA levels will impair insulin sensitivity[46] and vice versa, and the mechanism is thought to involve the operation of the Randle cycle[47].

It is therefore impossible to say at this stage whether insulin insensitivity or hypertriglyceridaemia is the dominant mechanism. It is also worth adding that raised triglyceride levels are frequently found as part of the other components of syndrome X, and may well contribute to the insulin insensitivity of these conditions as well as to the syndrome as a whole.

CENTRAL OBESITY

Although upper body or central obesity was a late addition to the list of features of syndrome X, the association between upper body obesity and certain cardiovascular risk factors including hypertension and diabetes was recognized more than 40 years ago by Vague[4]. He also observed that upper and lower body distributions of fat were features of the male and female sexes, respectively, although not exclusively. Later studies showed that an increased waist-to-hip ratio is a useful index of upper body obesity[48,49]. The technique of computed tomography (CT) scanning has been used to demonstrate an association between upper body obesity and increased visceral fat stores in women[50]. However, a further study using the same method in a group of obese subjects of both sexes found two subgroups with upper body obesity: (a) those subjects with predominantly increased abdominal subcutaneous fat, and (b) those with increased visceral fat[51]. Interestingly, only the latter group showed a positive association with both increased plasma triglyceride and blood glucose levels following an oral glucose load. Upper body obesity has also been shown to be independently associated with other features of syndrome X and NIDDM including hypertension[52], decreased plasma HDL cholesterol and increased plasma triglyceride levels[53].

Insulin insensitivity is a well-established feature of obesity[41], but there is evidence to suggest that the peripheral insulin insensitivity is more marked in obese subjects with upper versus lower body fat distribution[54]. Moreover, hepatic insulin extraction appears to be impaired in upper body obesity, which may contribute to the hyperinsulinaemia in this state[55].

Several epidemiological studies have suggested that upper body obesity may act as an independent risk factor for CAD[56]. Thus an increased waist-to-hip ratio was found to be a risk factor for CAD independent of body mass index (BMI) in a group of 800 males[57]. Similarly, central obesity as defined as an increased subscapular skin fold thickness was found to be related to an increased risk of CAD in both sexes independent of BMI in the Framingham study[58]. It is probable that central obesity is simply a marker for an underlying but linked risk factor for CAD, but this remains unclear.

The mechanisms dictating the pattern of fat distribution in obesity have yet to be determined. Bouchard and colleagues[59] studied obesity in pairs of identical twins. They found that the pattern of fat distribution, including intra-abdominal deposition, was similar within twin pairs, suggesting some genetic determination. Environmental factors such as diet and physical exercise are also likely to play a role in dictating the pattern of distribution[60]. However, the different prevalence rates of upper body obesity between sexes has also focused attention on the possible role of the sex hormones[61].

The mechanism by which central obesity could cause insulin insensitivity remains speculative. It has been postulated that omental and central adipocytes are metabolically more active than peripheral fat cells[61]. They release NEFA into the portal circulation and provide substrate for hepatic triglyceride synthesis. This hypothesis, however, remains to be proven.

OTHER CARDIOVASCULAR RISK FACTORS

The balance of evidence from recent epidemiological studies suggests that hyperinsulinaemia *per se* may act as independent risk factor for the development of CAD[62]. Observations from experimental studies support this proposition. In particular, Cruz and colleagues[63] showed that the chronic infusion of insulin into one femoral artery in the dog produced arterial wall cellular proliferation and lipid accumulation in the ipsilateral, but not contralateral, femoral artery. Hyperinsulinaemic pigs also have increased triglyceride content of the arteries[64]. Other studies have shown that insulin stimulates arterial smooth muscle cell proliferation[65] and promotes cholesterol synthesis and accumulation in rat aorta[66]. Other work supporting a direct atherogenic role for insulin has been previously summarized[15]. Thus hyperinsulinaemia may well make a significant contribution to the development of atherosclerosis and CAD in syndrome X.

Another potentially important but only recently defined CAD risk factor is an increase in the circulating levels of plasminogen activator inhibitor 1 (PAI-1) activity[67]. This factor inhibits the pathway of fibrinolysis and thus increases blood coagulability[68]. In a recent prospective study, elevated PAI-I levels predicted that progression of coronary artery atherosclerosis in patients with CAD and impaired glucose tolerance[69]. As recently summarized by Juhan-Vague and colleagues[67], elevated circulating PAI-1 levels have been found to be associated with many of the features of syndrome X, including central obesity, hypertriglyceridaemia, insulin insensitivity and fasting hyperinsulinaemia. In a previous study of Vague and colleagues[70], the only significant association that remained following multiple regression analysis was that between elevated insulin and PAI-1 levels. An association between PAI-1 and fasting plasma insulin levels has been reported by Kluft and colleagues[71], although it appeared to be secondary to an association between peripheral insulin insensitivity and PAI-1 levels. However, the association between elevated insulin and PAI-1 levels has not been consistent[72,73], although a correlation between split proinsulin products and PAI-1 levels has been described in NIDDM[73]. Irrespective of these inconsistencies, it is evident that elevated PAI-1 levels are associated with the principal features of syndrome X and may well be an additional feature of the syndrome. The mechanisms involved with the increase in PAI-1 levels in this syndrome remain unclear. As summarized by Juhan-Vague and colleagues[67], the evidence for a direct role of hyperinsulinaemia increasing PAI-1 is not strong. However, hyperinsulinaemia might exert an indirect effect by increasing circulating levels of VLDL triglyceride which have been shown to stimulate endothelial PAI-1 secretion; insulin insensitivity appears to be a prerequisite for such an effect. Further work is required to elucidate the relative importance of these putative mechanism(s).

AETIOLOGY OF SYNDROME X

The evidence presented suggests that hyperinsulinaemia plays a role in the development of the features of syndrome X. It has been proposed that the heterogeneity of metabolic defects underlying the different insulin insensitivity states argues against a key role for insulin insensitivity in the development of syndrome X[15]. We have emphasized that the full development of many, if not all, of the features of syndrome X requires the presence of both hyperinsulinaemia and insulin insensitivity. While hyperinsulinaemia appears to be crucial for the development of syndrome X, it must, with the singular exception of an insulinoma, develop secondary to a decrease in insulin sensitivity. In terms of aetiology, therefore, a decrease in insulin sensitivity must be the primary event in syndrome X.

The presence of a single genetic defect leading to the development of a particular pattern of insulin insensitivity and hence syndrome X has not been demonstrated and seems unlikely. This is because insulin sensitivity has been shown to vary markedly in the normal population[2], and is influenced by many different factors. Thus dietary composition and intake, physical exercise and endocrine status are all recognized determinants of insulin sensitivity[74–76]. There is almost certainly a number of genetic factors that might play a role. The Pima Indians are characterized by a marked decrease in insulin sensitivity due to at least in part, a significant genetic effect linked to the fatty acid binding protein[2] gene on chromosome 4[77]. In addition, metabolic studies in unaffected first-degree relatives from multiplex families with NIDDM have detected a primary defect in peripheral insulin sensitivity which is probably hereditary[78]. As well as genetic defects associated with a direct decrease in insulin sensitivity, it is probable that there will be other hereditary factors, for example determinants of body fat distribution, that will also exert a secondary influence on insulin sensitivity. Thus it is most likely that a

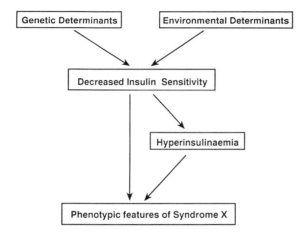

Figure 1 Simple model for the interaction of aetiological factors for syndrome X

combination of genetic and environmental factors influence the overall state of insulin sensitivity within an individual, and if this is particularly low and accompanied by persistent hyperinsulinaemia then the scene will be set for the development of syndrome X. This scenario is shown schematically in Figure 1.

Strong prospective evidence has now come from an 8-year follow-up study of 1125 Mexican–Americans and non-Hispanic whites[79]. Fasting insulin values at baseline were related to the incidence of hypertension on univariate analysis, and to the development of lowered HDL cholesterol, raised trigly-ceride and NIDDM on both univariate and multivariate analyses. Moreover, baseline insulin concentrations were highest in subjects who subsequently developed features of the metabolic syndrome, and this was not related to the degree of obesity at baseline.

There is one crucial consideration which has cast doubt over the role played by hyperinsulinaemia in the development of syndrome X. It has been pro-posed that the hyperinsulinaemia in this and related conditions, for example NIDDM, is an artefact and results from the cross-reactivity from other insulin-like molecules in the standard insulin assay. These other molecules are primarily split and intact proinsulin, which together have been shown to contribute about 26% and 60% of the total insulin-like molecules in healthy and NIDDM patients, respectively[80,81]. It is possible that these insulin-like molecules might also be involved in the pathogenesis of syndrome X. Thus an association between elevated levels of PAI-1 and proinsulin split products has been reported[73], while proinsulin has been shown to influence PAI-1 gene expression in endothelial cells[82]. Therefore, further studies using specific insulin assays are required to determine whether true hyperinsulinaemia

314 _____ M. Walker and K. G. M. M. Alberti

exists in syndrome X, and, if not, whether the apparent 'hyperinsulinaemia' is due to increased circulating levels of proinsulin and its split products. This area, however, does remain highly contentious as other workers have found that in NIDDM absolute hyperinsulinaemia does appear to be a feature (Reaven, personal communication).

TREATMENT

The cluster of disorders which comprise syndrome X forms a formidable array of cardiovascular risk factors and so warrants active intervention. Fortunately, there are treatment regimes which can influence virtually all of these risk factors. Thus weight loss will be beneficial, but perhaps more important is an increase in physical activity. Physical inactivity is a risk factor for hypertension, dyslipidaemia, and IGT and diabetes. A combined dietary and exercise programme is therefore indicated. This is not easy to implement long term although we have shown recently that sustained moderate weight loss over a 3- to 4-year period can restore some NIDDM subjects to a normal metabolic state[83]. In a long-term study in an East African Asian community we showed a substantial improvement in certain cardiovascular risk factors over a 6-year period following advice with regard to diet and exercise alone. There was a significant decrease in the prevalence of IGT and NIDDM, as well as in the lipid and blood pressure levels, accompanied by a small fall in weight[84]. Another possible approach is to use a triglyceride-lowering agent, which would also benefit glucose tolerance[45]. A medication is required that will produce a marked and specific improvement in insulin action; such an agent would allow us to test the hypothesis that an improvement in insulin sensitivity benefits all components of syndrome X.

REFERENCES

1 Avogaro P, Creapaldi G. Essential hyperlipemia, obesity and diabetes (Abstract) *Diabetologia* 1965; **1**: 137.
2 Reaven GM. Role of insulin resistance in human disease. *Diabetes* 1988; **37**: 1595–607.
3 Zimmet P. Non-insulin-dependent (type 2) diabetes mellitus: does it really exist? *Diabetic Med* 1989; **6**: 728–35.
4 Vague J. The degree of masculine differentiation of obesities: a factor determining predisposition to diabetes atherosclerosis, gout, and uric calculous disease. *Am J Clin Nutr* 1956; **4**: 20–34.
5 Logan RL, Riemersma RA, Thomson M, et al. Risk factors for ischaemic heart-disease in normal men aged 40: Edinburgh–Stockholm study. *Lancet* 1978; **i**: 949–55.
6 Zimmet P, King HOM, Bjorntorp PA. Obesity, hypertension, carbohydrate

disorders and the risk of chronic diseases: is there epidemiological evidence for integrated prevention programme? *Med J Aust* 1986; **145**: 256–62.

7 Pyorala K, Savolainen E, Kaukola S, Haapakoski J. Plasma insulin as coronary heart disease risk factor: relationship to other risk factors and predictive value during 9½ year follow-up of the Helsinki Policemen Study population. *Acta Med Scand Suppl* 1985; **701**: 38–52.

8 Ferrannini E, Haffner SM, Mitchell BD, Stern MP. Hyperinsulinaemia: the key feature of a cardiovascular and metabolic syndrome. *Diabetologia* 1991; **34**: 416–22.

9 Jarrett RJ. Epidemiology of macrovascular disease and hypertension in diabetes mellitus In: *International Textbook of Diabetes Mellitus* (eds KGMM Alberti, RA DeFronzo, H Keen, P Zimmet) Wiley, Chichester, 1992, pp 1459–1470.

10 Howard BV. Lipoprotein metabolism in diabetes mellitus. *J Lipid Res* 1987; **28**: 613–28.

11 Kannel WB, Gordon A, Schwartz MJ. Systolic versus diastolic blood pressure and risk of coronary heart disease. *Am J Cardiol* 1971; **27**: 335–46.

12 Modan M, Halkin H, Almog S, et al. Hyperinsulinemia: a link between hypertension obesity and glucose intolerance. *J Clin Invest* 1985; **75**: 809–17.

13 Manicardi V, Camellini L, Belloidi G, Cascelli C, Ferrannini E. Evidence for an association of high blood pressure and hyperinsulinaemia in obese man. *J Clin Endocrinol Metab* 1986; **62**: 1302–4.

14 Zavaroni I, Mazze S, Dall'Aglio E, et al. Prevalence of hyperinsulinemia in patients with high blood pressure. *J Int Med* 1992; **231**: 235–40.

15 DeFronzo RA, Ferrannini E. Insulin resistance: a multifaceted syndrome responsible for NIDDM, obesity, hypertension, dyslipidaemia and atherosclerotic cardiovascular disease. *Diabetes Care* 1991; **14**: 173–94.

16 Rowe JW, Young JB, Minaker KL, et al. Effect of insulin and glucose infusions on sympathetic nervous system activity in normal man. *Diabetes* 1981; **30**: 219–25.

17 Young JB, Landsberg L. Effect of oral sucrose on blood pressure on the spontaneously hypertensive rat. *Metabolism* 1981; **30**: 421–4.

18 Hwang IS, Ho H, Hoffman BB, Reaven GM. Fructose-induced insulin resistance and hypertension in rats. *Hypertension* 1987; **10**: 512–16.

19 DeFronzo RA, Cooke C, Andres R, Falcona GR, Davis PJ. The effect of insulin in renal handling of sodium, potassium, calcium and phosphate in man. *J Clin Invest* 1975; **55**: 845–55.

20 Saad M, Knowler W, Pettitt DJ, et al. Insulin and hypertension relationship to obesity and glucose intolerance in Pima Indians. *Diabetes* 1990; **39**: 1430–5.

21 Alberti KGMM, Dowse G, Finch C, et al. Is blood pressure related to peripheral insulin levels? A community study in Mauritius. *Diabetes* 1989; **39** (Suppl 1): 92A.

22 Asch S, Wingard DL, Barrtt-Connor EL. Are insulin and hypertension independently related? *Ann Epidemiol* 1991; **1**: 231–44.

23 Fujita N, Baba T, Tomiyama T, Kodama T, Kako N. Hyperinsulinaemia and blood pressure in patients with insulinoma. *Br Med J* 1992; **304**: 1157.

24 Jarrett RJ. In defence of insulin: a critique of syndrome X. *Lancet* 1992; **340**: 469–71.

25 Ferrannini E, Buzzigoli G, Bonadona R, et al. Insulin resistance in essential hypertension. *N Engl J Med* 1987; **317**: 350–7.

26 Ramaiya KL, Mgonda Y, Swai ABM, McLarty DG, Alberti KGMM. Insulin sensitivity in non-obese untreated hypertensive African subjects with normal glucose tolerance in Dar es Salaam, Tanzania. *Diabetic Med* 1992; **9**: 44A.

27 Shen D-C, Shein S-M, Fuh M, Chen Y-DI, Reaven GM. Resistance to insulin-

stimulated glucose uptake in patients with hypertension. *J Clin Endocrinol Metab* 1988; **66**: 580–3.

28 Doria A, Fioretto P, Avogado A, et al. Insulin resistance is associated with high sodium–lithium countertransport in essential hypertension. *Am J Physiol* 1991; **261**: E684–E691.

29 Catalano C, Winocour PH, Thomas TH, et al. Erythrocyte sodium–lithium countertransport activity and total body insulin-mediated glucose disposal in normoalbuminuric normotensive type 1 (insulin-dependent) diabetic patients. *Diabetologia* 1993; **36**: 52–6.

30 Mahnensmith RL, Aronson PS. The plasma membrane sodium–hydrogen exchanger and its role in physiological and pathophysiological processes. *Circ Res* 1985; **56**: 773–88.

31 Bruner HR, Change P, Wallach R, Sealey JE, Laragh JH. Angiotensin II vascular receptors: their avidity in relationship to sodium balance, the autonomic nervous system and hypertension. *J Clin Invest* 1972; **51**: 58–67.

32 Carlson LA, Bottiger LE. Risk factors for ischaemic heart disease in men and women. *Acta Med Scand* 1985; **218**: 207–11.

33 Fontbonne A, Eschwere E, Cambien F, et al. Hypertriglyceridaemia as a risk factor of coronary heart disease mortality in subjects with impaired glucose tolerance or diabetes. *Diabetologia* 1989; **32**: 300–4.

34 Miller NE, Thelle DS, Forde OH, Mjos OD. The Tromso Heart Study. High density lipoprotein and coronary heart disease: a prospective case–control study. *Lancet* 1977; **i**: 37–42.

35 Kannel WB. Lipids, diabetes, and coronary heart disease: insights from the Framingham Study. *Am Heart J* 1985; **110**: 1100–7.

36 Greenfield M, Kolterman O, Olefsky J, Reaven GM. Mechanism of hypertriglyceridaemia in diabetic patients with fasting hyperglycaemia. *Diabetologia* 1980; **18**: 441–6.

37 Olefsky JM, Fazrquhar JW, Reven GM. Reappraisal of the role of insulin in hypertriglyceridaemia. *Am J Med* 1974; **57**: 551.

38 Gibbons F. Assembly and secretion of hepatic very-low-density lipoprotein. *Biochem J* 1990; **268**: 1–13.

39 Abbott WGH, Lillioja S, Young AA, et al. Relationships between plasma lipoprotein concentrations and insulin action in an obese hyperinsulinaemic population. *Diabetes* 1987; **36**: 897–904.

40 Groop LC, Bonadonna RC, DelPrato S, et al. Glucose and free fatty acid metabolism in non-insulin-dependent diabetes mellitus. *J Clin Invest* 1989; **84**: 205–13.

41 Groop LC, Saloranta C, Shank M, et al. The role of free fatty acid metabolism in the pathogenesis of insulin resistance in obesity and noninsulin-dependent diabetes mellitus. *J Clin Endocrinol Metab* 1991; **72**: 96–107.

42 Golay A, Zech L, Shi M-Z, et al. High density lipoprotein (HDL) metabolism in noninsulin-dependent diabetes mellitus: measurement of HDL turnover using tritiated HDL. *J Clin Endocrinol Metab* 1987; **65**: 512–17.

43 Thiebaud D, DeFronzo RA, Jacot E, et al. Effect of long chain triglyceride infusion on glucose metabolism in man. *Metabolism* 1982; **31**: 1128–36.

44 Fulcher GR, Walker M, Catalano C, Agius L, Alberti KGMM. Metabolic effects of suppression of nonesterified fatty acid levels with Acipimox in obese NIDDM subjects. *Diabetes* 1992; **41**: 1400–8.

45 Jones IR, Swai A, Taylor R, et al. Lowering of plasma glucose concentrations with bezafibrate in patients with moderately controlled NIDDM. *Diabetes Care* 1990; **13**: 855–63.

46 Walker M, Fulcher GR, Catalano C, et al. Physiological levels of plasma non-esterified fatty acids impair forearm glucose uptake in normal man. *Clin Sci* 1990; **79**: 167–74.
47 Randle PJ, Hales CN, Garland PB, Newsholme EA. The glucose fatty-acid cycle: its role in insulin sensitivity and the metabolic disturbances of diabetes mellitus. *Lancet* 1963; **i**: 785–9.
48 Kessebah AH, Vydelingum N, Murray R, et al. Relation of body fat distribution to metabolic complications of obesity. *J Clin Endocrinol Metab* 1982; **54**: 254–60.
49 Björntorp P. Regional patterns of fat distribution. *Ann Intern Med* 1985; **103**: 994–5.
50 Ashwell M, Cole TJ, Dixon AK. Obesity: new insights into the anthropometric classification of fat distribution shown by computed tomography. *Br Med J* 1985; **290**: 1692–4.
51 Fujioka S, Matsuzawa Y, Tokunaga K, Tarui S. Contribution of intra-abdominal fat accumulation to the impairment of glucose and lipid metabolism in human obesity. *Metabolism* 1987; **36**: 54–9.
52 Kandi H, Matsuzawa Y, Kotani K, et al. Close correlation of intra-abdominal fat accumulation to hypertension in obese women. *Hypertension* 1990; **16**: 484–90.
53 Després J-P. Lipoprotein metabolism in visceral obesity. *Int J Obes* 1991; **15** (Suppl 2): 45–52.
54 Kissebah AH. Insulin resistance in visceral obesity. *Int J Obes* 1991; **15** (Suppl 2): 109–15.
55 Peiris AN, Mueller RA, Smith GA, Struve MF, Kessebah AH. Splanchnic insulin metabolism in obesity: influence of body fat distribution. *J Clin Invest* 1986; **78**: 1648–57.
56 Larsson B. Obesity, fat distribution and cardiovascular disease. *Int J Obes* 1991; **15** (Suppl 2): 53–7.
57 Larson B, Svardsudd K, Welin L, et al. Abdominal adipose tissue distribution, obesity and risk of cardiovascular disease and death: a 13-year follow-up of participants in the study of men born in 1913. *Br Med J* 1984; **288**: 1401–4.
58 Kannel WB, Adrienne Cupples L, Ramaswami R, et al. Regional obesity and risk of cardiovascular disease: the Framingham Study. *J Clin Epidemiol* 1991; **44**: 183–90.
59 Bouchard C, Tremblay A, Despres J-P, et al. The response of long-term overfeeding in identical twins. *N Engl J Med* 1990; **322**: 1477–82.
60 Seidell JC. Environmental influences on regional fat distribution. *Int J Obes* 1991; **15** (Suppl 2): 31–5.
61 Björntorp P. Adipose tissue distribution and function. *Int J Obes* 1991; **15** (Suppl 2): 67–81.
62 Jarrett RJ. Is insulin atherogenic? *Diabetologia* 1988; **31**: 71–5.
63 Cruz AB, Amatuzio DS, Grande F, Hay LJ. Effect of intraarterial insulin on tissue cholesterol and fatty acids in alloxan-diabetic dogs. *Circ Res* 1961; **9**: 39–43.
64 Falholt K, Alberti KGMM, Heding LG. Aorta and muscle metabolism in pigs with peripheral hyperinsulinaemia. *Diabetologia* 1985; **28**: 32–7.
65 Pfeifle B, Ditschuneit H. Effect of insulin on growth of cultured human arterial smooth muscle cells. *Diabetologia* 1981; **20**: 155–8.
66 Stout RW. The effect of insulin on the incorporation of sodium ($1-^{14}C$) acetate into the lipids of the rat aorta. *Diabetologia* 1971; **7**: 367–72.
67 Juan-Vague I, Alessi MC, Vague P. Increased plasma plasminogen activator inhibitor 1 levels: a possible link between insulin resistance and atherothrombosis. *Diabetologia* 1991; **34**: 457–62.

68 Kruithof EKO. Plasminogen activator inhibitor type 1: biochemical, biological and clinical aspects. *Fibrinolysis* 1988; **2** (Suppl 2): 59–70.
69 Bavenholm P, Efendic S, Wiman B, et al. Relationship of insulin response to glucose challenge to severity and rate of progression of coronary atherosclerosis in young survivors of myocardial infarction (Abstract), *Eur Heart J* 1990; **11** (Suppl 178): 7.
70 Vague P, Juhan-Vague I, Aillaud MF, et al. Correlation between blood fibrinolytic activity, plasminogen activator inhibitor level, plasma insulin level and relative body weight in normal and obese subjects. *Metabolism* 1986; **35**: 250–3.
71 Kluft C, Potter van Loon BJ, de Maat MPM. Insulin resistance and changes in haemostatic variables. *Fibrinolysis* 1992: **6** (Suppl 3): 11–16.
72 Sundell IB, Nilsson TK, Hallmans G, Hellsten G, Dahlen GH. Interrelationships between plasma levels of plasminogen activator inhibitor, tissue plasminogen activator, lipoprotein(a), and established cardiovascular risk factors in a North Swedish population. *Atherosclerosis* 1989; **80**: 9–16.
73 Nagi DK, Hendra TJ, Ryle AJ, et al. The relationships of concentrations of insulin, intact proinsulin and 32–33 split proinsulin with cardiovascular risk factors in type 2 (non-insulin-dependent) diabetic subjects. *Diabetologia* 1990; **33**: 532–7.
74 Kemmer FW, Berger M. Exercise. In: *International Textbook of Diabetes Mellitus* (eds KGMM Alberti, RA DeFronzo, H Keen, P Zimmet) Wiley, Chichester, 1992, pp 725–45.
75 Beck-Nielson H. Clinical disorders of insulin resistance. In: *International Textbook of Diabetes Mellitus* (eds KGMM Alberti, RA DeFronzo, H Keen, P Zimmet) Wiley, Chichester, 1992, pp 531–50.
76 Björntorp P. Biochemistry of obesity in relation to diabetes. In: *International Textbook of Diabetes Mellitus* (eds KGMM Alberti, RA DeFronzo, H Keen, P Zimmet) Wiley, Chichester, 1992, pp 551–68.
77 Prochazka M, Lillioja S, Knowler WC, Tait J, Bogardus C. Confirmation of genetic linkage between markers on chromosome 4q and a gene for insulin resistance in obese Pima Indians. *Diabetes* 1992; **41**: 9A.
78 Eriksson J, Franssila-Kallunki A, Ekstrand A, et al, Early metabolic defects in persons at increased risk for non-insulin-dependent diabetes mellitus. *N Engl J Med* 1989; **321**: 337–43.
79 Haffner SM, Valdex RA, Hazuda HP, et al. Prospective analysis of the insulin-resistance syndrome (syndrome X). *Diabetes* 1992; **41**: 715–22.
80 Sobey WJ, Beer SF, Carrington CA, et al. Sensitive and specific two-site immunoradiometric assays for human insulin, proinsulin, 65–66 split, and 32–33 split proinsulin. *Biochem* 1989; **260**: 535–41.
81 Temple RC, Clark PMS, Nagi DK, et al. Radioimmunoassay may overestimate insulin in non-insulin-dependent diabetics. *Clin Endocrinol* 1990; **32**: 689–92.
82 Schneider DJ, Nordt TK, Sobel BE. Stimulation of proinsulin of expression of plasminogen activator inhibitor type 1 in endothelial cells. *Diabetes* 1992; **41**: 890–5.
83 Akinmokun A, Harris P, Home PD, Alberti KGMM. Is diabetes always diabetes? *Diabetes Res Clin Pract* 1992; **305**: 1057–62.
84 Ramaiya KL, Swai ABM, Alberti KGMM, McLarty D. Life style changes decrease rate of glucose intolerance and cardiovascular (CVD) risk factors: a six year intervention study in a high risk Hindu Indian subcommunity. *Diabetologia* 1992; **35**: 60A.

Chapter Seventeen

Towards Prevention of Non-insulin-dependent Diabetes Mellitus

Angela Spelsberg and JoAnn E. Manson

Department of Medicine, Harvard Medical School and Brigham and Women's Hospital, and Department of Epidemiology, Harvard School of Public Health, Boston, Massachussetts, USA

INTRODUCTION

NON-INSULIN-DEPENDENT DIABETES MELLITUS: A PUBLIC HEALTH PROBLEM

Non-insulin-dependent diabetes mellitus (NIDDM) represents one of the most prevalent chronic diseases worldwide, afflicting individuals in developed as well as in developing societies. More than 12 million prevalent cases of NIDDM are estimated in the USA and at least half are undiagnosed[1]. NIDDM has become the seventh leading cause of death and the third leading cause by disease in the USA[2]. The National Health and Nutrition Examination Survey (NHANES, 1976–1980) determined a prevalence rate of diagnosed

Causes of Diabetes. Edited by R. D. G. Leslie
© 1993 John Wiley & Sons Ltd

and undiagnosed diabetes (by National Diabetes Data Group criteria) among American whites aged 20–74 years of 5.2% in men and 6.7% in women[3]. For African–Americans, prevalence estimates were almost twice the rates of whites: 8.9% for black males and 10.2% for black females. In both races, diabetes prevalence increases with age, reaching 18% in whites aged 65–74 years and 26% in blacks of that age group. In numerous populations world-wide, the disease has achieved epidemic dimensions[4]; in some South Pacific island populations such as the Nauru Indians, NIDDM prevalence (by World Health Organization criteria) is 24.3% in age groups older than 20 years, and among native American Indians such as the Pima Indians, the corresponding NIDDM prevalence is 25.5% among those older than 25 years[5]. Of particular importance in implicating environmental factors in the genesis of NIDDM are the observed increases in NIDDM rates among migrant populations previously considered to be resistant to diabetes, such as Japanese–Americans or Chinese–Mauritians who have been recently exposed to a more Westernized life style[4]. The striking increases in NIDDM prevalences among those migrant populations are shown in Table 1.

The impact of NIDDM on morbidity and mortality, as well as the economic costs attributable to the disease, are substantial in both industrialized and developing countries. In the USA, 144 000 deaths were attributed to NIDDM in 1986, representing 6.8% of all US deaths[10]. Also, morbidity among persons with NIDDM, including hypertension, cardiovascular disease, cerebrovascu-

Table 1 Age-standardized comparisons of diabetes prevalence in migrant populations and native populations residential in the homeland

Source of data	Age (years)	Sex	Year(s) of study	Prevalence (%)
Chinese				
Taiwan				
Rural	≥40	M, F	1984	5.1
Urban[6]	≥40	M, F	1984	8.1
Singapore[7]	≥30	M	1975–1985	6.0
	≥30	F	1975–1985	5.4
Mauritius[8]	≥30	M	1986	14.7
	≥30	F	1986	10.7
Japanese				
Hiroshima[9]	40–96	M	1975	5.3
	40–96	F	1975	8.7
American–Japanese				
Hawaii[9]	40–96	M	1975	14.2
	40–96	F	1975	11.1

lar disease, peripheral vascular disease, nephropathy, skin ulcer, limb ampu-
tation and visual disorders (glaucoma, cataract, blindness), was substantially
higher than among non-diabetics. The relative prevalence of these conditions,
comparing persons with NIDDM with non-diabetics, ranged from 2.5 (hypertension) to 10.3 (blindness)[10]. A total of 951 000 persons were declared
permanently disabled because of NIDDM or related conditions in 1986.
Health care expenditures for NIDDM patients during 1986 were calculated
to be $11.56 billion, of which $6.83 billion was spent on general treatment or
unspecified complications, $3.85 billion for circulatory disorders, $0.39 billion
for visual disorders, $0.24 billion for neuropathy, $0.15 billion for skin ulcers,
and $0.10 billion for nephropathy. The annual health care expenditure per
case averaged $1274 for men below 65 years, $1475 for women below 65
years, $2206 for men above 65 years, and $3073 for women above 65 years.
Taking into account the additional costs of lost productivity, NIDDM
accounted for total economic costs of $19.8 billion in the USA in 1986[10].
Current combined direct and indirect costs of NIDDM in the USA have been
estimated to be as high as $40 billion annually[11].

Non-white populations appear to carry a heavier burden of morbidity than
whites. The onset of NIDDM is at earlier ages among African–Americans,
Mexican–Americans, Pima Indians and the inhabitants of the island communities of the Pacific region, than among whites[3,4,12]. In Pacific and migrant
Asian Indian and American Indian populations, NIDDM is frequently found
in early adulthood, 20–30 years before the typical onset of NIDDM in white
populations[12]. Consequently, complications of the disease are seen at relatively young ages. Currently, data on complications of NIDDM in non-white
populations are sparse. Studies of retinopathy in Pacific islanders found a
prevalence of 25% of retinal microangiopathic changes among Nauru and
Kiribati Micronesians with NIDDM[12], and it was speculated that, due to early
onset of NIDDM in these populations, these developing countries will face
substantial economic and social costs related to diabetes.

In contrast to microangiopathy, atherosclerotic diseases such as coronary
artery disease (CAD) appear to be rare in non-white NIDDM patients,
except among the New Zealand Maori[13]. The relatively short exposure to
Westernized lifestyle and low levels of the traditional cardiovascular risk
factors in the South Pacific Indian populations, native American Indians,
Mexican–Americans and Japanese–Americans could explain the apparently
low prevalence of CAD and CAD-related deaths compared to white
populations[12]. However, with continuing Westernization, the cardiovascular
risk profile in these populations may approach the pattern already seen in the
New Zealand Maori and in Caucasian populations. Among African–
Americans with NIDDM, the prevalence of myocardial infarction or angina
is 20–30% lower than in white diabetic subjects[14]. Hypertension, however,
appears to be more common among African–American diabetic subjects than

among Caucasian diabetic subjects in each age group below 65 years. Further, microvascular complications such as visual impairment and end-stage renal disease are increased up to four-fold in black patients with NIDDM compared to whites[3].

Death certificate data in the USA in 1978 showed a lower prevalence (45%) of ischaemic heart disease among deceased blacks in whom diabetes was the underlying or contributing cause of death than among whites (55%). Cerebrovascular disease, other circulatory diseases, renal disease, infections and neoplasms, however, were more frequently reported on death certificates among diabetic blacks than whites. Despite lower rates of atherosclerotic disease among diabetics in Pacific populations than in the USA age-standardized death rates attributable to NIDDM among Nauruans and other Pacific populations are more than twice those in the USA[14-16].

NIDDM: A PREVENTABLE CONDITION?

Despite strong genetic influences, NIDDM should be regarded as a potentially preventable disease. The pathogenesis of NIDDM suggests that

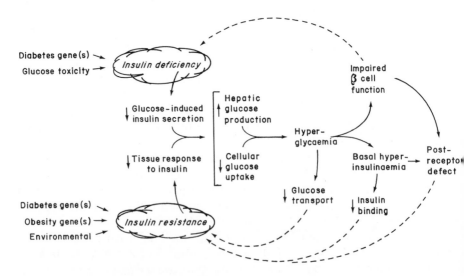

Figure 1 Pathogenetic sequence of events leading to the development of glucose intolerance, insulin resistance and impaired insulin secretion in NIDDM. Note that whether the primary defect that initiates the glucose intolerance resides in the β cell or in peripheral/hepatic tissues, development of insulin resistance eventually will ensue or become aggravated, respectively. By the time that overt fasting hyperglycaemia (>140 mg/dl) develops, both impaired insulin secretion and severe insulin resistance are present. Broken arrows represent positive feedback loops that result in self-perpetuation of primary defects. (Reproduced from De Fronzo[61]. Copyright ©1988 by the American Diabetes Association, Inc.)

environmental factors have a major role in the development of NIDDM (Figure 1). Valuable insights into the genetic–environmental interaction in the aetiology of NIDDM derive from studies of high-risk populations such as the Pima and the Nauru Indians, as well as migrant populations, including Japanese–Americans, Asian Indians in Fiji, Chinese and Creoles in Mauritius and Bangladeshi migrants to the UK[4]. In particular, those populations that had been considered 'immune' to NIDDM, e.g. the Japanese and Chinese, illustrate the powerful impact of modern lifestyle factors on the risk of developing chronic non-communicable diseases in populations traditionally free from these diseases (see Table 1). At present, epidemiological evidence on modifiable determinants of NIDDM is based primarily on descriptive and analytical observational studies; randomized trial data are scant. Epidemiological research concerning NIDDM clearly is in an early developmental stage[4]. However, in view of the immense public health implications of the disease and its complications, the initiation of preventive measures appears to be justified for the few strong risk factors currently recognized: obesity, physical inactivity and dietary factors. Current epidemiological knowledge concerning these determinants will be discussed in the following sections and will be evaluated in their public health context.

MODIFIABLE DETERMINANTS FOR NIDDM IN WOMEN AND MEN

OBESITY

Biological Mechanisms

Several biological mechanisms have been proposed to link obesity and NIDDM. Obesity has been demonstrated to be associated with insulin resistance, i.e. a decreased ability of the body to respond to the action of insulin[17], and a reduced number of insulin receptors[18]. It is widely believed that the insulin-resistant state induces compensatory hyperinsulinaemia and that impaired glucose tolerance (IGT) and NIDDM finally develop with an exhaustion of β cell function[17]. However, a recent study among Pima Indians and Caucasians revealed a 50% greater plasma insulin response to an oral glucose load among Pimas that could not be explained by confounding factors such as level of obesity, age, sex, insulin resistance or plasma glucose concentrations[19]. This finding raised the possibility of a primary hyperinsulinaemia causing insulin resistance by down-regulation of insulin receptor and postreceptor action and, finally, the development of overt diabetes in those individuals with a probable genetic defect of insulin secretion and/or action[18]. The major site of insulin resistance in obese NIDDM patients is the skeletal muscle, and deposition of glucose as glycogen is abnormally low in these subjects[20] owing to a reduced activity of glycogen synthase[21]. The metabolic insulin resistance observed in obesity, with increased fat oxidation and glucose–fat–substrate competition, may lead to the impairment of non-oxidative glucose uptake in muscle tissue. The observation that less than 10% of obese white individuals develop NIDDM strongly suggests that interactions between different environmental factors, e.g. exposure to overeating, physical inactivity or obesity, in combination with genetic defects, may account for the final disturbance of insulin secretion[20].

Epidemiological Evidence

Results from cross-cultural, migrant and analytical studies indicate that obesity is a strong risk factor for NIDDM and IGT[8,22-37] (Table 2).

The evidence is based primarily on the fact that the majority of persons with NIDDM are obese, that populations in which the prevalence of NIDDM is high have a higher degree of obesity than lower-risk populations[25], and that obesity is associated with insulin resistance[38]. Ecological and analytical epidemiological data have reflected the complexity of the association between obesity and NIDDM. Studies of Pacific migrant populations have suggested that different levels of obesity do not fully explain the high variability of diabetes prevalence in these Pacific populations[12]. A cross-sectional comparison of Melanesians, migrant Asian Indians in Fiji and Micronesians showed a significant positive association between body mass index (BMI) and the prevalence of NIDDM in Micronesian men, and in women of all three ethnic groups, but not in Melanesian or Indian men after adjusting for age[26]. In a study among Japanese migrants in Hawaii, higher prevalences of diabetes were observed among migrants than among Japanese living in Hiroshima across all weight categories; NIDDM rates among migrants approached those of natives of the host country[9]. Cross-sectional data in Pima Indians, who have the highest diabetes incidence and prevalence rates worldwide, have not consistently shown a significant association between obesity and NIDDM[27]; longitudinal data, however, confirmed a positive relationship in Pima Indians[28].

Most prospective cohort studies have demonstrated that obesity is an independent strong predictor of NIDDM in men and women[28-37]. In a Swedish study comprising a birth cohort of men born in 1913, the relative risk of developing NIDDM after 13.5 years of observation was 21.7 among those in the highest BMI quintile compared to men in the lowest BMI quintile[32,37]. In the Nurses' Health Study, the investigators followed 113 861 US white female nurses for 8 years and detected a strong continuous relationship between obesity and risk of NIDDM[36]. Obese women in the highest BMI categories (BMI $\geq$ 29 kg/m^2) had a 20–60-fold increased diabetes risk compared to lean women (BMI < 22 kg/m^2). Also, weight change since the age of 18 years was an important, although less strong, predictor of NIDDM in this cohort of women. The risk of NIDDM among women with a weight gain of 10–20 kg after the age of 18 was 4.6 times higher than in women with stable weight; the risk increased substantially when weight gain was more pronounced[36]. In turn, clinical studies of weight loss in NIDDM patients have demonstrated improved glucose tolerance and insulin resistance[39–43]. In the Nurses' Health Study, a subgroup of women with a BMI > 27 kg/m^2 at entry and who lost 5–20 kg in the subsequent 4 years of the study had a 30% reduction in risk of NIDDM compared to women whose weight did not change more than 1 kg (age-adjusted relative risk $= 0.7$, 95% confidence interval 0.5–1.1)[36]. Other prospective studies have also shown a positive, but weaker, association between obesity and NIDDM[28,33–35]. This may in part be related to a smaller number of study participants, thereby requiring broader categorization of BMI categories and limiting the ability to detect an effect at very high levels of BMI. Some prospective studies have not observed an independent association of obesity and NIDDM[44,45]. The totality of available evidence, however, supports an independent role of obesity in the development of NIDDM, although the strength of the association appears to be influenced by genetic factors and is subject to variation both within and between populations.

BODY FAT DISTRIBUTION

A similarly complex picture emerges concerning the role of body fat distribution and the risk of NIDDM. It has been speculated that insulin resistance is primarily modulated by abdominal obesity[46], which reflects increased omental fat. Intra-abdominal visceral fat is more sensitive than other fat cells to lipolytc stimuli; the resulting elevations in portal concentrations of free fatty acids may produce insulin resistance in the liver and adverse metabolic effects including glucose intolerance[47]. A centralized fat distribution, in particular the accumulation of intra-abdominal fat as measured by truncal skinfold thickness and/or waist-to-hip ratio (WHR), has been found to be an independent predictor of NIDDM in both women and men regardless of BMI[48,49]. The available epidemiological evidence is summarized in Table 3.

The Gothenburg Study demonstrated a 9.6-fold elevated risk of NIDDM among men in the highest WHR category compared to men in the lowest category in univariate analyses. No risk elevation was observed in the lowest WHR category despite increasing BMI values. After controlling for BMI, still a significant positive association was seen between 2-hour blood glucose concentration and WHR; however, the positive relationship between WHR and risk of NIDDM over 13.5 years was no longer significant[32,37]. Similar findings were obtained in the follow-up study of Swedish women in Gothenburg[50]. In a cross-sectional analysis of the TOPS (Take Off Pounds

Table 2 Association between obesity and risk of NIDDM: epidemiological studies

Source of data	Age (years)	Sex	Year(s) of study	Comparison groups	Association RRᵃ Highest/Lowest
Ecologic					
Central and South America, Uruguay, East Pakistan, Malaya[25]	>3	M, F	1966–1970	All weight groups	N/A#
Cross-sectional					
Melanesians	≥20	M	1980	Tertiles of BMI[b]	0.9
Indians	≥20	M	1980	Tertiles of BMI	1.6
Micronesians[26]	≥20	M	1981	Tertiles of BMI	3.6
Melanesians	≥20	F	1980	Tertiles of BMI	5.6
Indians	≥20	F	1980	Tertiles of BMI	3.0
Micronesians[26]	≥20	F	1981	Tertiles of BMI	3.8
American–Japanese	40–59	M	1976	Tertiles of BMI	2.8[d]
Japanese	40–59	M	1975	Tertiles of BMI	0.2[c]
American–Japanese	60–96	M	1976	Tertiles of BMI	1.4
Japanese	60–96	F	1975	Tertiles of BMI	1.7[d]
American–Japanese	40–59	F	1976	Tertiles of BMI	1.8
Japanese	40–59	F	1975	No NIDDM cases in comparison group	–

American–Japanese	60–96	F	1976	Tertiles of BMI	2.2
Japanese[9]	60–96	F	1975	Tertiles of BMI	0.4
US whites	20–74	M, F	1976–80	PDW[e] categories	2.8
US blacks[3]	20–74	M, F	1976–80	PDW categories	2.9
Prospective cohort					
Mexican Americans[4]	25–64	M, F	1979–87	Quartiles of BMI	1.97[f]
Pima Indians[27]	≥5	M, F	1972–87[g]	BMI > 27 vs < 27	2.9
Pima Indians[28]	35–64	F	1965–80	BMI > 25 vs < 25	1.5
Bedford Study[29]		M, F	1962–72	BMI tertiles	2.1
Swedish men[30]	40–49	M	1960–70	Cohort relative weight ≥ 130% vs < 100%	24.0
Birth Cohort, Gothenburg, Sweden[32,37]	54	M	1963–77	BMI quantiles	21.7
Israeli men[34]		M	1967–72	BMI > 24 vs < 24	2.5
Zutphen Study[88]	41–60	M	1960–85	BMI quantiles	2.4
US Nurses[36]	30–55	F	1976–84	BMI deciles	60.9

[a]RR = relative risk, adjusted for age and some other potential confounding variables.
[b]BMI = body mass index: weight (kg) divided by the square of height (m^2).
#N/A: Not available; correlation coefficient for mean percent of standard weight and prevalence of diabetes (r = 0.89).
[c]Comparison between medium versus lowest category.
[d]Comparison between highest versus medium BMI tertile.
[e]PDW = per cent desirable weight, based on 1959 Metropolitan Life Insurance tables.
[f]Comparison made between highest versus lowest three BMI quartiles.
[g]Median length of follow-up 3.3 years.

329328

328

Table 3 Association between increased abdominal fat (WHR) and risk of NIDDM: epidemiological studies

Source of data	Age (years)	Sex	Year(s) of study	Comparison groups	Association RR Highest/Lowest
Cross-sectional					
TOPS Baseline Survey[51]	20–70	F	1969	WHR tertiles	2.8[b]
Hindu Indians	25–74	M	1987	WHR tertiles	2.8
Muslim Indians	25–74	M	1987	WHR tertiles	5.8
Creole Mauritians[46]	25–74	M	1987	WHR tertiles	3.7
Chinese Mauritians[46]	25–74	M	1987	WHR tertiles	4.1
Hindu Indians	25–74	F	1987	WHR tertiles	8.9
Muslim Indians	25–74	F	1987	WHR tertiles	2.5
Creole Mauritians[46]	25–74	F	1987	WHR tertiles	5.6
Chinese Mauritians[46]	25–74	F	1987	WHR tertiles	9.8
Finnish Elderly	65–74	M	1986–88	WHR ≥ 0.98 vs < 0.98	1.4
Population[52]	65–74	M, F	1986–88	WHR ≥ 0.89 vs < 0.89	1.95
Prospective cohort					
Mexican–Americans[4]	25–64	M, F	1979–87	Quartiles of centrality index[a]	1.83
Birth Cohort, Gothenburg, Sweden[32,37]	54	M	1963–77 (13.5 years)	WHR quintiles	9.6
Zutphen study[88]	41–60	M	1960–85	Subscapular skinfold > 10 mm vs < 10 mm	2.4

[a]Centrality index: ratio of subscapular to triceps skinfold; comparisons made between highest versus lowest three quartiles.
[b]Adjusted for both age and BMI.

Sensibly) cohort[51], a positive relation between upper body fat accumulation (indicated by upper tertiles of WHR, or neck and bust girth values) and risk of NIDDM was observed. This finding was corroborated among a representative sample of 1300 Finnish women and men aged 65–74 years. A BMI of $\geq$ 25 kg/m^2 in women and $\geq$ 27 kg/m^2 in men and a WHR $\geq$ 0.89 in women and $\geq$ 0.98 in men were all associated with a two-fold increase in prevalence of NIDDM and IGT[52]. However, as with overall obesity, differences in body fat distribution could not fully explain the observed differences in NIDDM prevalence between ethnic groups[53]. A recent study of NIDDM and IGT prevalence among four ethnic groups in the Pacific (Hindu and Muslim Asian Indians, Creoles of predominantly African origin and Chinese Mauretanians) found an independent strong effect of WHR among Hindu, Creole and Chinese women that exceeded the effect of BMI, whereas among men BMI was more important. The reverse was true for Muslim Asian Indian men and women[46]. In summary, increased abdominal fat has recently emerged as an independent and strong risk factor for NIDDM and IGT. The impact of this finding, including possible determinants of WHR and potential preventive measures, remains to be elucidated[12]. Recent studies have suggested a possible role of cigarette smoking, alcohol consumption and sedentary lifestyle, in addition to age and BMI, as determinants of abdominal adiposity. In the Rancho Bernardo Study, an increase of WHR with age and BMI was seen among 685 men and 943 women[54]. An independent association of WHR with smoking, alcohol consumption and sedentary lifestyle was observed in men, and with smoking and alcohol consumption in women. A similar association of abdomen-to-hip ratio with cigarette smoking and alcohol and an inverse relation with physical activity was reported among men in the Normative Aging Study[55]. Also, European men were found to have increased abdominal fat accumulation with cigarette smoking and physical inactivity[56].

DIETARY FACTORS

In view of the importance of obesity as a risk factor for NIDDM, an understanding of the role of diet as a determinant of both obesity and NIDDM is crucial. Cross-sectional and migrant studies have suggested a positive correlation between the prevalence of diabetes and total fat intake, animal fat intake and protein consumption[25]. In contrast, total carbohydrate consumption appears to be inversely related to NIDDM prevalence[25]. Japanese–Americans living in Hawaii were found to have a two-fold increase in animal fat and simple carbohydrate ingestion and nearly twice the NIDDM prevalence of their Japanese peers ($p < 0.01$)[9]. In a recent cross-sectional study of dietary habits assessed by 24-hour recall and the prevalence of IGT and NIDDM determined by oral glucose tolerance test in previously undiagnosed 1317 Hispanic and non-Hispanic whites in Colorado, the investigators found a positive association between high fat and low carbo-hydrate intake and glucose intolerance[57]. After adjustment for age, sex, ethnicity, BMI and energy intake, the risk of NIDDM increased by 45% with every 40 g per day increment in total fat intake, and by 31% with every 90 g per day decrease in carbohydrate intake; however, the estimates were not statistically significant[57]. In Pacific populations, the overall change of dietary habits with a more Westernized lifestyle towards a high-calorie, refined carbohydrate, high-fat and low-fibre diet has been proposed as a potential cause of the dramatic increase in NIDDM rates in these populations[12]. No specific dietary component, however, has been identified as a predominant determinant of diabetes in these regions[12]. The potential for confounding, in particular by total caloric intake, BMI or level of physical activity in ecological studies limits the interpretation of these findings. Table 4 provides an overview of the different findings from ecological, cross-sectional, as well as prospective cohort studies.

Clinical and animal studies have revealed several plausible biological mechanisms by which increased dietary fat may play an important role in the genesis of NIDDM. Ingestions of high-fat diets in animal studies produced an altered fat distribution, as well as an increase in total body weight and a higher proportion of body fat for a given body weight[58,59], which have all been related to unfavourable effects on glucose tolerance[60]. Obese non-diabetic and obese NIDDM individuals were shown to have elevated fasting levels of circulating free fatty acids (FFA)[61]. Intracellular FFA oxidation is a powerful inhibitor of glycogen storage and glucose oxidation in the cell. In obese non-diabetics and obese NIDDM patients, increased postabsorptive plasma FFA levels and a weakened antagonistic effect of insulin on lipid oxidation have been demonstrated[62,63]. Therefore, an elevated rate of FFA oxidation, either directly induced by a high-fat diet or mediated through the development of obesity, is theoretically able to induce all major intracellular abnormalities of glucose metabolism of NIDDM[17]. However, the use of plasma FFA concentrations as a marker for individual fatty acid intake is controversial. More data are needed to determine which fatty acid measure-ments in plasma or tissue reflect dietary intake of a specific fatty acid. At present, it seems that the measurement of fatty acids in adipose tissue provides a good estimate of long-term dietary fat ingestion because of the slow fatty acid turnover in adipose tissue[64].

There have been only a few prospective studies of diet and risk of NIDDM, showing inconsistent relationships between certain dietary factors, such as increased meat and animal fat intake[65,66], or decreased total caloric intake[67]. None of the prospective studies revealed an increased risk of NIDDM with sugar, saturated fat intake or other specific nutrients. The Nurses' Health Study analysed information obtained by a semi-quantitative food frequency questionnaire among 84360 US nurses followed for 6 years[68]. Diets higher in

Table 4 Association between dietary factors and risk of NIDDM: epidemiological studies

Source of data	Age (years)	Sex	Year(s) of study	Study description	Association
Ecological					
Central and South America, Uruguay, East Pakistan, Malaya[25]	>34	M, F	1966–70	Prevalence of diabetes, diet surveys in nine populations	↑ Risk with high fat, high protein, low carbohydrate intake
American–Japanese Japanese[9]	40–96 40–96	M M	1976 1975	Prevalence of diabetes and dietary history	↑ Risk with high fat, high animal protein; high simple sugar intake
Cross-sectional					
Hispanic and non-hispanic whites[57]	30–74	M, F	1984–88	Prevalence of NIDDM and IGT, 24-hour diet recall	↑ Risk with high fat, low carbohydrate intake
Pacific islanders[12]	≥20	M, F	1976–81	Prevalence of NIDDM, dietary survey	↑ Risk with high fat, low carbohydrate intake
Prospective cohort					
Seventh-day Adventist[65]	≥30	M	1969–88		↑ Risk with high meat intake
Seventh-day Adventist[65]	≥30	F	1969–88		No associations
Swedish Women, Gothenburg[67]	40–59	F	1975–87		↑ Risk with decreased caloric intake
Zutphen Study[88]	41–60	M	1960–85		No associations
US Nurses'[68]	30–55	F	1980–86		↓ Risk with: potassium, magnesium, vegetable fat

vegetable fat, magnesium and potassium were each associated with a reduction in risk of clinical diabetes. Animal studies and clinical studies in humans of magnesium, potassium and calcium intakes have suggested that these nutrients increase insulin secretion and reduce blood sugar concentrations[68]. Again, sugar, total fibre and carbohydrate intake were not related to an increased risk of NIDDM. A significant inverse relation between daily alcohol consumption and diabetes risk was observed in obese women (BMI $\geq$ 29 kg/m^2) as well as, although less pronounced, in leaner women. The association between the ratio of polyunsaturated to saturated fat intake (P : S) and diabetes risk was borderline significant (p = 0.07): women in the highest P : S ratio quintile had a 33% reduction in risk of NIDDM compared to women in the lowest quintile. Compared to the powerful impact of obesity in this cohort, the importance of dietary factors in the development of NIDDM appeared to be minor. However, in the same cohort, specific dietary factors were demonstrated to influence the risk of obesity. Among these factors were protein, animal fat, total fat and sucrose intake, whereas vegetable fat, dietary fibre, and alcohol showed an inverse relationship with BMI[69]. It seems plausible that these dietary factors may influence the development of NIDDM through the promotion of obesity.

PHYSICAL ACTIVITY

Biological Mechanisms

Several known biological mechanisms could explain a beneficial effect of physical activity in reducing the risk of NIDDM. Skeletal muscle represents the predominant site of insulin resistance in NIDDM[17], and exercise training has been shown to improve insulin sensitivity in these tissues[70,71]. Exercise has a favourable effect on glucose tolerance and insulin sensitivity both in patients with pre-existing NIDDM and non-diabetics—an effect that can persist up to 72 hours after cessation of exercise[72–74]. In clinical trials, obese individuals with impaired glucose tolerance have been found to have lower insulin levels and improved glucose metabolism after moderate exercise regimens, even without weight loss[75–76]. In addition to independent effects of exercise on insulin resistance, studies among non-diabetics suggest that the addition of exercise to caloric restriction will facilitate loss of adipose tissue and will assist in maintenance of reduced body weight[77].

Epidemiological Evidence

The potential beneficial effects of physical activity on the development of NIDDM have been investigated in only a few epidemiological studies[49]. Support for the benefits of exercise on NIDDM risk is provided by descriptive comparisons of active rural versus more sedentary urban high-risk Pacific populations, as well as cross-sectional and longitudinal studies of active compared to sedentary individuals within both developing and developed societies[12,26,46,78–84] (Tables 5 and 6).

In Melanesian and Indian Fijian males, the prevalence of NIDDM among men classified as sedentary was more than twice the rate in those classified as exercising moderately to heavily[78]. The same association was observed among migrant Asian Indians, African Creoles and Chinese Mauretanians[46]. Not all cross-sectional studies, however, have shown a significant association between glucose tolerance and physical activity[79,80]. Few prospective cohort studies have been conducted on physical activity and risk of NIDDM. These prospective studies have consistently shown a marked decrease in NIDDM risk in physically active individuals compared with their sedentary peers[81–83] (see Table 5). In a prospective study of 5990 male alumni of the University of Pennsylvania during 14 years of follow-up, leisure-time activity was inversely associated with the risk of NIDDM; for every 500 kcal increment of energy expenditure, a 6% reduction in diabetes risk was observed after adjustment for age, BMI and other variables[81]. The strongest protective effect was observed among those at highest risk for NIDDM (men with high BMI, history of hypertension or family history of diabetes). Risk reductions with physical activity were also found among 87 253 women in the Nurses' Health Study. During 8 years of follow-up, women who exercised vigorously at least once per week had an age-adjusted relative risk of NIDDM of 0.67 (95% confidence interval (CI) 0.60–0.75; $p < 0.001$) compared to women exercising less than once weekly; a significant 16% reduction in NIDDM risk persisted after additional adjustment for BMI[82]. Finally, in a study of 21 271 US male physicians, the age-adjusted relative risk of NIDDM was again found to decrease with increasing frequency of exercise[83]. Compared to men exercising vigorously less than once per week, the relative risk was 0.77 for vigorous exercise once weekly, 0.67 for two to four times per week, and 0.58 for five times or more per week ($p_{trend} = 0.0002$). The reduction in risk of NIDDM remained significant after adjustment for both age and BMI (relative risk (RR) = 0.71; 95% CI 0.56–0.91) for an exercise frequency of at least once per week compared to less than once weekly. Risk reductions were particularly pronounced among obese men (BMI > 26.4 kg/m^2)[83]. In conclusion, the consistently observed reductions in risk of NIDDM among physically active compared to sedentary individuals in all the prospective studies[81–83] and most of the cross-sectional investigations[8,26,46,78,84] indicate that physical inactivity imposes a substantial risk for the development of NIDDM and that regular vigorous exercise is protective against NIDDM. However, at present, data are limited with respect to the intensity, frequency and duration of exercise that will be most effective in reducing the occurrence of NIDDM.

Table 5 Association between physical inactivity and risk of NIDDM: cross-sectional epidemiological studies

Source of data	Age (years)	Sex	Year of study	Comparison groups	Association RR $\frac{\text{Most sedentary}}{\text{Most active}}$	Potential confounding variables controlled in analysis
Cross-sectional						
Melanesians	≥20	M	1980	Inactive vs active[a]	2.7	Age
Indians	≥20	M	1980	Inactive vs active	2.0	
Micronesians[26]	≥20	M	1982	Inactive vs active	1.4	
Melanesians	≥20	F	1980	Inactive vs active	2.4	Age
Indians	≥20	F	1980	Inactive vs active	0.9	
Micronesians[26]	≥20	F	1981	Inactive vs active	2.4	
Hindu Indians	25–74	M	1987	Activity tertiles	1.46	Age, BMI, family history of diabetes
Muslim Indians	25–74	M	1987	Activity tertiles	1.47	
Creole Mauritians[46]	25–74	M	1987	Activity tertiles	2.60	
Chinese Mauritians[46]	25–74	M	1987	Activity tertiles	0.93	
Hindu Indians	25–74	F	1987	Activity tertiles	2.57	Age, BMI, family history of diabetes
Muslim Indians	25–74	F	1987	Activity tertiles	1.01	
Creole Mauritians[42]	25–74	F	1987	Activity tertiles	1.42	
Chinese Mauritians[42]	25–74	F	1987	Activity tertiles	0.27	
US college alumni[84 b]	40–80	F	1982	Non-athletes vs athletes	3.41	Age

[a] Activity scores 1 and 2 combined = inactive; activity scores 3 and 4 combined = active.
[b] Retrospective cohort.

Table 6 Association between physical activity and risk of NIDDM: prospective epidemiological studies

Source of data	Age (years)	Sex	Year of study	Comparison groups	Association RR $\frac{\text{Active}}{\text{Sedentary}}$	Potential confounding variables controlled in analysis
Prospective cohort[a] University of Pennsylvania alumni[83]	39–68	M	1962–76	Each 500 kcal/week increase in physical activity index	0.94	Age, BMI, history of hypertension, parental history of diabetes
US Nurses[82]	34–59	F	1980–88	Vigorous exercise less than once weekly	0.84	Age, BMI, family history of diabetes, history of hypertension
US Physicians[83]	40–84	M	1980–88[b]	Vigorous exercise less than once weekly	0.71	Age, BMI, history of hypertension

[a]Participants in each of the prospective cohort studies were predominantly white.
[b]Median length of follow-up 5 years.

OTHER MODIFIABLE DETERMINANTS

Cigarette Smoking

A possible association between cigarette smoking and diabetes is suggested by findings that smoking decreases fasting insulin levels and causes a transient increase in blood glucose levels after an oral glucose load[85]. Smoking is also associated with a higher WHR[86], which may increase the risk of NIDDM. Epidemiological data on this subject have been limited, however. During a 12-year follow-up period among women in the Nurses' Health Study, current smokers had an increased risk of NIDDM, and a statistically significant dose–response trend was observed. Among women who smoked ⩾25 cigarettes per day, the relative risk of NIDDM was 1.42 (95% CI 1.18–1.72) compared to non-smokers, after adjustment for age, BMI, family history of diabetes, physical activity and other risk factors[87]. In a 25-year prospective study among middle-aged Dutch men, those who smoked > 20 cigarettes per day had a relative risk of diabetes of 3.3 (95% CI 1.4–7.9), after controlling for age, subscapular skinfold thickness, resting heart rate, alcohol and energy intake[88]. Control for relative weight, family history of diabetes, and physical activity were not complete, however. In two other relatively small studies, no relation between smoking and diabetes was observed[89,90]. The available data suggest that cigarette smoking may be an additional modifiable risk factor for NIDDM. The adverse health effects of smoking are already so great with respect to other health outcomes, however, that major public health interventions to prevent and discourage smoking are undebatably warranted.

PARITY

Parity has been proposed as a possible determinant of geographic, ethnic and social class differences in the prevalence of diabetes among women[91]. As reviewed in a recent report[92], most previous studies of parity and NIDDM have not controlled for obesity. Further, among women of diverse socio-economic backgrounds, differences other than parity may explain the variations in NIDDM risk. Although a recent study of white women of high socio-economic status in California suggested a modest increase in NIDDM and IGT risk with increasing parity, the association was non-linear and excess risk was found predominantly in a small subgroup of women with six births or more[91]. Other recent studies that included control for obesity have not corroborated an association between parity and NIDDM[92,93]. It is unlikely that parity has an important impact on the incidence of NIDDM in the USA and other industrialized countries, where few women have more than six children.

CONTRACEPTIVE AND POSTMENOPAUSAL HORMONE THERAPY

Exogenous oestrogen therapy has been implicated in the genesis of diabetes because oestrogens have been shown to have an insulin antagonistic effect, to be associated with elevated levels of contra-insulin hormones including growth hormone and glucocorticoids, and to lead to alterations in intestinal glucose absorption[94]. Current use of oral contraceptives increases serum glucose and insulin levels after a standard glucose challenge[95]. The long-term effects of past oral contraceptive use are largely unknown, however. Although a modest deterioration in glucose tolerance assessed by intravenous testing has been observed after 18 months of progestogen or combination-type oral contraceptives[96], only a marginal elevation in risk of NIDDM (RR = 1.10) was observed in the Nurses' Health Study among women who had used oral contraceptives in the past, as compared with never users[97]. The effect of non-contraceptive oestrogen therapy on the risk of NIDDM is even less clear. In the Nurses' Health Study—to our knowledge the only prospective large-scale study that has investigated this relationship—no increase in risk of clinical NIDDM was observed among current or past users of post-menopausal hormones, as compared with women who had never used these hormones[98]. On the basis of available literature on contraceptive and non-contraceptive oestrogen therapy, it appears unlikely that these hormones materially augment the risk of NIDDM in women.

EFFICACY OF POTENTIAL INTERVENTION STRATEGIES

CONTROL OF OBESITY

Although obesity represents one of the most prevalent public health problems in industrialized countries, research on the prevention of obesity, as well as the potential benefits and risks of weight loss strategies among the obese, have been limited. At present, there seems to be little doubt that overweight individuals have increased risk for morbidity and mortality; it cannot be concluded, however, that weight loss will reduce these increased risks[99]. Paradoxically, most epidemiological studies even suggest that weight loss is associated with increased mortality, a phenomenon most likely due to the underlying causes of weight loss such as severe illness or psychosocial stresses[99]. In obese NIDDM patients, weight loss has been shown to improve glucose tolerance and insulin resistance[39-43]. Based on data from the Nurses' Health Study at least 90% of NIDDM cases among US white women may be

338 _____ A. Spelsberg and J. E. Manson

attributable to overweight (BMI > 22 kg/m²)[36]. To our knowledge, no long-term large-scale follow-up studies or long-term randomized trials have assessed the benefits of sustained weight reduction in obese individuals or obese NIDDM patients. These studies are urgently needed to address these issues.

INCREASE OF PHYSICAL ACTIVITY

Increased physical activity has been related to an improvement in insulin resistance and glycaemic control in both diabetic and non-diabetic obese individuals[72,100]. Skeletal muscle appears to be the primary site of impaired insulin action[17,38]; stimulation of muscle blood flow has been shown to be an important determinant of glucose uptake in the muscle after administration of insulin[17]. Regular exercise augments muscular blood flow and may thereby improve insulin sensitivity of muscle tissue. At present, it remains unclear whether such improvements in insulin sensitivity require regular and sustained physical training or can be achieved with moderate levels of activity[100]. In addition to favourable independent effects on insulin sensitivity, exercise is clearly beneficial by facilitating weight loss and maintaining reduced body weight[83,101]. In view of the proportion (60%) of US adults estimated to be sedentary[102], the potential public health impact of an increased physical activity level in the general population could be enormous. Based on data from the Physicians' Health Study[83], at least 25% of NIDDM cases could be prevented by an increase in physical activity.

TARGETED INTERVENTION

HIGH-RISK GROUP-TARGETED PRIMARY PREVENTION

Although epidemiological research concerning the primary prevention of NIDDM remains at a relatively early stage, particularly compared to cardiovascular research[4], the evidence discussed above already offers important pathways for primary intervention strategies. Epidemiology and public health may be viewed as two sides of a coin: epidemiological evidence on one side elucidates causal mechanisms of exposure–disease relationships, and public health on the other side applies the evidence for successful intervention measures. In the case of NIDDM, the focus of early intervention can be based on the following facts: (1) we can identify certain high-risk groups, e.g. certain ethnic groups, persons with a family history of diabetes who carry a genetic susceptibility, ageing individuals, sedentary individuals and the large obese proportion of the population; (2) both obesity and lack of physical activity have emerged as important and modifiable risk factors for NIDDM. In prospective studies, a large proportion of NIDDM cases in women and men were found to be attributable to overweight and physical inactivity [36,83].

These data strongly support the need for public health intervention even at the present early stage of NIDDM research.

ARGUMENTS FOR A POPULATION-BASED STRATEGY

It is well established that obesity and physical inactivity are closely related to other disease entities, such as cardiovascular diseases and hypertension. Insulin resistance has been postulated as the common underlying cause of several metabolic disorders, including obesity, hypertension and atherosclerotic disease[38]. Further, the prevalence of both obesity and sedentary lifestyle is high according to cross-sectional data in the US population[3], as well as worldwide. In view of this knowledge, an extension of the research activities to include randomized trials of promising primary intervention strategies, as well as further observational, clinical and laboratory research, are urgently needed and recommended[4,22]. We propose that the anticipated global benefits of weight reduction and increased physical activity, not only for prevention of NIDDM, but also cardiovascular diseases, hypertension and certain cancers[103–105], should argue for a population-based rather than high-risk intervention strategy. Currently, a large-scale trial of dietary fat reduction, supplementation with calcium and vitamin D, and hormonal replacement therapy in relation to risk of cardiovascular diseases, osteoporosis, breast cancer and other major illnesses in postmenopausal women (the Women's Health Initiative) is in preparation in the USA. The trial will also provide data on the role of dietary fat reduction, weight loss and exercise in the prevention of NIDDM. Intervention studies such as this will be most powerful tools to demonstrate the benefits and possible adverse effects of different dietary, exercise and weight loss regimens on long-term disease prevention. Although studies in high-risk populations for certain diseases do offer the advantage of greater efficiency, nearly the entire population of the USA and most other industrialized countries can be considered at high risk of NIDDM, hypertension, atherosclerotic disease and other health conditions linked to obesity, physical inactivity and insulin resistance. The mutual occurrence of the potentially modifiable risk factors such as obesity and physical inactivity and the link between these risk factors and NIDDM, as well as several related disease entities, in the general population justify, in our view, population-based primary intervention as a public health priority even at this early stage of our knowledge.

CONCLUSIONS

NIDDM represents one of the most prevalent chronic diseases worldwide. The impact of NIDDM on morbidity and mortality, as well as the economic costs attributable to the disease, are substantial both in industrialized and developing countries. Despite strong genetic influences, NIDDM should be regarded as a potentially preventable disease. At present, epidemiological evidence strongly supports the initiation of preventive measures for the few modifiable determinants currently recognized: obesity, physical inactivity and dietary factors. Cigarette smoking may be an additional modifiable risk factor for NIDDM. In prospective studies, it has been estimated that 25% of NIDDM cases could be attributed to physical inactivity in the white US male population, and 90% of NIDDM cases among US white women may be attributable to overweight. Nearly the entire population of the USA and most other industrialized countries can be considered at high risk of NIDDM and other health conditions linked to obesity, physical inactivity and insulin resistance. An extension of the research activities to include randomized trials of primary prevention strategies for these determinants, as well as further observational, clinical and laboratory research, are urgently needed and recommended.

REFERENCES

1 Harris MI. Prevalence of noninsulin-dependent diabetes and impaired glucose tolerance. In: *Diabetes in America: Diabetes Data Compiled 1984* (ed National Diabetes Data Group) US Department of Health and Human Services publication (PHS) 85–1468, National Institutes of Health, Bethesda, 1985, VI, pp 1–31.

2 National Center for Health Statistics. Table B. Advance Report of final mortality statistics, 1984. *Monthly Vital Statistics Report* Vol 35, No 6, Suppl 2. US Department of Health and Human Services publication (PHS) 86–1120, Public Health Service, Hyattsville, MD, 26 September 1986.

3 Harris MI. Noninsulin-dependent diabetes mellitus in black and white Americans. *Diabetes Metab Rev* 1990; **6**: 71–90.

4 Stern MP. Kelly West lecture. Primary prevention of type II diabetes mellitus. *Diabetes Care* 1991; **14**: 399–410.

5 World Health Organization Study Group on Diabetes Mellitus: *Technical Report Series No 727*, WHO, Geneva, 1985.

6 Tai TY, Yang CL, Chang CJ, et al. Epidemiology of diabetes mellitus among adults in Taiwan, R.O.C. In: *Epidemiology of Diabetes Mellitus: Proceedings of the International Symposium on Epidemiology of Diabetes Mellitus* (eds S Vannasaeng, W Nitianant, S Chandraprasert) Crystal House, Bangkok, 1987, pp 42–8.

7 Thai AC, Yeo PPB, Lun KC, et al. Changing prevalence of diabetes mellitus in Singapore over a 10-year period. In: *Epidemiology of Diabetes Mellitus: Proceedings of the International Symposium on Epidemiology of Diabetes Mellitus* (eds S Vannasaeng, W Nitianant, S Chadraprasert) Crystal House, Bangkok, 1987, pp 63–7.

8 Dowse GK, Gareeboo H, Zimmet PZ, et al. High prevalence of NIDDM and impaired glucose tolerance in Indian, Creole, and Chinese Mauritians. *Diabetes* 1990; **39**: 390–6.

9 Kawate R, Yamakido M, Nishimoto Y, et al. Diabetes mellitus and its vascular complications in Japanese migrants on the island of Hawaii. *Diabetes Care* 1979; **2**: 161–70.

10 Huse DM, Oster G, Killen AR, Lacey MJ, Colditz GA. The economic costs of non-insulin-dependent diabetes mellitus. *JAMA* 1989; **262**: 2708–13.

11 Bransome ED. Financing the care of diabetes mellitus in the US. *Diabetes Care* 1992; **15**: 1–5.

12 Zimmet P, Dowse G, Finch C, Serjeantson S, King H. The epidemiology and natural history of NIDDM: lessons from the South Pacific. *Diabetes Metab Rev* 1990; **6**: 91–124.

13 Prior IAM. Cardiovascular epidemiology in New Zealand and the Pacific. *NZ Med J* 1974; **80**: 245–52.

14 Schooneveldt M, Songer T, Zimmet P, Thoma K. Changing mortality patterns in Nauruans: an example of epidemiological transition. *J Epidemiol Community Health* 1988; **42**: 89–95.

15 Kuberski TT, Bennett PH. Diabetes mellitus as an emerging public health problem on Guam. *Diabetes Care* 1980; **3**: 235–41.

16 Crews D, McKeen P. Mortality related to cardiovascular disease and diabetes mellitus in a modernising population. *Soc Sci Med* 1982; **16**: 175–81.

17 DeFronzo RA, Bonadonna RC, Ferrannini E. Pathogenesis of NIDDM: a balanced overview. *Diabetes Care* 1992; **15**: 318–68.

18 Lyen KR. The insulin receptor. *Ann Acad Med Singapore* 1985; **14**: 364–71.

19 Lillioja S, Nyoba BL, Saad MF, et al. Exaggerated early insulin release and insulin resistance in a diabetes-prone population: a metabolic comparison of Pima Indians and Caucasians. *J Clin Endocrinol Metab* 1991; **73**: 866–76.

20 Beck-Nielsen H, Vaag A, Damsbo P, et al. Insulin resistance in skeletal muscles in patients with NIDDM. *Diabetes Care* 1992; **15**: 418–29.

21 Schulman D, Rothman DL, Jue T, et al. Quantitation of muscle glycogen synthesis in normal subjects and subjects with non-insulin-dependent diabetes by ^{13}C nuclear magnetic resonance spectroscopy. *N Engl J Med* 1990; **322**: 223–8.

22 King H, Dowd JE. Primary prevention of type 2 (non-insulin-dependent) diabetes mellitus. *Diabetologia* 1990; **33**: 3–8.

23 World Health Organization Expert Committee on Diabetes Mellitus: Second Report. *Technical Report Series No 646*, WHO, Geneva, 1980.

24 Morris RD, Rimm DL, Hartz AJ, Kalkhoff RK, Rimm AA. Obesity and heredity in the etiology of non-insulin-dependent diabetes mellitus in 32,662 adult white women. *Am J Epidemiol* 1989; **130**: 112–21.

25 West KM, Kalbfleisch JM. Influence of nutritional factors on prevalence of diabetes. *Diabetes* 1971; **20**: 99–108.

26 King H, Zimmet P, Raper LR, Balkau B. Risk factors for diabetes in three Pacific populations. *Am J Epidemiol* 1984; **119**: 396–409.

27 Saad MF, Knowler WC, Pettitt DJ, et al. The natural history of impaired glucose tolerance in Pima Indians. *N Engl J Med* 1988; **319**: 1500–6.

28 Knowler WC, Pettitt DJ, Savage PJ, Bennett PH. Diabetes incidence in Pima Indians: contributions of obesity and parental diabetes. *Am J Epidemiol* 1981; **113**: 144–56.

29 Keen H, Jarrett RJ, McCarthey P. The ten-year follow-up of the Bedford Survey (1962–1972). *Diabetologia* 1982; **22**: 73–8.

30 Westlund K, Nicolaysen R. Ten-year mortality and morbidity related to serum cholesterol. *Scand J Clin Lab Invest* 1972; **30** (Suppl): 1–24.

31 Modan M, Karasik A, Halkin H, et al. Effect of past and concurrent body mass

index on prevalence of glucose intolerance and type 2 (non-insulin-dependent) diabetes and on insulin response: the Israel study of glucose tolerance, obesity and hypertension. *Diabetologia* 1986; **29**: 82–9.

32 Olsson LO, Larsson B, Svärdsudd K, et al. The influence of body fat distribution on the incidence of diabetes mellitus: 13.5 years of follow-up of the participants in the study of men born in 1913. *Diabetes* 1985; **34**: 1055–8.

33 Wilson PW, McGee L, Kannel WB. Obesity, very low density lipoproteins, and glucose intolerance over fourteen years: the Framingham Study. *Am J Epidemiol* 1981; **114**: 697–704.

34 Medalie JH, Hermann JB, Goldbourt U, Papier CM. Variations in incidence of diabetes among 10,000 adult Israeli males and the factors related to their development. *Adv Metab Disord* 1978; **9**: 93–110.

35 Butler WJ, Ostrander LD Jr, Carman WJ, Lamphier DE. Diabetes mellitus in Tecumseh, Michigan: prevalence, incidence, and associated conditions. *Am J Epidemiol* 1982; **116**: 971–80.

36 Colditz GA, Willett WC, Stampfer MJ, et al. Weight as a risk factor for clinical diabetes in women. *Am J Epidemiol* 1990; **132**: 501–13.

37 Olsson LO, Larsson B, Björntorp P, et al. Risk factors for type 2 (non-insulin-dependent) diabetes mellitus: thirteen and one-half years of follow-up of the participants in the study of men born in 1913. *Diabetologia* 1988; **31**: 798–805.

38 DeFronzo RA, Farrannini E. Insulin resistance: a multifaceted syndrome responsible for NIDDM, obesity, hypertension, and atherosclerotic valvular disease. *Diabetes Care* 1991; **14**: 173–94.

39 Doar JWH, Thompson ME, Wilde CE, et al. Influence of treatment with diet alone on oral glucose tolerance test and plasma sugar and insulin levels in patients with maturity onset diabetes. *Lancet* 1975; **i**: 1263–7.

40 Berger M, Baumhoff EE, Gries FA. Weight reduction and glucose intolerance in obesity (In German). *Deutsch Med Wochenschr* 1976; **101**: 307–12.

41 Henry RR, Wiest-Kent TA, Scheaffer L, Koltermann OG, Olefsky JM. Metabolic consequences of very-low-calorie diet in obese non-insulin-dependent diabetic and nondiabetic subjects. *Diabetes* 1986; **35**: 155–64.

42 Henry RR, Brechtel G, Griver K. Secretion and hepatic extraction of insulin after weight loss in obese non-insulin-dependent diabetes mellitus. *J Clin Endocrinol Metab* 1988; **66**: 979–86.

43 Henry RR, Gumbiner B. Benefits and limitations of very-low-calorie diet therapy in obese NIDDM. *Diabetes Care* 1991; **14**: 802–823.

44 O'Sullivan JB. Population retested for diabetes after 17 years: new prevalence study in Oxford, Massachusetts. *Diabetologia* 1969; **5**: 211–214.

45 Jarrett RJ, Keen H, McCartney P. Worsening to diabetes in persons with impaired glucose tolerance: ten years of experience in the Bedford and Whitehall Studies. In: *Advances in Diabetes Epidemiology* (ed E Eschwege) Elsevier, Amsterdam, 1982, pp 95–102.

46 Dowse GK, Zimmet PZ, Gareboo H, et al. Abdominal obesity and physical activity as risk factors for NIDDM and impaired glucose tolerance in Indian, Creole, and Chinese Mauretanians. *Diabetes Care* 1991; **14**: 271–82.

47 Bolinder J, Kager L, Östman J, Arner P. Differences at the receptor and postreceptor levels between human omental and subcutaneous adipose tissue in the action of insulin on lipolysis. *Diabetes* 1983; **32**: 117–23.

48 Barrrett-Connor E. Epidemiology, obesity, and non-insulin-dependent diabetes mellitus. *Epidemiol Rev* 1989; **11**: 172–81.

49 Jarrett RJ. Epidemiology and public helath aspects of non-insulin-dependent diabetes mellitus. *Epidemiol Rev* 1989; **11**: 151–71.

50 Lundgren H, Bengtsson C, Blohme G, Lapidus L, Sjöström L. Adiposity and adipose tissue distribution in relation to incidence of diabetes in women: results from a prospective population study in Gothenburg, Sweden. *Int J Obes* 1989; **13**: 413–23.

51 Freedman DS, Rimm AA. The relation of body fat distribution, as assessed by six girth measurements, to diabetes mellitus in women. *Am J Public Health* 1989; **79**: 715–21.

52 Mykkänen L, Laakso M, Uusitupa M, Pyörälä K. Prevalence of diabetes and impaired glucose tolerance in elderly subjects and their association with obesity and family history of diabetes. *Diabetes Care* 1990; **13**: 1099–105.

53 Haffner SM, Stern MP, Hazuda HP, Pugh J, Patterson JK. Role of obesity and fat distribution in non-insulin-dependent diabetes mellitus in Mexican Americans and non-Hispanic whites. *Diabetes Care* 1986; **9**: 153–61.

54 Laws A, Terry RB, Barrett-Connor E. Behavioral covariates of waist-to-hip ratio in Rancho Bernardo. *Am J Public Health* 1990; **80**: 1358–62.

55 Troisi RJ, Weiss ST, Segal MR, et al. The relationship of body fat distribution to blood pressure in normotensive men: the Normative Aging Study. *Int J Obes* 1990; **14**: 515–25.

56 Seidell JC, Cigolini M, Deslypere J, et al. Body fat distribution in relation to physical activity and smoking habits in 38-year-old European men: the European fat distribution study. *Am J Epidemiol* 1991; **133**: 257–66.

57 Marshall JA, Hamman RF, Baxter J. High-fat, low-carbohydrate diet and the etiology of non-insulin-dependent diabetes mellitus: the San Luis Valley Diabetes Study. *Am J Epidemiol* 1991; **134**: 590–603.

58 Danforth E. Diet and obesity. *Am J Clin Nutr* 1985; **41**: 1132–45.

59 Storlien LH, James DE, Burleigh KM, et al. Fat feeding causes widespread in vivo insulin resistance, decreased energy expenditure, and obesity in rats. *Am J Physiol* 1986; **251**: E576–83.

60 Leibel RL, Edens NK, Fried SK. Physiological basis for the control of body fat distribution in humans. *Annu Rev Nutr* 1989; **9**: 417–43.

61 DeFronzo RA. Lilly Lecture. The triumvirate: β-cell, muscle, liver. A collusion responsible for NIDDM. *Diabetes* 1988; **37**: 667–87.

62 Lillioja S, Bogardus C, Mott DM, et al. Relationship between insulin mediated glucose disposal and lipid metabolism in man. *J Clin Invest* 1985; **75**: 1106–15.

63 Groop LC, Saloranta C, Shank M, et al. The role of free fatty acid metabolism in the pathogenesis of insulin resistance in obesity and noninsulin-dependent diabetes mellitus. *J Clin Endocrinol Metab* 1991; **72**: 96–107.

64 Hunter D. Biochemical indicators of dietary intake. In: *Nutritional Epidemiology* (ed WC Wilett) Oxford University Press, New York, 1990, pp 191–9.

65 Snowden DA, Phillips RL. Does a vegetarian diet reduce the occurrence of diabetes? *Am J Public Health* 1985; **75**: 507–12.

66 Tsunehara CH, Leonetti DL, Fujiimoto WY. Diet of second-generation Japanese–American men with and without non-insulin-dependent diabetes mellitus. *Am J Clin Nutr* 1990; **52**: 731–8.

67 Lundgren H, Bengtsson C, Blohme G, Lapidus L, Sjöström L. Dietary habits and incidence of non-insulin-dependent diabetes mellitus in a population study of women in Gothenburg, Sweden. *Am J Clin Nutr* 1989; **49**: 708–12.

68 Colditz GA, Manson JE, Stampfer MJ, et al. Diet and risk of clinical diabetes in women. *Am J Clin Nutr* 1992; **55**: 1018–23.

69 Colditz GA, Wilett WC, Stampfer MJ, et al. Patterns of weight change and their relation to diet in a cohort of healthy women. *Am J Clin Nutr* 1990; **51**: 1100–5.

70 Mondon CE, Dolkas CB, Reaven GM. Site of enhanced insulin sensitivity in exercise-trained rats. *Am J Physiol* 1980; **239**: E169–77.

71 Dahm GL, Sinha MK, Caro JF. Insulin receptor binding and protein kinase activity in muscles of trained rats. *Am J Physiol* 1987; **252**: E170–5.

72 Schneider SH, Amorosa LF, Khachadurian AK, Ruderman NB. Studies on the mechanism of improved glucose control during regular exercise in type 2 (non-insulin-dependent) diabetes. *Diabetologia* 1984; **26**: 355–60.

73 Koivisto VA, Yki-Jarvinen H, DeFronzo RA. Physical training and insulin sensitivity. *Diabetes Metab Rev* 1986; **1**: 445–81.

74 Burstein R, Polychronakos C, Toews CJ, et al. Acute reversal of the enhanced insulin action in trained athletes: association with insulin receptor changes. *Diabetes* 1985; **34**: 756–60.

75 Björntorp P, DeJounge K, Sjostrom L, Sullivan L. The effect of physical training on insulin production in obesity. *Metabolism* 1970; **19**: 631–8.

76 Soman VR, Koivisto VA, Deibert D, Felig P, DeFronzo RA. Increased insulin sensitivity and insulin binding to monocytes after physical training. *N Engl J Med* 1979; **301**: 1200–4.

77 Stern JS, Titchenal CA, Johnson PR. Does exercise make a difference? In: *Recent Advances in Obesity Research.* London, England: John Libbey & Co Ltd; 1987, pp 337–49.

78 Taylor R, Ram P, Zimmet P, Raper LR, Ringrose H. Physical activity and prevalence of diabetes in Melanesian and Indian men in Fiji. *Diabetologia* 1984; **27**: 578–82.

79 King H, Taylor R, Koteka G, et al. Glucose tolerance in Polynesia: population-based surveys in Rarotonga and Niue. *Med J Aust* 1986; **145**: 505–10.

80 Jarrett RJ, Shipley MJ, Hunt R. Physical activity, glucose tolerance and diabetes mellitus: the Whitehall Study. *Diabetic Med* 1986; **3**: 549–51.

81 Helmrich SP, Ragland DR, Leung RW, Pfaffenbarger RS. Physical activity and reduced occurrence of non-insulin-dependent diabetes mellitus. *N Engl J Med* 1991; **325**: 147–52.

82 Manson JE, Rimm EB, Stampfer MJ, et al. Physical activity and incidence of non-insulin-dependent diabetes mellitus in women. *Lancet* 1991; **338**: 774–8.

83 Manson JE, Nathan DM, Krolewski AS, et al. A prospective study of exercise and incidence of diabetes among U.S. male physicians. *JAMA* 1992; **268**: 63–7.

84 Frisch RE, Wyshak G, Albright TE, Albright NL, Schiff I. Lower prevalence of diabetes in female former college athletes compared with nonathletes. *Diabetes* 1986; **35**: 1101–5.

85 Janzen L, Berntorp K, Hanson M, Lindell SE, Trell E. Glucose tolerance and smoking: a population study of oral and intravenous glucose tolerance test in middle-aged men. *Diabetologia* 1983; **25**: 86–8.

86 Shinokata H, Muller DC, Andres R. Studies in the distribution of body fat. *JAMA* 1989; **261**: 1169–73.

87 Rimm EB, Manson JE, Stampfer MJ, et al. A prospective study of cigarette smoking and the risk of diabetes in women. *Am J Public Health* 1993; **83**: 211–14.

88 Feskens EJ, Kromhout D. Cardiovascular risk factors and the 25-year incidence of diabetes mellitus in middle-aged men: the Zutphen Study. *Am J Epidemiol* 1989; **130**: 1101–8.

89 Medalie JH, Papier CU, Goldbourt U, Herman JB. Major factors in the development of diabetes mellitus in 10,000 men. *Arch Intern Med* 1975; **135**: 811–17.

90 Wilson PWF, Anderson KM, Kannel WB. Epidemiology of diabetes mellitus in the elderly. *Am J Med* 1986; 80 (Suppl 5A): 3–9.

91 Kritz-Silverstein D, Barrett-Connor E, Wingard D. The effect of parity on the later development of non-insulin-dependent diabetes mellitus or impaired glucose tolerance. *N Engl J Med* 1989; **321**: 1214–19.
92 Manson JE, Rimm EB, Colditz GA, et al. A prospective study of parity and the subsequent development of non-insulin-dependent diabetes mellitus. *Am J Med* 1992; **93**: 13–18.
93 Collins VR, Dowse GK, Zimmet PZ. Evidence against association between parity and NIDDM from five population groups. *Diabetes Care* 1991; **14**: 975–81.
94 Goldman JA, Ovardia JL. The effect of estrogen on intravenous glucose tolerance in women. *Am J Obstet Gynecol* 1969; **103**: 172–8.
95 Eschwege E, Fontbonne A, Sinon D, et al. Oral contraceptives, insulin resistance and ischemic vascular disease. *Int J Gynecol Obstet* 1990; **31**: 263–9.
96 Goldman JA. Intravenous glucose tolerance after 18 months on progestogen or combination-type oral contraceptives. *Israel J Med Sci* 1978; **14**: 324–7.
97 Rimm EB, Manson JE, Stampfer MJ, et al. Oral contraception use and the risk of clinical diabetes in a large prospective study of women. *Diabetologia* 1992; **35**: 967–72.
98 Manson JE, Rimm EB, Colditz GA, et al. A prospective study of postmenopausal estrogen therapy and subsequent incidence of non-insulin-dependent diabetes mellitus. *Ann Epidemiol* 1992; **2**: 665–73.
99 Technology Assessment Conference Pannel. Methods for voluntary weight loss and control: Technology Assessment Conference statement. *Ann Intern Med* 1992; **116**: 942–9.
100 Holloszy JO, Schultz J, Kusnierkiewizc J, Hagberg JM, Ehsani AA. Effects of exercise on glucose tolerance and insulin resistance: brief review and some preliminary results. *Acta Med Scand* 1987; **711**: 55–65.
101 Wood PD, Stefanick ML, Williams PT, Haskell WL. The effects on plasma lipoproteins of a prudent weight-reducing diet, with or without exercise, in overweight men and women. *N Engl J Med* 1991; **325**: 461–6.
102 Hughes T, Capell F, Benn S, et al. Sex-, age-, and region-specific prevalence of sedentary lifestyle in selected states in 1985: the behavioral factor surveillance system. *MMWR* 1987; **36**: 195–204.
103 Slattery ML, Schumacher MC, Smith KR, West DW, ABD-Elgha'ny N. Physical activity, diet, and the risk of colon cancer in Utah. *Am J Epidemiol* 1988; **128**: 989–95.
104 Whittemore AF, Wu-Williams AH, Lee M, et al. Diet, physical activity, and colorectal cancer among Chinese in North America and China. *J Natl Cancer Inst* 1990; **82**: 915–22.
105 Gerhardsson M, Floderus B, Norell SE. Physical activity and colon cancer risk. *Int J Epidemiol* 1988; **17**: 743–8.

Index

Index compiled by Campbell Purton